"Whether you come to this elevated and expanded edition of *Medical Medium* as a new reader or as a seasoned follower of the book series, know this: there's already a track record established of the power of healing this book has provided. People from around the world who've tried everything medical research and science had to offer have found this information to be a sanctuary. They've found that it has allowed them to rise out of the ashes."

— Anthony William, Medical Medium

Praise for ANTHONY WILLIAM

"Anthony doesn't offer gimmicks or fads to finding ultimate health. His recommended foods and cleansing programs are simple and delicious and THEY WORK! If you're done living with pain, fatigue, brain fog, intestinal disorders, and a myriad of other nasty ailments, drop everything and read this (and his other) books. He will quickly bring health and hope back into your life."

— Hilary Swank, Oscar-winning actress

"Celery juice is sweeping the globe. It's impressive how Anthony has created this movement and restored superior health in countless people around the world."

— Sylvester Stallone

"Anthony's understanding of foods, their vibrations, and how they interact with the body never ceases to amaze. Effortlessly he explains the potential harmony or disharmony in our choices in a way anyone can understand. He has a gift. Do your body a favor and treat yourself."

— Pharrell Williams, 13-time Grammy-winning artist and producer

"I've been drinking celery juice every morning for the last six months and feel great! I've noticed a huge difference in my energy levels and digestive system. I even travel now with my juicer so I don't miss out on my daily celery juice!"

— Miranda Kerr, international supermodel, founder and CEO of KORA Organics

"Anthony has turned numerous lives around for the better with the healing powers of celery juice."

— Novak Djokovic, #1-ranked tennis champion in the world

"Anthony is a trusted source for our family. His work in the world is a light that has guided many to safety. He means so much to us."

— Robert De Niro and Grace Hightower De Niro

"While there is most definitely an element of otherworldly mystery to the work he does, much of what Anthony William shines a spotlight on—particularly around autoimmune disease— feels inherently right and true. What's better is that the protocols he recommends are natural, accessible, and easy to do."

— Gwyneth Paltrow, Oscar-winning actress, #1 *New York Times* best-selling author, founder and CEO of GOOP.com

"All great gifts are bestowed with humility. Anthony is humble. And like all the right remedies, his are intuitive, natural, and balanced. These two make for a powerful and effective combination."

— John Donovan, CEO of AT&T Communications

"Anthony William is truly dedicated to sharing his knowledge and experience to spread the word of healing to all. His compassion and desire to reach as many people as he can to help them heal themselves is inspiring and empowering. Today, in a world of obsession with prescription medication, it is so refreshing to know that there are alternative options that truly work and can open a new door to health."

— Liv Tyler, star of *9-1-1: Lone Star*, *Harlots*, the *Lord of the Rings* trilogy, *Empire Records*

"Anthony's knowledge on the food we consume, the impact it has on our body, and our overall well-being has been a game changer for me!"

— Jenna Dewan, star of *Soundtrack*, *World of Dance*, *Step Up*

"Anthony is a wonderful person. He identified some long-term health issues for me, he knew what supplements I needed, and I felt better immediately."

— Rashida Jones, Grammy-winning director of *Quincy*, producer and star of *Angie Tribeca*, star of *Parks and Recreation* and *The Office*

"Resonance is a powerful thing in life, as is self-empowerment. Wonderfully enough, Anthony William, his books, and his CELERY JUICE call-to-action have hit both of those notes with me. The reinforcement from Anthony that our bodies are capable of incredible healing and resilience is a much-needed message. Too often, I want quick fixes that ultimately lead to more problems. Real nutrition is the best medicine, and Anthony inspires us all to fuel our body, mind, and spirit with nature's bounty; it's powerful medicine straight from the Source."

— Kerri Walsh Jennings, 3-time gold medal–winning and 1-time bronze medal–winning Olympic volleyball player

"Anthony is a magician for all my label's recording artists, and if he were a record album, he would far surpass Thriller. His ability is nothing short of profound, remarkable, extraordinary, and mind-blowing. He is a luminary whose books are filled with prophecies. This is the future of medicine."

— Craig Kallman, Chairman and CEO, Atlantic Records

"I refer to Anthony William's books constantly for the most insightful wisdom and recipes to restore energy and good health. Interested in the unique and powerful qualities of each food he describes, I'm inspired to consider how I can enhance the ritual of cooking and eating for the sake of wellness each day."

— Alexis Bledel, Emmy-winning star of *The Handmaid's Tale*, *Gilmore Girls*, *Sisterhood of the Traveling Pants*

"Anthony's books are revolutionary yet practical. For anybody frustrated by the current limits of Western medicine, this is definitely worth your time and consideration."

— James Van Der Beek, creator, executive producer, and star of *What Would Diplo Do?* and star of *Pose* and *Dawson's Creek*, and Kimberly Van Der Beek, public speaker and activist

"Anthony is a great man. His knowledge is fascinating and has been very helpful for me. The celery juice alone is a game changer!"

— Calvin Harris, producer, DJ, and Grammy-winning artist

"I am so grateful to Anthony. After introducing his celery juice protocol into my daily routine, I have seen a marked improvement in every aspect of my health."

— Debra Messing, Emmy-winning star of *Will & Grace*

"My family and friends have been the recipients of Anthony's inspired gift of healing, and we've benefited more than I can express with rejuvenated physical and mental health."

— Scott Bakula, executive producer and star of *NCIS: New Orleans*; Golden Globe–winning star of *Quantum Leap* and *Star Trek: Enterprise*

"Anthony has dedicated his life to helping others find the answers that we need to live our healthiest lives. And celery juice is the most accessible way to start!"

— Courteney Cox, star of *Cougar Town* and *Friends*

"Anthony is not only a warm, compassionate healer, he is also authentic and accurate, with God-given skills. He has been a total blessing in my life."

— Naomi Campbell, model, actress, activist

"Anthony's extensive knowledge and deep intuition have demystified even the most confounding health issues. He has provided a clear path for me to feel my very best— I find his guidance indispensable."

— Taylor Schilling, star of *Orange Is the New Black*

"We are incredibly grateful for Anthony and his passionate dedication to spreading the word about healing through food. Anthony has a truly special gift. His practices have entirely reshaped our perspectives about food and ultimately our lifestyle. Celery juice alone has completely transformed the way we feel and it will always be a part of our morning routine."

— Hunter Mahan, 6-time PGA Tour–winning golfer

"Anthony William is changing and saving the lives of people all over the world with his one-of-a-kind gift. His constant dedication and vast amount of highly advanced information have broken the barriers that block so many in the world from receiving desperately needed truths that science and research have not yet discovered. On a personal level, he has helped both my daughters and me, giving us tools to support our health that actually work. Celery juice is now a part of our regular routine!"

— Lisa Rinna, star of *The Real Housewives of Beverly Hills* and *Days of Our Lives*, *New York Times* best-selling author, designer of the Lisa Rinna Collection

"Anthony is a truly generous person with keen intuition and knowledge about health. I have seen firsthand the transformation he's made in people's quality of life."

— Carla Gugino, star of *Jett*, *The Haunting of Hill House*, *Watchmen*, *Entourage*, *Spy Kids*

"I've been following Anthony for a while now and am always floored (but not surprised) at the success stories from people following his protocols . . . I have been on my own path of healing for many years, jumping from doctor to doctor and specialist to specialist. He's the real deal and I trust him and his vast knowledge of how the thyroid works and the true effects food has on our body. I have directed countless friends, family, and followers to Anthony because I truly believe he possesses knowledge that no doctor out there has. I am a believer and on a true path to healing now and am honored to know him and blessed to know his work. Every endocrinologist needs to read his book on the thyroid!"

— Marcela Valladolid, chef, author, television host

"What if someone could simply touch you and tell you what it is that ails you? Welcome to the healing hands of Anthony William—a modern-day alchemist who very well may hold the key to longevity. His lifesaving advice blew into my world like a healing hurricane, and he has left a path of love and light in his wake. He is hands down the ninth wonder of the world."

— Lisa Gregorisch-Dempsey, *Extra* Senior Executive Producer

"Anthony William's God-given gift for healing is nothing short of miraculous."

— David James Elliott, *Spinning Out, Trumbo, Mad Men, CSI: NY*; star for ten years of *JAG*

"I am a doctor's daughter who has always relied on Western medicine to ameliorate even the smallest of woes. Anthony's insights opened my eyes to the healing benefits of food and how a more holistic approach to health can change your life."

— Jenny Mollen, actress and *New York Times* best-selling author of *I Like You Just the Way I Am*

"Anthony William is a gift to humanity. His incredible work has helped millions of people heal when conventional medicine had no answers for them. His genuine passion and commitment for helping people is unsurpassed, and I am grateful to have been able to share a small part of his powerful message in Heal."

— Kelly Noonan Gores, writer, director, and producer of the *Heal* documentary

"Anthony William is one of those rare individuals who uses his gifts to help people rise up to meet their full potential by becoming their own best health advocates . . . I witnessed Anthony's greatness in action firsthand when I attended one of his thrilling live events. I equate how spot-on his readings were with a singer hitting all the high notes. But beyond the high notes, Anthony's truly compassionate soul is what left the audience captivated. Anthony William is someone I am now proud to call a friend, and I can tell you that the person you hear on the podcasts and whose words fill the pages of best-selling books is the same person who reaches out to loved ones simply to lend support. This is not an act! Anthony William is the real deal, and the gravity of the information he shares through Spirit is priceless and empowering and much needed in this day and age!"

— Debbie Gibson, Broadway star, iconic singer-songwriter

"I had the pleasure of working with Anthony William when he came to Los Angeles and shared his story on Extra. What a fascinating interview as he left the audience wanting to hear more . . . people went crazy for him! His warm personality and big heart are obvious. Anthony has dedicated his life to helping people through the knowledge he receives from Spirit, and he shares all of that information through his Medical Medium books, which are life changing. Anthony William is one of a kind!"

— Sharon Levin, *Extra* Senior Producer

"Anthony William has a remarkable gift! I will always be grateful to him for discovering an underlying cause of several health issues that had bothered me for years. With his kind support, I see improvements every day. I think he is a fabulous resource!"

— Morgan Fairchild, actress, author, speaker

"I love Anthony William! My daughters Sophia and Laura gave me his book for my birthday, and I couldn't put it down. The Medical Medium has helped me connect all the dots on my quest to achieve optimal health. Through Anthony's work, I realized the residual Epstein-Barr left over from a childhood illness was sabotaging my health years later. Medical Medium has transformed my life."

— Catherine Bach, *The Young and the Restless*, *The Dukes of Hazzard*

"My recovery from a traumatic spinal crisis several years ago had been steady, but I was still experiencing muscle weakness, a tapped-out nervous system, as well as extra weight. A dear friend called me one evening and strongly recommended I read the book Medical Medium by Anthony William. So much of the information in the book resonated with me that I began incorporating some of the ideas, then I sought and was lucky enough to get a consultation. The reading was so spot-on, it has taken my healing to an unimagined, deeper, and richer level of health. My weight has dropped healthily, I can enjoy bike riding and yoga, I'm back in the gym, I have steady energy, and I sleep deeply. Every morning when following my protocols, I smile and say, 'Whoa, Anthony William! I thank you for your restorative gift . . . Yes!'"

— Robert Wisdom, *Ballers*, *The Alienist*, *Rosewood*, *Nashville*, *The Wire*, *Ray*

"In this world of confusion, with constant noise in the health and wellness field, I rely on Anthony's profound authenticity. His miraculous, true gift rises above it all to a place of clarity."

— Patti Stanger, host of *Million Dollar Matchmaker*

"I rely on Anthony William for my and my family's health. Even when doctors are stumped, Anthony always knows what the problem is and the pathway for healing."

— Chelsea Field, *NCIS: New Orleans*, *Secrets and Lies*, *Without a Trace*, *The Last Boy Scout*

"Anthony William brings a dimension to medicine that deeply expands our understanding of the body and of ourselves. His work is part of a new frontier in healing, delivered with compassion and with love."

— Marianne Williamson, #1 *New York Times* best-selling author of *Healing the Soul of America*, *The Age of Miracles*, and *A Return to Love*

"Anthony William is a generous and compassionate guide. He has devoted his life to supporting people on their healing path."

— Gabrielle Bernstein, #1 *New York Times* best-selling author of *The Universe Has Your Back*, *Judgment Detox*, and *Miracles Now*

"Information that WORKS. That's what I think of when I think of Anthony William and his pro-found contributions to the world. Nothing made this fact so clear to me as seeing him work with an old friend who had been struggling for years with illness, brain fog, and fatigue. She had been to countless doctors and healers and had gone through multiple protocols. Nothing worked. Until Anthony talked to her, that is . . . from there, the results were astounding. I highly recommend his books, lectures, and consultations. Don't miss this healing opportunity!"

— Nick Ortner, *New York Times* best-selling author of *The Tapping Solution for Manifesting Your Greatest Self* and *The Tapping Solution*

"Esoteric talent is only a complete gift when it's shared with moral integrity and love. Anthony William is a divine combination of healing, giftedness, and ethics. He's a real-deal healer who does his homework and shares it in true service to the world."

— Danielle LaPorte, best-selling author of *White Hot Truth* and *The Desire Map*

"Anthony is a seer and a wellness sage. His gift is remarkable. With his guidance I've been able to pinpoint and address a health issue that's been plaguing me for years."

— Kris Carr, *New York Times* best-selling author of *Crazy Sexy Juice,*
Crazy Sexy Kitchen, and *Crazy Sexy Diet*

"Twelve hours after receiving a heaping dose of self-confidence masterfully administered by Anthony, the persistent ringing in my ears of the last year . . . began to falter. I am astounded, grateful, and happy for the insights offered on moving forward."

— Mike Dooley, *New York Times* best-selling author of *Infinite Possibilities* and scribe of *Notes from the Universe*

"Whenever Anthony William recommends a natural way of improving your health, it works. I've seen this with my daughter, and the improvement was impressive. His approach of using natural ingredients is a more effective way of healing."

— Martin D. Shafiroff, financial advisor, past recipient of #1 Broker in America ranking by WealthManagement.com and #1 Wealth Advisor ranking by Barron's

"Anthony William's invaluable advice on preventing and combating disease is years ahead of what's available anywhere else."

— Richard Sollazzo, M.D., New York board-certified oncologist, hematologist, nutritionist, and anti-aging expert and author of *Balance Your Health*

"Anthony William is the Edgar Cayce of our time, reading the body with outstanding precision and insight. Anthony identifies the underlying causes of diseases that often baffle the most astute conventional and alternative health-care practitioners. Anthony's practical and profound advice makes him one of the most powerfully effective healers of the 21st century."

— Ann Louise Gittleman, *New York Times* best-selling author of over 30 books on health and healing and creator of the highly popular Fat Flush detox and diet plan

"As a Hollywood businesswoman, I know value. Some of Anthony's clients spent over $1 million seeking help for their 'mystery illness' until they finally discovered him."

— Nanci Chambers, co-star of *JAG*; Hollywood producer and entrepreneur

"I had a health reading from Anthony, and he accurately told me things about my body only known to me. This kind, sweet, hilarious, self-effacing, and generous man—also so 'otherworldly' and so extraordinarily gifted, with an ability that defies how we see the world— has shocked even me, a medium! He is truly our modern-day Edgar Cayce, and we are immensely blessed that he is with us. Anthony William proves that we are more than we know."

— Colette Baron-Reid, best-selling author of *Uncharted* and TV host of *Messages from Spirit*

"Any quantum physicist will tell you there are things at play in the universe we can't yet understand. I truly believe Anthony has a handle on them. He has an amazing gift for intuitively tapping into the most effective methods for healing."

— Caroline Leavitt, *New York Times* best-selling author of *With or Without You, Is This Tomorrow*, and *Pictures of You*"

MEDICAL MEDIUM

ALSO BY ANTHONY WILLIAM

*Medical Medium Life-Changing Foods: Save Yourself and the Ones You Love
with the Hidden Healing Powers of Fruits & Vegetables*

*Medical Medium Thyroid Healing: The Truth behind Hashimoto's, Graves',
Insomnia, Hypothyroidism, Thyroid Nodules & Epstein-Barr*

*Medical Medium Liver Rescue: Answers to Eczema, Psoriasis, Diabetes, Strep,
Acne, Gout, Bloating, Gallstones, Adrenal Stress, Fatigue, Fatty Liver,
Weight Issues, SIBO & Autoimmune Disease*

*Medical Medium Celery Juice: The Most Powerful Medicine
of Our Time Healing Millions Worldwide*

*Medical Medium Cleanse to Heal: Healing Plans for Sufferers of Anxiety, Depression,
Acne, Eczema, Lyme, Gut Problems, Brain Fog, Weight Issues, Migraines, Bloating,
Vertigo, Psoriasis, Cysts, Fatigue, PCOS, Fibroids, UTI, Endometriosis & Autoimmune*

All of the above are available at your local bookstore, or may be ordered by visiting:

Hay House USA: www.hayhouse.com®

Hay House Australia: www.hayhouse.com.au

Hay House UK: www.hayhouse.co.uk

Hay House India: www.hayhouse.co.in

MEDICAL MEDIUM

Secrets Behind Chronic and Mystery
Illness and How to Finally Heal

Revised & Expanded Edition

ANTHONY WILLIAM

HAY HOUSE, INC.
Carlsbad, California • New York City
London • Sydney • New Delhi

Published in the United States by: Hay House, Inc.: www.hayhouse.com®
Published in Australia by: Hay House Australia Pty. Ltd.: www.hayhouse.com.au
Published in the United Kingdom by: Hay House UK, Ltd.: www.hayhouse.co.uk
Published in India by: Hay House Publishers India: www.hayhouse.co.in

Indexer: J S Editorial, LLC
Cover design: David Somoroff & Vibodha Clark
Interior design: Julie Davison
Revised edition: Nick C. Welch
Interior graphics: Vibodha Clark

The Library of Congress has cataloged the previous edition as follows:

William, Anthony.
 Medical medium : secrets behind chronic and mystery illness and how to finally heal / Anthony William.
   pages cm
 ISBN 978-1-4019-4829-0 (hardback)
 1. Self-care, Health. 2. Holistic medicine. 3. Mind and body. 4. Healing. I. Title.
 RA776.95.W55 2015
 613.2--dc23
                    2015015291

Hardcover ISBN: 978-1-4019- 6287-6
E-book ISBN: 978-1-4019-6292-0
Audiobook ISBN: 978-1-4019-6293-7

10 9 8 7 6 5 4 3 2
1st edition, March 2021

Printed in the United States of America

SUSTAINABLE FORESTRY INITIATIVE
Certified Chain of Custody
Promoting Sustainable Forestry
www.sfiprogram.org
SFI-01268
SFI label applies to the text stock

For Indigo, Ruby, and Great Blue

CONTENTS

"This book has something for everyone, regardless of what food program, diet, or nutritional belief system you may practice. It's for anyone who wants access to the most advanced knowledge about healing available.

The information here is neutral, independent. It's about practitioners and healers getting ahold of this knowledge, learning how to help more people. It is about you getting ahold of this knowledge and learning how to heal yourself. It is about the truth.

The truth about the world, ourselves, life, purpose— it all comes down to healing. And the truth about healing is now in your hands."

— Anthony William, Medical Medium

FOREWORD

How do you know what you know?

Most of the things you know, you've learned—from your caregivers, from your friends, at school, in books, and in the streets. These are the things you know that you know.

But inside of you there are other types of knowing. There is, for example, the knowing that you are, that you exist. That you are you. This knowing you are born with.

There is another type of knowing that is hard to talk about, because most people take it for granted. This is the knowing that your body has of how to function. Without you being a cardiologist, your heart knows how to pump blood. Without you being a gastroenterologist, your gut knows how to digest food and absorb it.

Then there is the knowing that comes as a feeling, such as your gut instinct or intuition. This knowing is highly intelligent and kind of magic. It lets you know things without ever having seen or heard of them—and it may save your life. This is the kind of knowledge that people advise you to trust. But where does it come from? And how does it let you know about things? Who decides when this knowing will communicate with you?

As a man of science, I have been taught to the point of indoctrination that I must only trust what I can observe, measure, test, and reproduce. But as a man with a heart, I cannot measure the love I feel for my wife and kids—yet it is more real than any cell I ever studied under a microscope, and so much more important.

From time immemorial there have been accounts of people who have extraordinary abilities—different kinds of knowing with almost miraculous qualities. Savants who know things that computers have difficulty coming up with. Prodigies in every area of the human realm, such as music, art, and sports, to name just a few.

Lately I have become aware of some individuals who communicate with those who have crossed over to the other side. These crossover mediums are sweeping the country with their fascinating messages that people swear could only come from their deceased loved ones. One of my all-time favorite books is Brian Weiss's *Many Lives, Many Masters*. Dr. Weiss hypnotizes patients, who then regress to past lives and even to spaces in between lives where spiritual masters relay extraordinary messages.

These sessions have a profound healing effect on the people who experience them.

And then there are the healers. Men and women—some of them famous—with the ability to make the blind see, the crippled walk, and the sick fully recover. These healers are the ones I am most fascinated with. Maybe a little because of envy. I would love to be given the gift of healing fully with my touch. I would go on a healing spree, starting at the children's hospitals.

Whenever I hear about anyone with a special healing-related ability, I immediately want to meet them, make them part of my network, experience their gift for myself, refer patients to them, and hopefully learn the ability myself. That is how I got in touch with Anthony William.

A few years ago, I was having abdominal pains daily and went for a sonogram in which we saw a tumor in my liver. A follow-up MRI confirmed it, as well as swollen inguinal lymph nodes. I became alarmed and scheduled a biopsy of one of the lymph nodes, and while waiting for the procedure day, I was given Anthony's number. I got an appointment fast, and within the first minute of our consultation, he told me about my liver—and went so far as to correctly predict the biopsy results. More importantly, he prescribed a regimen of supplements and foods that immediately resolved my abdominal pains, which were completely unrelated to my liver tumor (a benign old cyst previously undiscovered).

Since then, I have consulted with Anthony about my wife and kids and always received advice that worked. I have also sent many of my curious and open-minded patients to him and have gotten wonderful feedback from each and every one of them. Where his knowing comes from is for you to interpret. It is my belief that it comes from the same frequency as intuition, just at a stronger volume. In fact, Anthony himself describes it as a voice that speaks into his ear.

When Anthony told me he had written a book, I was jumping with excitement. Finally I could hear from someone with an uncanny healing ability about how this works, about his personal history and experience. And when I read the book I was blown away. It is well written, sincere, interesting, humble, fascinating. I could not put it down, and I am so happy for you, because you are about to have that same experience. A journey into the mind and soul of a true healer, this is better than space travel.

I hope you enjoy this book as much as I did.

With much love,
Alejandro Junger, M.D.
New York Times best-selling author
of *Clean, Clean Eats,* and *Clean Gut*

Answers for Our Time

You are holding the book that started it all—a fresh, upgraded, timely edition of the title where I first opened the door to anyone and everyone with healing knowledge from above to help the wider masses get answers, heal, and reclaim their lives.

Whether you come to this elevated and expanded edition of *Medical Medium* as a new reader or as a seasoned follower of the book series, know this: there's already a track record established of the power of healing this book has provided. People from around the world who've tried everything medical research and science had to offer have found this information to be a sanctuary. They've found that it has allowed them to rise out of the ashes.

Year after year since this book first entered the world, I've had the opportunity to publish book after book, each new volume in the Medical Medium series geared to help people reach a new level of healing and awakening. Each book has a purpose in entering the world at the time it does. The latest book, *Cleanse to Heal*, was published in the historic spring of 2020—a moment when the world was greatly in need of its antiviral cleanses. And this new edition of *Medical Medium*, the first book in

the series, is in your hands at this particular moment for a reason.

I've always taught you the tools for dealing with viruses. For more than 35 years, I've been teaching people about viruses. Doctors, professionals in health, countless others—I've been teaching them about how viruses work in the body, how we can protect ourselves, and how we can rid viruses to heal and overcome our symptoms and conditions. When the first edition of *Medical Medium* reached the public, viruses were not yet on medical communities' radar as a driving cause of the epidemic of chronic illness that has developed over the last 70 years. And yet, thanks to countless readers who reclaimed their health and vitality by applying the Medical Medium protocols in these chapters—and thanks to the doctors who saw the truth here, too—this information started to take root. The publication of this book started an awakening that viruses are very much responsible for so much of what we suffer from today.

From the beginning, I've given you the information you need to protect yourself and your family, to make yourself stronger, so threats like viruses can't take you down. This has always been one of the foundations of Medical Medium information.

Our current moment calls for a return to the foundation. This moment calls for you to receive access to the most timely—and timeless—healing information possible. As always, it's not only about viruses. It's also about the other threats in our environment, which we can only guard against when we hold the right knowledge.

In these pages, you'll find the timeless Medical Medium healing fundamentals that this book has always offered, along with fresh information specifically geared to our time. If you've already read the first edition of *Medical Medium*, know that this new edition is worth a cover-to-cover read so you don't miss out on any of the new healing insights.

Here are a few highlights:

- **The truth about how COVID connects to chronic illness**

  You'll find this information in Chapter 3, "Epstein-Barr Virus, Chronic Fatigue Syndrome, and Fibromyalgia," although it's critical reading for *anyone*.

- **Refreshed supplement lists, with dosages, for chronic symptoms and conditions**

  Because supplement availability and quality can change over time, the supplement protocols at the end of each chapter in Part II and Part III have been refreshed. You'll find that these protocols now correspond with this book's companion, *Cleanse to Heal*. You'll also find a new chapter in Part IV that includes critical guidance

about applying supplements, as well as instructions for immune support through Medical Medium Zinc Shock Therapy and Medical Medium Vitamin C Shock Therapy.

- **Medical Medium 28-Day Healing Cleanse recipes**

  Now you can turn to full-color recipes to support and motivate you through the Medical Medium 28-Day Healing Cleanse (which, by the way, is an antiviral cleanse—as is any Medical Medium cleanse).

- **Expanded soul-healing and spiritual support from above**

  You have a special purpose here on earth. Even in the face of great uncertainty and change, we all need you to hang in there with us, keep a light heart, and find ways to connect with your purpose. The expanded offerings in Chapter 24, "Soul-Healing Meditations and Techniques," Chapter 25, "Essential Angels," and Chapter 26, "Keep the Faith," are here for you. You can apply these powerful techniques— which don't even require you to leave bed—when you need to connect with peace, grounding, and wholeness.

Never forget the power of your steps toward healing. Whenever you work to take care of yourself, your own pursuit of truth and vitality helps free others. The change this book has already brought can help you connect with what I mean:

Because of this book, Epstein-Barr virus (EBV) testing is becoming a regular practice in both the conventional and alternative worlds of medicine as doctors start to connect their patients' mysterious symptoms with EBV. That's thanks to the hundreds of thousands of patients who have brought this information to their doctor's office and asked for help regarding what they've learned here. Readers continue to introduce more and more health-care providers to this book, and it has prompted a new movement to look for the deeper causes of chronic illness—and to take EBV seriously. Prior to the publication of *Medical Medium*, EBV was practically a non-concern. Medical communities didn't understand what the virus could do—because, for example, medical research and science were unaware that EBV creates symptoms that lead to neurological problems. Now EBV testing and awareness are becoming everyday at the doctor's office. Research and science are finally starting to find a link between Epstein-Barr virus and dozens of conditions.

This book has also prompted medical research and science to start to remove Lyme disease from the bacterial category and, for now, place it in the autoimmune category. While labeling Lyme as autoimmune still does not represent a full understanding of Lyme symptoms, this recategorization is a way for medical research and science to admit, "We don't understand this as well as we thought we did"—and that's a major shift toward progress.

Again, this is a testament to how readers went into action with the information in Chapter 16, "Lyme Disease." It's thanks to people who read here in *Medical Medium* that Lyme disease is viral, not bacterial, who brought that information to their doctors, and who applied the healing protocols here and got results. It's also thanks to the doctors who have educated themselves with this material as they work to help patients. Many doctors have even applied the healing protocols in their own lives.

Another important change: this book has brought a newfound understanding of what toxic heavy metals can really do—the conditions they can cause and contribute to when they're inside our body. The relationship between toxic heavy metals and viruses, too, is starting to gain awareness thanks to all those who have read Medical Medium information and decided to make change in the world.

These are only a few of the changes we're starting to see as the truths here reach more and more people. I'm here as a messenger, to offer living words from above with answers to what challenges health most today. With this new edition, the potential for progress is even greater.

You deserve answers. You deserve to have the knowledge and tools to protect yourself and your loved ones. Always remember: your work toward healing has greater meaning than you could ever know.

Many blessings,
Anthony William, Medical Medium

"You are holding the book that started it all—a fresh, upgraded, timely edition of the title where I first opened the door to anyone and everyone with healing knowledge from above to help the wider masses get answers, heal, and reclaim their lives."

— Anthony William, Medical Medium

Introduction

Have you tried everything, gone everywhere, and your health still isn't where you want it to be? Do you want reassurance that you haven't imagined, caused, or created your suffering?

Are you frightened by the rise of diseases such as cancer? Are you seeking tools for prevention?

Do you want to lose weight? To look and feel younger? Have more energy? To help a loved one who's ailing? To safeguard your family's well-being?

Do you want to feel like yourself again? To regain mental clarity and balance? To gain spiritual support and tap into your soul's potential?

Do you want to rise up and meet the challenges of the 21st century?

Do you feel confused by the contradictory health information out there and just want one clear guide with the real answers that have helped millions?

Then this book is for you. You will not find these answers anywhere else.

With every passing year, these answers reach more people. This information spreads in the world, sometimes misinterpreted and often not cited back to the Medical Medium book series or to my lectures throughout the years. Know that what you are reading here is the original source.

This book is unlike anything you've read. You won't find citation after citation, references to study after study, because this is still fresh, unique, ahead-of-its-time information that comes from above. In places where the information you read here sounds like it may already exist from other sources, the truths and facts actually come from Spirit of Compassion, a source I'll explain more in Chapter 1, "Origins of the Medical Medium." In the instance where Spirit referred me to an earthly source for a particular study to offer historical context, you'll see the footnote. Science has discovered some of what I write about here, and has yet to discover much of it. Everything I share in these pages comes from a higher authority, the Spirit of Compassion, that wants everyone to heal and live up to their potential.

This book unveils many of Spirit's most precious medical truths. It's the answer for anyone who's suffering from a chronic condition or a mystery illness that doctors haven't been able to resolve.

It's not just a book for people who are limited in their daily lives by symptoms and conditions, though. It's a book for every person on the planet.

Health trends and fads come and go, and then may come back around again, depending on how much financial backing and promotion breathes life back into them. When one is popular, it's hugely persuasive for people's consciousness. Then the new attraction comes along, the old one fades, and we're too distracted by the shiny new packaging to realize it contains the same misconceptions all over again. With each decade that goes by, we forget about the medical mistakes of the previous period, and history repeats itself.

Unlike other books in the health industry that repackage the same old theories with catchy new names, the pages that follow contain healing guidance that Spirit of Compassion is revealing for the first time. When the first edition of this book reached the masses years ago, it created a new movement—an eye-opening to what causes chronic illness. While this elevated and expanded edition of *Medical Medium* is built on the same foundation as the first edition, it also contains fresh and timely information and support. That's why it's critical that this new edition is released—so it can further educate medical communities and give people a fighting chance for their health freedom.

THE QUICKENING

Spirit of Compassion calls our current era the *Quickening*. Never before has civilization changed at such a fast pace.

Technology has revolutionized virtually everything about our lives. We live in a period of breathtaking wonder and opportunity.

It's also an era of danger. By the time we mentally process something that's just happened, it's already old news. We're in such a rush that we always feel the need to be a step ahead. Along with up-to-the-minute information at our fingertips come greater demands, responsibilities—and health pitfalls. Lightning-fast advances sometimes come at the price of unconsidered vulnerabilities.

These changes affect all of humankind—and womankind especially bears the brunt. It's women who face the greatest expectations in our current day, women whose bodies so often get pushed to the brink. And chronic illness has become such a widespread issue—for women, for men, and for children.

If we don't interrupt the constant flow of misinformation, if we don't recognize what our foremothers and forefathers have gone through and redirect our course, then the generations to come will have to endure unnecessary suffering. To keep up with the changing times—to survive—we must learn to adapt. The only way to do that is to protect our health.

The popular approach right now in books, articles, social media, and podcasts about chronic illness is to advise people to eliminate what are theorized to be inflammatory foods from their diets while making theoretical improvements to gut health—and that's as far as it goes. The information out there doesn't explain what actually causes autoimmune disorders or chronic conditions, or how to rid yourself of the real root problems. That is why people stay sick.

But there are genuine explanations for the conditions that leave medical communities in a stagnant place and leave patients without answers. The *illusion* is that there is movement in medical communities' understanding of chronic illness. The reality is that appearance of advancement often comes from false leads and guessing games—and people are still suffering. That stagnation doesn't need to hold you back anymore. There are powerful methods to deal with the challenges we face in the modern era.

This book is the guide to truly freeing yourself. I've written it so you can truly heal—and keep yourself from getting sucked into the trends and fads and mistakes and half-truths and errors and distractions and deceptions about health and wellness. Spirit of Compassion has provided this information so we can help today's children grow into healthy adults.

I'm in no way anti-science. I don't question that the earth is round, or that the earth is billions of years old, or the value of the scientific method. What Spirit of Compassion reveals in this book is being read here, and as a result, becoming recognized by the scientific community, more and more each day.

If you or a loved one is sick, do you feel you have 20 or 30 or 50 years to wait for answers? Can you bear to watch your daughter or son grow up to face the same health issues that you have, and the same limits of medicine?

That's why it's time this elevated and expanded edition of this book reached the public—so *you* can read it now.

HOW TO USE THIS BOOK

You may be reading this book for any number of reasons. Perhaps a doctor has handed you a diagnosis, and you want to know what's really behind the label. Maybe you have symptoms you don't know how to name, and you're searching for answers. Maybe you're a health-care professional, or the loved one of someone who's sick, and you want to know the best way to provide care. Or you may have a general interest in optimal health and well-being, and you want to learn how to tap into your best self and your purpose in life.

This book has something for everyone, regardless of what food program, diet, or nutritional belief system you may practice. It's for anyone who wants access to the most advanced knowledge about healing available.

Here's how it works: In Part I, "Where It All Begins," you'll learn about my connection with Spirit of Compassion and my life's work of helping people recover from the mystery factors keeping them sick so they can come back to life and prevent further health issues. I also discuss *mystery illness*, and why it's much more pervasive than anyone realizes.

Validation and knowledge are two of the most powerful tools for recovery, so the chapters in the middle two sections are devoted to explaining the real stories behind dozens of ailments.

Part II, "The Hidden Epidemic," is all about the Epstein-Barr virus, an overlooked pathogen that's secretly behind debilitating conditions such as fibromyalgia, chronic fatigue syndrome, multiple sclerosis, rheumatoid arthritis, thyroid disorders, and more. Epstein-Barr's various strains and stages are plaguing people, especially women, in so many different ways—it's the mystery illness of mystery illnesses. You'll also find critical answers here about how COVID connects to chronic illness.

Part III, "Secrets Behind Other Mystery Illnesses," moves on to other health conditions that are widely misunderstood and includes descriptions of their surprising and varied causes. None of this information can wait another moment to reach more people.

At the end of each chapter in both Parts II and III, you'll also find targeted healing suggestions, including recommended foods and supplements for specific illnesses. (Before applying supplements, make sure to read Chapter 21.)

Then turn to Part IV, "How to Finally Heal," where I disclose the true secrets to vibrant health. These are more big pieces of the puzzle missing from the health world today. Part IV is about recovery, prevention, self-discovery, and healing the soul—so whether your focus is overcoming illness, going from good health to great, or tapping into your true self, you'll find resources here. These resources include tips for optimal digestion, a healing cleanse, hidden ingredients that can hinder your health, insights into the most healing foods on the planet, options for detoxification, and instructions for spiritual techniques like healing injuries from emotional hardships through unique meditations and calling upon angels for support.

THE TRUTH ABOUT HEALING

The word *quicken* doesn't just mean "become faster." It also means "spring to life." Historically, it referred to the first signs of movement a fetus showed in the womb.

Which is to say, this time of the Quickening isn't just about life speeding up. It's also about rebirth.

A new world is emerging. If we're to keep up—and not fall prey to the dangers that accompany rapid change—we must adapt.

Every word of this book is devoted to helping you with that process.

I'm about getting people better. Before the Medical Medium book series was published, I had already helped tens of thousands of people fully recover from what ailed them, stave off further illness, and live vibrant lives, which was why I wanted to share this success with the wider world. Now that these books have gone into the wider world, millions of people have been changing their lives with information from above.

You'll see me use the term *medical communities* often throughout the book. By this I mean the conventional and alternative medical communities, as well as the newer fields of integrative and functional medicine. I don't take sides with any of them; I also don't point fingers. I support the work they do. Doctors continually reach out to me to discuss the information in the Medical Medium books and talk about how to apply it in their practices, because they're seeing it help others. The information here is neutral, independent. It's about practitioners and healers getting ahold of this knowledge, learning how to help more people. It is about *you* getting ahold of this knowledge and learning how to heal yourself. It is about the truth.

Aren't we all looking for truth? Truth about our world, the universe? Truth about ourselves? About life? About why we are here? About our purpose?

When we're sick, we question ourselves. We feel cut off from life, from what we were put on earth to do. We doubt basic truths, like the body's ability to heal, because we haven't yet connected to what's really behind our illnesses. We go from doctor to doctor, medical community to medical community, looking for an answer. We lose faith in life itself.

When we become well, doubt melts away. We have energy to devote to our true purpose. We watch ourselves transform, and we believe in the good in life again. We get reacquainted with our path in this world. We find our way back home with peace in our heart and soul.

The truth about the world, ourselves, life, purpose—it all comes down to healing.

And the truth about healing is now in your hands.

"If we don't interrupt the constant flow of misinformation, if we don't recognize what our foremothers and forefathers have gone through and redirect our course, then the generations to come will have to endure unnecessary suffering. To keep up with the changing times —to survive—we must learn to adapt. The only way to do that is to protect our health."

— Anthony William, Medical Medium

PART I

WHERE IT ALL BEGINS

"I've devoted my life to this work.
I'm here as a messenger. It's who I am.

People told me as a child that I have a gift. As the years
went by, Spirit of Compassion made something perfectly
clear: the gift was never mine. It's for the ones in need,
the ones who struggle, suffer, and are searching
for answers. This gift is for you."

— Anthony William, Medical Medium

CHAPTER 1

Origins of the Medical Medium

When this book was first published, I revealed truths you couldn't learn anywhere else. You wouldn't hear them from your doctor, read them in other books, or find them on social media.

These are prophecies that had not yet surfaced, and that I was bringing to light for the first time.

Since the initial publication of *Medical Medium*, how medical communities view symptoms, conditions, illness, and disease has finally started to change due to the original and unique information in this book and the rest of this series. The information here has propelled both alternative and conventional medicine in a new direction. It has opened the door for medical communities to finally start awakening to the widespread effect of viruses on the global population. This book has become a reference guide in doctor's offices around the world.

I'm not a physician. I have no medical training. Yet I can tell you things about your health that no one else can. I can give you advanced medical information that's decades ahead of medical research and science so you can finally get clarity on chronic and mystery illnesses that doctors often misdiagnose, treat incorrectly, or tag with certain labels even when they don't truly understand what causes the symptoms.

Since I was a young child, I've been helping individuals heal with the insights I'm about to share. Now, it's time for you to learn how to use these powerful healing tools and secrets.

It's how Spirit of Compassion has told me it's meant to be.

AN UNEXPECTED GUEST

My story begins when I'm four years old.

As I'm waking up one Sunday morning, I hear an elderly man speaking.

His voice is just outside my right ear. It's very clear.

He says, "I am the Spirit of the Most High. There is no spirit above me but God."

I'm confused and alarmed. Is someone else in my room? I open my eyes and look around, but don't see anybody. *Maybe some-one's talking or playing a radio outside,* I think.

I get up and walk to the window. There are no people—it's too early in the morning. I have no idea what's going on, and I'm not sure I want to.

I run downstairs to be with my parents and feel safe. I don't say anything about the voice. But as the day goes on, a feeling builds up—that I'm being watched.

In the evening I settle into my chair at the dinner table. With me are my parents, my grandparents, and some other family members.

As we're eating, I suddenly see a strange man standing behind my grandmother. He has gray hair and a gray beard, and is wearing a brown robe. I assume he's a family friend who's come to join our meal. Instead of sitting down with us, though, he keeps standing behind my grandmother . . . and looking only at me.

When none of my family reacts to his presence, I slowly realize that I'm the only one who sees him. I look away to see if he'll disappear. When I look back, he's still there staring at me. His mouth doesn't move, but I can hear his voice by my right ear. It's the same voice I heard when waking up. This time he says, in a calming tone, "I am here for you."

I stop eating.

"What's wrong?" my mom asks. "You're not hungry?"

I don't answer, just keep looking at the man, who lifts his right arm and waves for me to come over to my grandmother.

Feeling an undeniable instinct to follow his instruction, I climb out of my chair and walk to Grandma.

He takes my hand and puts it on my grand-mother's chest while she's eating.

Grandma backs away with a start. "What are you doing?" she asks.

The gray man looks at me. "Say 'lung cancer.'"

I'm at a loss. I don't even know what *lung cancer* means.

I try to say it, but it comes out as a mumble.

"Do it again," he tells me. "Lung."

"Lung," I say.

"Cancer."

"Cancer," I say.

My entire family is staring at me now. I'm still focused on the gray man.

"Now say, 'Grandma has lung cancer.'"

"Grandma has lung cancer," I say.

I hear a fork clatter on the table.

The gray man pulls my hand from Grandma and gently places it at my side. Then he turns and starts climbing steps that weren't there before.

He looks back at me and says, "You will hear from me all the time, but you may never see me again. Not to worry." He continues climbing until he steps through the ceiling of my house—and now *does* disappear.

My grandmother stares at me. "Did you say what I thought you said?"

There's a panic at the table. What just happened doesn't make sense for a number of reasons—starting with the fact that, as far as we know, Grandma is fine. She hasn't noticed any problems or seen any doctors.

The next morning I wake up . . . and hear the voice again: "I am the Spirit of the Most High. There is no spirit above me but God."

Just like the previous morning, I look around but don't see anyone.

From that day on the same thing happens every morning, without fail.

Meanwhile, my grandmother is shaken by what I said to her. Even though she feels fine, she makes an appointment for a general checkup.

A few weeks later she visits her doctor—and a chest X-ray reveals that she has lung cancer.

THE VOICE

As the mysterious visitor continues to greet me every morning, I start to pay attention to what he sounds like.

His crystal-clear voice is somewhere between baritone and tenor—a bit on the low side, but not *very* low. It has depth and resonance. Even though he's near my right ear, his speech has the stereo effect of surround sound. The visitor is loudest in the morning.

It's hard to gauge his age. Sometimes he sounds like an exceptionally strong, healthy 80-year-old, matching the gray man I saw at dinner. At other times he sounds thousands of years old.

You might say he has a soothing voice. Yet constantly hearing a voice is hard to get used to. The voice isn't internal. It is not thoughts I'm thinking. It is not my own inner voice. I can separate my own thoughts from the voice I hear. It's a voice that comes from an outside source directly above my right ear, as if someone were standing next to me. I can't will it to go away.

I can physically block it. When I put my hand in front of my ear, I can make the voice sound very faint. As soon as I move my hand away, he's at full volume again.

I ask him to stop talking to me. At first I'm polite about it. Then I'm not.

It doesn't matter what I say, though. He talks whenever he wants to.

SPIRIT OF COMPASSION, SPIRIT OF THE MOST HIGH

I start calling the voice by name, Spirit of the Most High. Sometimes I call him *Spirit* for short, or *Most High.*

By age eight I hear Spirit continually throughout the day. He tells me about the physical health of anyone I encounter.

No matter where I am or what I'm doing, I'm told about the aches, pains, and illnesses of whoever's nearby, and also what the person needs to do to become better. The relentlessness of this ongoing and intimate information is extremely stressful.

I ask Spirit to stop telling me these things I don't want to know.

"We're not here on this earth very long," Spirit says. "We can't waste any time." He tells me that he's trying to teach me as much as possible in the short time we have together, and that we can't spare a moment.

Hearing this devastates me. Somehow I believed that life is so long that it feels like we live forever. I feel my childhood slipping away with the grim reality of this truth Spirit has just shared. When I tell Spirit this job is too demanding, he ignores me.

I learn that I *can* engage in some conversation with him, though. I'm old enough to pose some fundamental questions, so I ask, "Who are you? *What* are you? Where did you come from? And why are you here?"

Spirit replies, "First I will tell you what I am not.

"I am not an angel. And I am not a person. I was never a human being. I am not a ghost or a 'spirit guide,' either.

"I am a *word*."

I blink fast, trying to take this in. All I can think to ask is, "Which word?"

Spirit replies, "Compassion."

I'm not sure how to respond. But I don't need to. Spirit keeps talking. "I am literally the living essence of the word *compassion*. I sit at the fingertip of God."

"Spirit, I don't understand. Are *you* God?"

"No," the voice replies. "At the fingertip of God sits a word, and that word is compassion. I am that word. A living word. The closest word to God."

I shake my head. "How can you be just a word?"

"A word is an energy source. Certain words hold great power. God pours light into words such as I and instills us with the breath of life. I am *more* than a word."

"Is there anyone else like you?" I ask.

"Yes: Faith. Hope. Joy. Peace. And more. They are all living words, but I sit above all of them, because I am the closest to God."

"Do these words speak to people, too?"

"Not as I do to you. These words are not heard by the ear. They live in each person's heart and soul. As do I. Words such as *joy* and *peace* do not stand alone in the heart. They require compassion to be complete."

"Why can't peace be enough by itself?" I ask. Many times since Spirit entered my life, I've wished for peace and quiet.

"Compassion is the understanding of suffering," Spirit replies. "There is no peace, joy, or hope until those who suffer are understood. Compassion is the soul of these words; without it, they are empty. Compassion fills them with truth, honor, and purpose.

"*I* am compassion. And no other sits above me but God."

Trying to make sense of this, I ask, "Then what is God?"

"God is a word. God is *love*, which is above all other words. God is also *more* than a word. Because God loves all. God is the most powerful source of existence.

"People can love. But people do not love all others unconditionally. God does."

It's too much for me to process. I end the conversation with one personal question: "Do you talk to anyone else?" *Because if you do,* I'm thinking, *I'm going to seek them out so I don't have to feel so alone.*

"The angels and other Godly beings look to me for guidance. I provide all who care to listen with the lessons and wisdom of God," says Spirit of the Most High, who I realize is Spirit of Compassion. "But on earth, I speak directly only to you."

ME AND MY SHADOW

As you might imagine, this is a lot to absorb at age eight.

Being able to hear a voice from above clearly at all times, and freely engage in conversation with it, is a different experience entirely from those who call themselves mediums. What distinguishes it further is that the voice speaks outside the ear, so that it's an independent source separate from my thoughts. It's essentially having someone follow me around everywhere—someone who keeps telling me things I really don't want to hear about the health of everyone around me.

The upside is, Spirit of Compassion provides me with medical information that's incredibly advanced—decades ahead of its time—more advanced than any medical community or health source for chronic illness. Plus I'm regularly informed about my *own* health, which is a great rarity.

Spirit of Compassion shares much more than only health and medical information. He provides me with insights into how the world works on a level beyond what anyone knows about the planet, the universe, and life beyond Planet Earth. Spirit tells me about ancient civilizations and what sits undiscovered at the bottom of our oceans. He tells me about worldly deceptions created by people of evil nature and about deceptions of global industries that affect the population's health. He tells me about environmental shifts, what the planet is up against, and future setbacks that could affect many people.

These are all things I cannot change. Spirit teaches me that we don't have control over the free will of those who wreak havoc on this planet out of greed and game. Where I *can* make a difference is helping people find answers, gain health benefits, and get their lives back—so they can lead happier, healthier lives and at least have peace within themselves.

Although by this point, I know that Spirit of the Most High is the living essence of the word *compassion*, it can be hard for me to stay open to the name Spirit of Compassion. I witness Spirit's level of compassion for others, for their suffering and struggles and what they need. Where is the compassion for me, I wonder, when I have to take on such responsibility at such a young age? I want some of Spirit of Compassion's focus and loving nature for my childhood self; I want restorative time with Spirit, and that's very limited. Anyone who's with me, Spirit's focus is on them. The more people I'm around, the more is required of me. Even when I get alone time with my parents, Spirit of Compassion prompts me to focus on what's going on with them.

Only periodically do I catch short moments of one-on-one time with Spirit of Compassion for comfort and reassurance that he cares about me. Spirit does assure me that he has compassion for me, although as an eight-year-old, I don't have the perspective and acceptance yet to see or feel that fully. What I feel is a weight on my shoulders on an hour-by-hour, sometimes second-by-second, basis. Depending on how much work is involved in having to see the world's suffering and focus on everyone besides myself at any given moment, I switch off on what I call Spirit. Some days, I'm more open and call him Spirit of Compassion. Other days—when the inner struggle of hearing a voice and the harsh reality of spending my waking hours with that voice focused on everybody around me weighs heavily—I call him Spirit of the Most High.

Spirit tries to influence me to use my free will wisely. When I'm still eight years old, I spend a week building a dam in a stream by my house. Spirit tells me it's a bad idea, that it will flood the neighbor's lawn.

"It'll be fine," I say.

Then a downpour comes, the stream rises—and it floods the neighbor's lawn. As the man from the house yells at me, I hear in my ear, "I told you. You didn't listen to me."

Spirit is constantly watching my every move and telling me what I should and shouldn't do. It makes having any kind of normal childhood impossible. That same year I build the dam,

I know in great detail about the physical and emotional health of my friends and even my teacher—who's struggling through an awful relationship with her boyfriend. I absorb every bit of it, which is overwhelming and distressing.

That year, Spirit tells me that a classmate is coming down with meningitis. I tell the teacher, who calls the boy to her desk and asks, "Do you have meningitis?" He's never heard the word before and doesn't know what it means.

"Well, he's going to get it soon even if he doesn't have it this second," I say.

My teacher is alarmed at such a serious accusation, so she calls our parents and sends us both to the school nurse. When the nurse takes our temperatures, they come back normal. Soon my classmate's parents and my mom arrive. Along with my teacher, we all head to the principal's office, where a big discussion begins. "Does he have meningitis?" the adults ask each other. "Where would he get it?"

"No," they agree. "We don't have any idea how he could have gotten it."

"Well," I say, echoing my earlier words, "I believe he's going to come down with it."

My mom knows my history, so she recognizes this is very possible and sticks up for me. "There's a good chance this will happen."

The other adults question me. "Were you around anyone who had meningitis?"

I tell them no. Soon the meeting ends and my classmate, teacher, and I return to class.

The next day, my classmate isn't in school. The teacher was informed that he's in the hospital with a temperature of 104 degrees and a case of meningitis.

With experiences like this, it's getting to the point where I'm lacking the time and energy to focus on myself. I even find it possible to lose myself with the amount of incoming information and detail about everyone else's lives.

As I feel my freedom disappear, Spirit gives me words of hope and kindness yet is always honest and forthcoming. Spirit tells me to expect worse—and that we will get through it. "Your biggest challenges are yet to come."

"What do you mean?" I ask.

"Only one or two people per century are given this gift," he says. "It is not a typical intuitive or psychic ability. It is something that most fail to survive. You will find it almost unbearable not to be able to live like a normal person, never mind a normal teenager.

"Eventually you will see almost nothing but the suffering of others. You will somehow have to find a way of becoming comfortable with that. Otherwise, the chances are you will end your life."

READING BODIES

Spirit of Compassion becomes both my best friend and my albatross. I appreciate that he's training me for a job God has chosen for me. Still, the responsibility is immense.

One day he tells me to go to a large, beautiful cemetery near my home. "I want you to stand over that grave," he says, "and figure out how the person died."

That's quite a request to make of an eight-year-old.

At this point, though, I've been so bombarded with the health information of both friends and strangers that I try to view this as just one more case.

And with Spirit's help, I'm able to do what he asks.

This adds another dimension to the gift: not only does Spirit verbally inform me of what's wrong with someone's health, he also helps me visualize physical scans of the person's body.

I spend years of my childhood in different cemeteries performing this exercise with hundreds of corpses. I become so good at it that I can almost instantly sense if someone's died of heart attack, stroke, cancer, liver disease, car accident, suicide, or murder.

Along with this, Spirit teaches me to look very deeply into the bodies of the living. He promises that once this training is concluded, I'll be able to scan and see inside *anyone* with extreme accuracy.

Whenever I get tired or want to do something more fun, Spirit tells me, "Someday you'll be performing scans on people that will mean the difference between life and death. You will be able to tell if a person's lungs are about to collapse, or an artery is about to clot and shut down someone's heart."

Once, I reply, "Who cares? Why does it matter? Why should *I* care?"

"You *must* care," Spirit responds. "What all of us do here on earth matters. The good works you perform matter to your soul. You must take this responsibility seriously."

SELF-HEALING

At age nine, while other children are riding bikes and playing baseball, I'm constantly witnessing disease in the people around me and listening to Spirit of Compassion tell me what's needed for them to get better. I'm learning what adults don't know to do for their health and exactly what actions they should take to heal.

At this point I'm so filled with health-related knowledge and training that it's hard not to start applying it.

One opportunity arises when I get sick myself. Eating out with my family one evening, I ignore Spirit's usual dietary recommendations and warnings and eat a dish that gives me food poisoning. I choose the dish because at this age, I have a sense of safety knowing that if I get sick, I have Spirit to help me. This is not a wise way of looking at things, I quickly learn. Spirit allows me to experience this key life lesson for myself: that having Spirit to help me doesn't mean I'm not going to experience discomfort or pain from my own poor decision.

When I fall ill from the food, I think, *Okay, it's food poisoning. I'm going to get over this in a day or two.* Then it persists, each day running into the next. Before I know it, almost two weeks have passed. I lie in bed in agonizing abdominal pain. My parents take me to the doctor's office and even the ER one night when it gets really bad, hoping for any form of relief, but the fever and the pain in my gut don't stop. Finally Spirit of Compassion cuts through my delirium and tells me I'm going to need a mono eating protocol to rid this specific strain of *E. coli* bacteria from my body. He gives me a direct order to go to my great-grandfather's house and pick a box of heirloom pears from his tree. Spirit says I'm to eat nothing but these ripe pears, and I'll heal.

I do as he says and recover rapidly.

FIRE HIM, GOD

At age 10, I try to go over Spirit's head and deal directly with his boss. I'm getting a little older; I've been in this for six years by this point. I decide it's finally time.

I figure I can't tell God what I want through prayer because Spirit of Compassion will hear me.

So I climb some of the highest trees I can find to get as close to God as possible and carve messages in their trunks.

One of the first messages is, "God, I love Spirit, but it's time we cut out the middle man."

This is followed by some serious questions:

"God, why do people have to be sick?"

"God, why can't *you* fix everybody?"

"God, why do *I* have to help people?"

While these seem to me very reasonable things to ask, I receive no answers.

So I find some even more dangerously tall trees, and I climb to the highest branches in hopes that my recklessness will get God's attention. This time I carve requests for direct action:

"God, please give me back silence."

"God, I don't want to hear Spirit anymore. Make him go away."

As I carve in the words "God, let me be free," I lose my foothold and almost slip off the branch. *Not* that *kind of free!* I think. I inch my way back down to safety, defeated.

None of these messages makes any difference. Spirit just keeps talking to me.

If he's aware of my attempts to subvert his authority, he's gracious enough not to mention it. There's more important work at hand.

FIRST CLIENTS

At age 11, I want to do something productive and fun that'll take my mind off the voice by my ear, so I get a job carrying clubs at a golf course that's a 10-mile bike ride from home.

My gift is not so easily abandoned, though. While caddying, I can't help telling golfers about their conditions. I often know about their stiff joints, bad knees, sore hips, hurt ankles, tendonitis, and more before they do.

So I say, "Your swing's a little off, but that's not surprising considering your carpal tunnel situation," or "You'd do better if you dealt with your inflamed left hip."

They look at me with amazement and ask, "How did you know that?"

Then they request advice on how to get better, and I tell them what to eat, what changes to make to their behavior, therapies to try, and so on. The recommendations Spirit offers are often head-turners, because these are still the earlier days, when even the slightest healing food advice is shocking.

After caddying for several years, I crave a change. I decide that if I'm going to share Spirit's recommendations for food and supplements for healing, I might as well work in a place that sells them. So I get a job as stock boy in a local supermarket.

The people who rely on Spirit of Compassion and me for help come by whenever they like, and I take time out of replenishing shelves to help them. The owner of the supermarket doesn't mind that my work for him is periodically interrupted, because I'm bringing in new customers.

Besides, I'm helping him, too.

Whenever someone asks how I know what I know, I answer, "Spirit of Compassion."

It's a little odd talking someone through their gastritis in a supermarket aisle. It's also difficult, because supplements are barely available yet and the variety of food with specific medicinal qualities is limited. Spirit keeps explaining that in a couple of decades, stores will supply many more options for people's health. In the meantime, he helps me get creative with healing plans—such as juicing celery for people's ailments, which I do right there in the store. I love being able to hand someone exactly what she needs to get better.

WITH GREAT POWER COMES GREAT GUILT

At age 14, I sometimes sit in a bus or a train, and there goes Spirit of Compassion again, bringing up some health issue with the guy in front of me, so I tap him on the shoulder to tell him about it. At times the response is gratitude. Other times the reaction is to accuse me of invading his privacy. "Do you know my doctor?" some people ask. "Did you get ahold of my medical records?" That's a lot of distrust and hostility to deal with—especially since we haven't yet entered the Internet and digital age, and medical records aren't computerized yet. They're all on paper, locked far away in doctor's offices.

As I grow older, I learn to be careful about who I try to help unasked. If I see someone regularly, I still feel impelled to share what I know. So I develop the habit of first asking Spirit of Compassion to read someone's emotional state to determine whether they're approachable. That cuts down on the number of uncomfortable situations.

If someone is a stranger, I'll usually keep whatever I'm seeing to myself. This becomes a burden, though. When I'm a teen, I start feeling even more accountable for my actions. So if someone is in danger of kidney disease, or has cancer, and I do nothing, part of me feels it's my fault if the person ends up seriously ill or dead. When this is multiplied hundreds of times a day, the sense of guilt and responsibility becomes overwhelming.

ESCAPE ATTEMPTS

As my teenage years continue, life becomes more difficult. For instance, most people watch television to relax and escape. But when I watch, I receive health information from Spirit of Compassion about everyone on the screen. Spirit prompts me to automatically scan the condition of every person I see who needs help, whether they know they have a condition or not. When that happens over and over, TV is draining, not fun.

It's even worse when I go to a movie theater. I'm uncontrollably scanning the health of every person in my row, the row in front of me, the row in back of me, and so on.

And that's not the end of it. I scan the health of the people *in the movie*. I'm able to determine the condition of each actor during the time the film was shot, as well as the health of the actor in the present moment. Imagine what it's like to be at a movie and get bombarded by medical information about the people around you and up on the big screen.

Considering the last thing most teens want is to feel different from everyone else, this period is especially rocky. My feelings of alienation and being overwhelmed by responsibility lead to some rebellious teen impulses. I pursue various ways to escape my "gift."

I start spending a lot of time in the woods. I find nature soothing, and especially appreciate the absence of other people. With the help of Spirit, I learn to identify different species of birds during the day. At night he teaches me the names of stars—both what scientists call them and the names God has given them. It's not fully an escape, though, because Spirit also teaches me how to recognize herbs and foods growing around me—mullein, yellow dock, plantain, dandelion, burdock root, wild rose hips and petals, wild apples, wild berries—and how to use them for healing.

I also develop an interest in repairing cars. I like fixing up mechanical objects because they don't require me to become emotionally involved. Even if I fail to repair a junker Chevy with a bad engine, I never feel remotely as awful as I do when I can't help people because they're in too advanced a stage of disease to be healed.

But this hobby doesn't go as planned, either. People start noticing what I'm doing and coming over: "Wow, that's amazing! Can you fix *my* car?" I don't have it in me to say no—especially since Spirit is doing the hardest part, which is figuring out what's wrong.

One day when I'm 15, my mother and I stop at a station to get gasoline. I walk into the garage and find a bunch of mechanics staring at a car as if they're trying to solve a puzzle.

"What's going on?" I ask.

One of the men says, "We've worked on this car for weeks. It should run perfectly. But we can't get it to start."

Spirit immediately tells me the solution. "Open up the wire harness in the back of the firewall," I pass along to the mechanics.

"Buried in dozens of other wires you'll find a white one that's broken. Put that wire together and the car will run fine."

"That's ridiculous!" says another of the men.

"What's the harm in checking?" asks the first one. So they go in—and sure enough, there's a white wire broken in half.

They look at me with their jaws hanging open.

"Are you the owner of this car?" asks the skeptical mechanic. "Or are you a friend of his?"

"No," I reply. "I just have a knack for these things."

In a minute they fix the wire and try the car again. It starts up perfectly.

One of the mechanics starts dancing around. Another calls it "a miracle."

Word gets around, and soon a bunch of garages in my town, and also several neighboring towns, use me as the go-to guy for troubleshooting seemingly unfixable vehicles. When I show up to assist on a job, the mechanics who called me—much older guys with years of experience—are always incredulous. "What's this fifteen-year-old doing here?" they all ask. When I get the job done, though, they change their minds.

So instead of escaping responsibility, I gain more. On top of healing people, I become a car doctor.

The last straw is when I realize how emotional people are about their cars. A lot of times, they're even more invested in their cars' well-being than in their own health. At that point cars stop being fun for me.

I try some other distracting activities. For example, I join a rock band, because loud music helps drown out Spirit's voice. Spirit does not appreciate this. He patiently waits until I'm finished making a racket, then resumes his commentary on the health of those around me.

Nothing really works to make my gift go away. It becomes increasingly clear that I'm stuck with Spirit and my ability—and can't escape the path that's been laid out for me.

STARTING TO COMMIT

By the time I'm a young man, thanks to my training with Spirit, I've indirectly scanned and received health information from Spirit of Compassion on thousands of people and helped hundreds along the way.

One day I think, *Okay, this is the hand I've been dealt. I have a special purpose. I just have to accept it—for now.*

I also think, *This can't possibly go on forever. At some point I'll have fulfilled my responsibilities and will be set free to live a normal life.* Spirit has never said any such thing to me, yet I need to believe it to keep going.

In my early 20s, I begin dedicating myself in earnest to what Spirit has repeatedly told me is my destiny. I wholeheartedly open my door to sick people who come and see me for help, discover the true root causes of their illnesses, and tell them what Spirit of Compassion says they need to do to become healthy.

And despite my griping about the various stresses I've endured, it's fulfilling work. It feels good to watch people heal and get their lives back.

In these early days, sometimes what I can do is so empowering that I let the feeling of being all-knowing go to my head.

A good example is the time my neighbor approaches me about his wife, who can't walk or use her legs. She's been to dozens of doctors, and none of them have helped. My neighbor tells her, "Look, Anthony seems to know a lot about this stuff. Let's take a chance."

When they ask me what the problem could be that doctors can't seem to find, I ask Spirit, who informs me that she has arsenic poisoning—traces of arsenic in her brain that have come from their well. Shortly after, a well water analysis confirms the presence of arsenic. Her doctor then performs a blood test, which shows unacceptable levels of arsenic in her blood. With Spirit's recommendations on how to remove the toxic heavy metal from her system, within a year she's able to walk again.

I'm in my garden pulling up some onions for a salad (it's one of my favorite herbs to grow) when my neighbor comes around. "I just want to thank you again, Anthony," he says. "We went all over the country to meet top experts, and they couldn't do a thing. It doesn't make any sense—somehow you knew exactly what was wrong and what she needed. I don't know how it's possible. You're not even a doctor."

I look at him with onions in my hand and say, "It's because I'm always right. I can fix any problem because there's nothing I'm wrong about. Just remember that—I'm always right and will always be right."

Then I turn around, walk a few feet, and turn back to say, "And don't forget it!" when I step on a rake that slaps me in the face so hard it knocks me out.

As I lie on the ground, my concerned neighbor rushes to my side and stands over me. In my dazed state I think he's my constant companion. "Spirit?" I ask.

Spirit of the Most High replies, "*I'm* always right. *You're* always wrong. Remember that. I'm always *right*. You're always *wrong*."

Whenever I get carried away, I think of that moment. It's a reminder that while some of the things I do as a healer with the power of Spirit might be considered miraculous, I'm still a regular guy who can miss the mark if I'm not listening to what Spirit has to say.

THE TURNING POINT

When I'm a young adult, Spirit assumes I've passed the crisis point that led others with my gift over the centuries to end their lives. He assumes I've accepted that using my abilities to heal people is what I'll do for the rest of my life.

Which goes to show that even Spirit of the Most High can't predict everything when it comes to free will.

One day in late fall, I'm at a retreat by the water with no one but the woman I plan to spend my life with and my dog, August (short for Augustine).

I've had August for a year and am very close to her. She replaced my family dog, who was with me for 15 years. Just like that dog, August is essential to my sanity.

We're sitting by a large, deep bay. The water is icy cold, and the current is strong.

It's our last day. With great reluctance, we start getting ready to leave the peaceful isolation of this place.

Suddenly, with no warning, my dog jumps into the bay. I sense she picked up on my feelings. This is her way of saying, "We don't have to go. Let's stay here and keep playing."

Unfortunately, both the cold and the current take hold of her. She immediately starts slipping from us.

We stand on the shore, screaming at August to come back. I throw stones into the water to try to lead my dog back to me. This is our special signal—whenever I splash stones in the shallows, she returns to shore. But today, the current pulls her farther and farther away.

August goes 50 feet out. I see her struggling to get back and losing the battle. Then the cold freezes her so thoroughly that she stops paddling . . . and goes straight down.

I toss off my jacket, boots, and pants, and jump into the freezing water.

I've swum 15 feet out when Spirit of the Most High says, "If you keep going, you are not going to make it."

"It doesn't matter!" I yell. "I'm not abandoning August. I have to save my dog."

I swim another 15 feet—and then the merciless cold takes over. My body goes numb.

Spirit says, "You've done it now. You cannot turn back, and you cannot go forward. This is it."

"Really? You rob me of a normal, peaceful life, I dedicate my whole being to your work of healing, and this is all I get from you? You say, 'This is it,' and leave us to die?"

All the angst and anger I've suppressed since I was four years old comes pouring out. I let Spirit have it about my years of pent-up frustration over this continual torture I've always had to accept as a "gift": being set apart from everyone else, knowing too much about everyone at way too early an age, and being told what I had to do with my life instead of given even the slightest choice.

I tell Spirit, "I put up with a lot—sacrificing my childhood, experiencing everybody's pain and suffering, taking responsibility for healing thousands of strangers, and draining myself physically and mentally every day. And now you're telling me I can't even protect my own family?

"No, dammit!" I shout as the freezing waves threaten to engulf me. "If this is how you want me to end, Spirit, so be it. I'm getting my dog back, or I'm going down with her."

A very long second passes. Numb and exhausted, I realize that I may have finally pushed things too far. A few more moments without help, and I'll be following my dog August into the depths below.

I turn my head toward the shore to get one last glimpse of the woman I planned to spend the rest of my life with.

Spirit says, "You need to swim out twenty more feet."

In shock, I shout, "How?"

To my great surprise, I feel renewed strength. I resume swimming. In my mind, I continue to yell at Spirit that I deserve to survive this *with* my dog. Otherwise we should both die.

Spirit says, "I will get you to your dog. In return, you must commit to me. We go through this life the way we're supposed to. You accept that it is by the holy power of God you are destined to do this work for the rest of your life."

"Okay!" I shout. "Deal. Let me find August, and I'll work for you with no complaints ever again."

I swim the additional 20 feet. Spirit says, "Hold your breath and go eight feet down, then open your eyes."

As I hold my breath, a surge of power courses through my body. All of a sudden I can feel my legs again.

I swim what feels like eight feet down, open my eyes—and see an angel.

I've never encountered an angel before. I'm seeing what looks like a woman who has no trouble breathing underwater, with a glorious source of light behind her, light radiating from her eyes, and huge, beautiful wings of light growing out of her back. There's no question she's a divine being.

And in her arms is August, surrounded by a beautiful, peaceful light. For a moment, it feels like time stands still. My vision is surprisingly clear underwater, and I have no fear or trouble holding my breath.

I grab my dog by her collar. Then *something* pushes me upward with her.

We both reach the surface of the water.

The bay is still icy cold, and the current is still trying to violently pull us away from land and life. The wind is blowing strong.

When I open my eyes again, I see Spirit for a moment standing right above the water. It's the only time I've seen Spirit since the first day he appeared to me at age four.

"We don't have much time," he says. "The angel is leaving."

Just as I register once again that all could have been lost, another surge of power charges through my body. As I start swimming back through the frigid waters—holding on to August, who seems lifeless—it feels almost as if I'm being pulled across the 50 feet to safety.

My dog and I soon make it back to shore— and to my future wife, who is crying with relief.

As I drag myself and my dog up to the rocky sand, I cry in agony—not because I'm feeling the initial stages of hypothermia, but because I'm afraid my dog is gone. All I can think is, *Let her still be alive.*

She opens her eyes, gasps for air, and comes to life. The sun appears from behind the clouds, and a streak of light races across the water and shines on my dog, August. I look at the light and say, "Spirit, thank you."

And I realize: this is the first time since Spirit entered my life that I've ever thanked him for anything. The battles I've waged with Spirit of the Most High since I was four years old have to end. It's time for me to acknowledge the cards I've been dealt.

Even before this point, people in need have been coming to me in droves.

With this pledge, I wholly dedicate myself to helping them, without reservation and for the rest of my life.

I don't have to pretend the abilities I've been granted are a problem-free blessing. Yet I stop complaining and finally accept who I am.

That's when I truly assume my role as the Medical Medium.

THE COMMITMENT

When I committed to what Spirit of Compassion wanted of me, he helped me develop a routine for fulfilling it as efficiently as possible.

I never had to be in the same room with a person to perform a scan, so I arranged to speak with people in need by phone. This allowed Spirit of Compassion to help anyone in the world, regardless of location, and it minimized the transition time. Spirit of Compassion helped tens of thousands of people this way.

When I performed a scan, Spirit of Compassion would create a very bright white light that let me see into the person. While that was critical for obtaining what Spirit needed from me as the Medical Medium, the intensity of the light created a kind of "snow blindness" that temporarily impaired my vision in the real world, and it accumulated as the day went on if Spirit wanted me to scan more and more people. When Spirit and I finished helping people for the day, it could take a little time for my sight to return to normal.

(As a side note, I bring my assistant with me whenever I go somewhere that will have a lot of people, because I may lose a substantial portion of my sight due to "automatic" scans. For example, whenever I have to fly somewhere, I end up inadvertently learning about the health conditions of everyone on my plane. By the time we land I could be partially blind, so I need my assistant to lead me around until the effect wears off.)

A deep and comprehensive view of a person's condition could sometimes take minutes. However, when doing this throughout the years, it would take 10 to 30 minutes or more to explain what discoveries were found as well as advice for healing and how to work with their doctor.

Sometimes Spirit of Compassion would need to spend time bolstering or "reconstructing" someone in need. That's because Spirit cares about more than just people's physical illnesses.

SOUL, HEART, AND SPIRIT

When Spirit of Compassion delivers information in a scan, we see beyond a person's physical health. I also witness the person's soul, heart, and spirit. These are three entirely different components of a person's being that are often considered one and the same.

Even if your soul's been battered and your heart is faint, your spirit can keep you physically going while you look for opportunities to heal. For example, sometimes Spirit of Compassion wants me to tell a very ill person to start walking, go out to watch birds, and look at sunsets. That helps the person regain her or his spirit, and that can be the start to rebuilding the heart and soul.

You'll find much more about your soul, heart, and spirit, as well as essential techniques to heal and reclaim these parts of yourself, in Chapter 24, "Soul-Healing Meditations and Techniques."

THE ONE AND ONLY MEDICAL MEDIUM

While there are obvious disadvantages to having a voice continually talking into my ear, there are also some advantages.

Because Spirit of Compassion is distinct and separate from me, it doesn't matter if on a given day I'm feeling upset or ill or bored. Spirit is unaffected by my emotions and will consistently provide powerful, advanced information—ahead of medical research and science—about chronic illness and how to heal. It's the same process as when I was a child. Regardless of what my life struggles are, even if I'm in no condition in the moment to process what Spirit of Compassion is telling me (for example, if I only had two hours of sleep because of certain challenges occurring in life), the information will still come through. Focusing and concentrating on the intricate specificities takes work.

I don't have to use my intuitive skills. I don't channel the information, either. Other mediums sometimes hear inner voices, but mine isn't internal. People seeking help ask me, "Should I take off my jewelry to allow you to get a better read?" It doesn't matter if they're wrapped in tinfoil; the information is still going to come through and they're going to get the answers they need to move forward.

I'm often asked if Spirit of Compassion can help me with my family, loved ones, and even myself to get physical and spiritual information. The answer is yes. Again, because Spirit is separate from me, all I have to do is ask, and he tells and shows me what is best to know. This is one of the things that makes this gift unique.

One day a skeptical reporter demands I give her an answer on the spot: "I want you to tell me where it hurts. Does it hurt in my toe? My leg? My stomach? Does it hurt in my arm? My butt? Do I even hurt at all? Let's see what your voice says."

Spirit of Compassion immediately tells me, "She *does* hurt. She hurts on the left side of her head. Chronic migraines torment her." I reach over, touch the left side of her head, and say, "Spirit tells me you hurt here." She starts crying.

That's the level of instant accuracy Spirit provides.

If I get a call at 2 A.M. from a mom whose daughter is about to go into emergency surgery and the mom wants to know if it's the right choice, I have to be able to help the doctor determine in that moment if that little girl merely has a bad case of food poisoning, or if her appendix is about to explode.

It's important to see whether someone's recovering or is bleeding internally, if a child's fever is due to the flu or meningitis, if someone is suffering from heat sickness or is about to have a stroke. Spirit of Compassion delivers this information every time so it can be conveyed to their doctor.

Padre Pio and Edgar Cayce, those famous mystical healers of the 20th century, were the only two medical seers in recent history who accessed the level of compassion that Spirit demands of me. Their work as compassionate healers was in some ways similar to mine. However, our strengths and gifts are unique to each of us.

To be a compassionate healer of any kind, you have to adapt to each unique symptom, condition, or emotional injury to alleviate that person's pain and suffering. Spirit tells me this compassion is the most important element in healing.

Spirit of Compassion still tells me that no other medium does what I do. No one else alive has a voice providing profound, advanced, on-target medical information with crystal clarity. Spirit of Compassion's information about chronic mystery illness changes people's lives in a way nothing else has in our modern history.

I've devoted my life to this work. I'm here as a messenger. It's who I am.

People told me as a child that I have a gift. As the years went by, Spirit of Compassion made something perfectly clear: the gift was never mine. It's for the ones in need, the ones who struggle, suffer, and are searching for answers. This gift is for you.

"Whatever you're facing, you're not alone in it —and it's not meaningless. Always remember: you have a life ahead of you, years to come. Everything can change in the days ahead."

— Anthony William, Medical Medium

CHAPTER 2

The
Truth about
Mystery Illness

If you feel that you've been searching for health answers for far too long, you're not alone.

On average, a person will seek my help after 10 years of doctor shopping, having visited 20 different doctors. Sometimes it's more like 50 to 100 health-care providers of all kinds in that time frame. One woman I spoke with had gone to almost *400* doctors in seven years.

These people may have gotten labels for their conditions—lupus, for example, or fibromyalgia, Lyme disease, multiple sclerosis (MS), chronic fatigue syndrome, migraines, thyroid disorder, rheumatoid arthritis, colitis, irritable bowel syndrome, celiac disease, insomnia, anxiety, depression, and many others—yet they couldn't get better.

Or maybe doctors couldn't find tags for the symptoms these people had and doled out that old, misbegotten chestnut of a diagnosis, "It's all in your head," or the more recent one getting popular with the newer generations, "You created your problem."

What these people were really dealing with was mystery illness.

A mystery illness isn't just an unidentified disease or symptom, and it's not just the news story about eight kids in the Midwest who are hospitalized for sudden, unexplained sickness. I've certainly had people come to me for answers in those situations, yet it's a fraction of what I've seen day in and day out, a tiny subset of the much larger category of mystery illness.

Limiting the definition of mystery illness to rare, acute diseases is not helpful. It tricks the public. It makes people think that the medical cases that stump doctors are minimal and affect only a minute portion of the population.

Truth is, millions of people suffer from mystery illness. A mystery illness is any condition or symptom that leaves anyone perplexed for any reason. It can be a mystery because there isn't a name for a given set of symptoms—and so it's written off as a sign of mental imbalance. A mystery illness can also be an established, chronic condition for which there's no effective treatment of the root cause (because medical communities don't yet understand it), or a condition that's frequently misdiagnosed.

We're talking not just about the conditions I listed above, but also type 2 diabetes, hypoglycemia, TMJ, menopause complications, ADHD, acne, eczema, psoriasis, Bell's palsy, neuropathy, leaky gut syndrome, heart palpitations, autoimmune disease, and more. These are merely labels, with no meaning behind them besides confusion and suffering. That makes them mystery illnesses.

And what *about* autoimmune disease—the mistaken theory that the body attacks itself? That a person's own immune system purposely harms that person's organs and glands? Not true. (More on that in later chapters.) It's another label that diverts from the truth that medical science has not yet figured out why people are in chronic pain. Autoimmune disease is mystery illness. When you scratch the surface, you find that "autoimmune" really means "cause unknown."

If you visit a physician and complain of skin rashes, then hear that you have eczema, that's just a tag—not an answer. You may receive prescriptions for medications and tips for what to put on your skin, yet no explanation of *why* you have it, or how you can heal from it. The doctor may say that eczema is the body attacking itself—that is, your immune system mistaking your skin for an invader and trying to destroy it.

That's misguided. *The body doesn't attack itself.*

The truth? Eczema is just a name for one particular mystery illness—mystery to medical research and science. The tag *I've-got-a-rash disease* would be more accurate—it reveals

as much as medical research has so far uncovered about the disorder.

There's a real explanation for eczema. The answer is in the Medical Medium book series.

Mystery illness is at an all-time high. With each new decade to come, the number of people suffering from autoimmune disorders and other chronic mystery illnesses will double or triple. It's time to expand the definition of mystery illness, to wake up to the fact that millions of people need answers.

In the chapters that follow, I'll reveal the true nature of dozens of these mystery illnesses and symptoms, and I'll tell you what steps you need to take to heal or protect yourself.

The mystery will be revealed.

HEALING MERRY-GO-ROUND

When people present their mystery symptoms to doctor after doctor with no progress, I call that the *healing merry-go-round*. As hard as you try to get off the ride, you just keep going in circles.

In most professions, the job is straightforward. That's not to say that people such as plumbers, mechanics, accountants, and lawyers have easy occupations. They don't. Yet they operate within sets of rules. The accountant who can't get her columns to balance will eventually figure out the mistake in the ledger and post a correcting journal entry. The plumber who comes to fix a malfunctioning dishwasher will, even if the source of the problem is confusing at first, eventually figure out that a certain part needs to be replaced—or if that doesn't work, he'll install a new appliance.

Even some aspects of medicine are clear-cut. When someone gets into a skiing accident, for example, there's no mystery about what caused the broken leg—and no mystery about how to fix it. With something like a bone fracture—where cause, effect, and treatment are well defined—it's like a ferry ride: There's an end to the trip, and it's somewhere different from where you started. Perhaps there's fog along the way that complicates the journey—a patient's fractures are splintered, or she gets a pen cap stuck in her cast—but there's an established Point A and Point B, and medical personnel are trained to carry the patient from one place to the other.

Medical science is incredibly advanced at physical body repair. It's developed life-saving technology that allows patients to make radical recoveries from car accidents, broken bones, heart transplants, and so much more. Where would we be without the dedicated people who perform routine procedures, emergency feats, and revolutionary surgeries every day?

In the 20th century, medical science made great breakthroughs in virology, too . . . but it all got swept under the carpet. Because there was no funding to take these discoveries to the next level, these amazing doctors were left in the lurch as their findings about certain viruses went largely ignored.

As the pandemic has since brought home, sometimes a virus is the very clear cause of suffering. That doesn't mean doctors understand any given virus fully yet. Identifying a viral infection doesn't make its full health effects, prevention, or treatment clear-cut. Viruses are complex. As a society, we're waking up to that more and more every day. It makes the tragedy of virology's lost breakthroughs more resonant than ever: if discoveries hadn't been suppressed in the past, the world would have answers today about how to deal with COVID.

The world would also have the answers it needs to end the epidemic of chronic mystery illness. With mystery illness, the causes of symptoms often aren't evident. There's no clear trigger, no clear explanation of someone's suffering. Doctors' training doesn't map out Point A and Point B. There's no rule book for them to follow. A skeptical physician may not even see a clear indication that someone *is* suffering—and so launch the patient on a continual search for validation that her or his condition is even real.

Often, you may get what seems to be an answer. You may be told you have *Candida* or leaky gut, or that your microbiome or microflora are off, or that you're lacking protein or in need of healthy fats, or that it's your hormones, or it's because of the fruit you ate— told *that's* why you have acne or low energy or bloating or hives or a little brain fog. Even though it may seem like an answer, it's still part of the merry-go-round.

So many people with chronic illnesses aren't getting better. Sometimes it doesn't feel so much like a *merry*-go-round as a *glum*-go-round.

It's time for that to change.

I'm here to tell you that the fact that there's no rule book for mystery illness doesn't have to be a bad thing. Take the legal profession, for example. Countless people become lawyers because they're drawn to justice. They enroll in law school, get jobs . . . and then the realization hits that the justice they can bring to their clients is limited. It's all within the confines of human-devised, and sometimes unjust, laws. Having rule books isn't always a good thing.

Because there's no rule book for mystery illness, there are also no limits to recovery— if you plug in to the truths I reveal in the pages to come. Healing is one of the greatest freedoms God offers us. Healing is the law of the universe, the light, or whatever you choose to call the higher source—not the law of humans—and so it grants true justice. Untethered by statute, healing from mystery illness can exceed imagination.

ADDICTED TO ANSWERS

The medical establishment is a bit of an addict—one that gets its fix from being the authority on health. So what can happen when neither alternative nor conventional doctors have the answers? Denial.

This denial may come in the form of mislabeling a condition instead of admitting, "I don't know." It may come in the form of prescribing drugs or diet belief systems that hinder instead of heal. Or sometimes a physician may express that denial as dismissal—and refer a patient to a psychiatrist to "help" the patient with symptoms the physician insists are psychosomatic.

As with any addiction, the first step is for medical communities to admit they have a problem.

Whether conventional or alternative, traditional or nontraditional, if medical communities don't admit that the epidemic of women flattened by fatigue, anxiety, and pain is real and that no one knows the true root cause, how are researchers ever going to find adequate funding to uncover the real cause of fibromyalgia, lupus, or endometriosis? If they did find funding, would any answers found still be suppressed? Would the *real* answers be reported? The same goes for every other mystery illness.

If you're suffering, do you feel like you have decades to suffer before solutions surface in medical communities?

Many mothers come to me explaining that 20 years earlier, they came down with mystery symptoms and were diagnosed with thyroid disorder, migraines, hormone imbalances, or MS. Now they're watching their daughters go through the same exact thing. When they first got their diagnoses, these women say to me, they never would have thought that after two decades, medicine wouldn't have cures for their conditions, or even adequate explanations. They couldn't have guessed that medical advances regarding chronic conditions would have moved at such a glacial pace. They couldn't have imagined they'd have to watch their daughters suffer just as they did.

It shouldn't take ages to discover the true reason for a person's aches and pains or to discern a reliable treatment for those underlying issues. Patients shouldn't feel like they are fumbling in the dark for answers.

It's time for medical research and science to be honest and open, to accept that the medical model needs to adapt and move forward, to make the same leaps and bounds regarding chronic illness that it's made in other areas, such as life-saving surgeries. If we're to avoid several more decades of nonsense names for disorders, or the mistake of putting everything under the "autoimmune" umbrella, then it's time for medicine to admit that diagnostic tests are sometimes inadequate or fallible, that doctors' training sometimes leaves them operating on guesswork alone.

It's time for the medical establishment to seek out the answers we'll explore in this book.

TYPES OF MYSTERY ILLNESS

Mystery illness falls into four categories.

The first type is *unnamed illness*. A person may go from doctor to doctor describing her or his symptoms, withstand test after test, and hear that nothing is wrong. The blood work, MRIs, ultrasounds, and other imaging and exams don't raise any red flags. Often the only explanation the patient receives for the aches and pains is that it's all in the patient's head—that she or he is a hypochondriac, anxious, depressed, overworked, or bored. This can be crazy-making to someone suffering from a legitimate disorder. And if a doctor does believe the patient's pain is real yet can't explain its cause, she or he may call it *idiopathic*—which is just a fancy word for "unknown."

Ineffective treatment is the second category of mystery illness. In this scenario, the medical establishment does have a name for a given set of symptoms, but no viable avenue for recovery. The prescribed treatment makes no difference in the patient's health, or it worsens the condition, or the patient is told that she or he is simply stuck with feeling this way for life. At best, a patient will receive medications that manage the symptoms—such as those of MS—but don't make the condition itself any better.

With the third type of mystery illness, *misdiagnosis,* the patient also receives a name for what ails her—except it's wrong. Sometimes diagnostic trends are responsible. For example, hormones have taken the blame for any number of women's ailments that have nothing to do with menopause, perimenopause, or even just hormonal imbalance. Practitioners want to help their patients, though, so if they hear of others giving certain labels to certain sets of symptoms, they may follow the movement. In fact, alternative doctors have recently gone down the hormone path, taking their cue from the past decades' hormone movement in conventional medicine. This is an example of how trends can cross over and blur the lines between alternative and conventional.

The fourth category of mystery illness is *not knowing the true cause.* You may get a diagnosis, you may get a treatment plan—and you still don't know the true cause of the problem. Autoimmune diseases and disorders are a prime example. Conventional medicine believes in the autoimmune theory: that these very real symptoms and conditions are caused by the body's own immune system attacking its organs and glands. Even alternative medicine believes in the autoimmune theory. Both of these medical models will resort to similar medications. In no case will an autoimmune diagnosis and treatment plan lead to a true understanding of what's really causing the problem, because the autoimmune theory is only a theory. Medical research and science still deem autoimmune "cause unknown" because they can't explain why your immune system would attack your body in the first place. The idea that your body can turn against you is merely an institutionalized belief. The truth is, your body never turns against you. Your body never attacks you. There's a very different answer to why autoimmune diseases and disorders occur. That answer is in this book.

On the journey to find answers, people might find themselves in all four of these categories at one point or another. At the first doctor, a patient may hear that her or his symptoms are psychosomatic and that she or he should take up exercise, meditation, or a hobby as a new focus and mood booster. The next practitioner may validate that there is a true problem, give a name like lupus to it, and then, with the best of intentions, offer a course of treatment that ends up being ineffective. Still not feeling well, the patient may turn to a third health professional, only to get a new diagnosis of MS—this time incorrect—along with "remedies" that take her or him in the opposite direction from healing. Determined not to give up, the patient may visit a fourth doctor. Whether that doctor calls the symptoms lupus, MS, or decides to label them ME/CFS, the patient will either hear "cause unknown" or a theory about why the illness occurs that still doesn't illuminate the *true* cause.

Not knowing why you're suffering is the basic reality of living with nearly any chronic symptom or condition, whether undiagnosed, misdiagnosed, ineffectively treated, or diagnosed accurately yet without accurate explanation of what's really behind your health issue. If chronic suffering were understood, the epidemic of mystery illness would not be plaguing the population the way it is today. That's why this book exists: to give you and your doctors answers to lupus, MS, and ME/CFS—along with dozens more mystery illnesses—so you can solve the mystery and reclaim your life.

FADS AREN'T THE FUTURE

Most fads in conventional and alternative medicine don't become popular because they work. They become popular because of vested interests—power and money behind them—that allow these trends to grow their bandwidth.

Maybe a particular car or phone or clothing brand becomes trendy because of its quality and usefulness, or because it's fun, although plenty of high-quality, useful products are never seen. These trends still take engines of power and money behind them. And so it goes with medical trends. Diagnoses and treatments don't gather steam because of their healing benefits. The theory or thought process or catchphrase behind a medical trend—whether alternative, conventional, functional, integrative, or holistic—along with the interest groups behind the trend, have far more power over someone's consciousness than the results or benefits.

Health and lifestyle trends, too, are a bait-and-switch. They attract followers very easily if the people presenting them provide the allure of vibrant well-being because they're 22 and it just so happens they haven't become ill yet. The image of someone strong and young is powerful; it's easy to believe everything they're doing must be the answer. In reality, these trends are time-wasting techniques for someone who's really struggling with a symptom or condition. They lead people to question their own commitment and capabilities. If they could just have stayed longer with that workout regimen, they tell themselves—or that protein powder routine or that diet that eliminated fruit—they could have achieved the results that were promised. For the record, there are plenty of 22-year-olds who are sick and suffering who don't get this kind of visibility. Whatever your age, the problem isn't you.

To understand how medical, health, and lifestyle trends work, imagine a restaurant that always serves a special turkey dinner the week of Thanksgiving. The dinner has gotten so much hype over the years that the buzz trumps the meal itself. No one notices that the restaurant has never actually served turkey—the kitchen has secretly been cooking goose instead. If the meat tastes different from what one diner expected, he won't say anything and will just figure his own perception is off. It's a classic bait-and-switch, just like many of these trends.

Medical, health, and lifestyle trends are like the emperor with no clothes. They try to distract from what they lack with false confidence and denial. That's because these trends can have a life force all their own. If a belief system finds some influencers who market it heavily and catchily, then as a few years pass, it can become a grizzly bear of power over common sense. This fad process is behind the mistaken belief that a no-carb diet will solve *Candida* issues, the incorrect conviction that Hashimoto's disease is a condition in which the body's own immune system attacks the thyroid, and the misguided attempts to treat Lyme disease with antibiotics.

Some trends aren't all bad. Let's look at what's going on with hypothyroidism. So many women are walking around with this condition, suffering, whether diagnostic tests have spotted it or not. A recent trend among sensitive integrative medical doctors is to recognize these women's symptoms as real, to validate that these women are neither hypochondriacs nor bored housewives. Such doctors will usually say, "It's not showing up on tests, but I think your thyroid is off," and then treat the disease with a combination of medication and diet.

This is progress for women who have felt continually disregarded. At the same time, hypothyroidism is still in its mystery phase—because the doctors still haven't pointed to the underlying cause of the thyroid disease. The patients' hypothyroidism isn't going away, regardless of the medication they're taking. Many patients don't know that the thyroid medicine does nothing for the thyroid itself, nor was it originally prescribed for the thyroid. It doesn't eliminate the hypothyroidism. The thyroid stays underactive; the medication only helps mask the symptoms.

The same goes for any number of conditions. Take the ones I listed at the beginning of this chapter: fibromyalgia, lupus, Lyme disease, MS, chronic fatigue syndrome, migraines, colitis, rheumatoid arthritis, irritable bowel syndrome, celiac disease, insomnia, anxiety, depression . . . It may seem like medical communities are addressing these illnesses because they have names, or because compelling theories surface about them, or because popular treatments are available. Yet it's important to understand that medical research and science are still in the Dark Ages when it comes to aches and pains and mystery disorders. You also have to know that misdiagnoses are rampant. There's still a lot of confusion in the medical world about what's causing what.

Which is all to say: trends aren't answers.

IT'S NOT IN YOUR HEAD

It's an all-too-common phenomenon, particularly for women: an actual, valid illness meets with skepticism, disregard, or misinformation from the establishment that's meant to have the answers. Doctors can't help that they don't know the causes of these debilitating mystery symptoms—or that they have the wrong culprit pegged for a particular disorder.

In some cases the funding just isn't there for the research that's needed, or fads take studies in the wrong direction. In other cases, it's only a matter of time (though sometimes decades) before the right diagnostic technology will be available.

Physicians have often been taught that in the absence of explanations, it's a genuine help to tell patients that their conditions are psychosomatic. The health-care establishment believes this will give patients some sort of wake-up call, which would be true . . . if the illnesses were just in people's heads. With each year that passes, the population gets sicker, and many doctors are noticing. Living with symptoms has become the new normal, especially in the reproductive system arena. This wake-up call has many doctors handing out diagnoses much more readily than doctors of even the recent past. They're faster these days to give someone a label for their condition, even if the label isn't right.

There are actual, physical roots to chronic mystery conditions; medical research and science just haven't discovered or accepted them yet. It can take years and tens of thousands of dollars before people dealing with mystery illness find the information from Spirit of Compassion that's in these books. Friends and family may have begged them to stop the search, urged them to accept their diagnoses and the hands they've been dealt. Still, something has pushed them forward: the primal will to survive, the determination to make the most of life, the instinct that they deserve to be healthy.

There aren't any words for the relief these people find, or how empowered they become, once they understand what was really behind their suffering.

Now it's your turn to learn: You are not to blame for your illness. It's not something you manifested or attracted or created. It's not your fault. You certainly don't deserve to feel unwell. You have a God-given right to heal.

If you've dealt with chronic illness—which means any symptom you're living with that you don't want—then I'm sure you've dealt with the people who say, "But you look perfectly healthy," or "You look good," or "You don't look sick," thinking they're being helpful. You've no doubt stopped giving an honest answer to, "How are you?" because you can't bear to hear, "You're *still* not better?" It's less emotionally damaging to pretend you're fine than to listen as someone insists that a particular therapy will solve all your problems—as though you haven't already gone to the ends of the earth trying to find answers. You've probably listened as countless people have described their family members' struggles with illness—as though those experiences trump your own.

When health issues haven't gotten in the way of your life yet, it's easy to spout theories about how those who are sick just need to change their mind-sets and think more positively. When you don't understand the true nature of someone's symptoms—aches and pains, fatigue, bloating, eczema, anxiety—it's easy to think it's because a person is holding herself or himself back with a fear of healing, or that she or he is a malingerer who secretly enjoys the attention this malady brings.

Anyone who's told you these are the reasons for your illness hasn't been there. They haven't stood in your shoes. These ideas make things so much worse for those who suffer from mystery illness. They cause people to feel ashamed of their problems and avoid asking for help—to feel like they have to hide their suffering out of worry they'll be called out as fakes, weaklings, or complainers.

Let's make it crystal clear: Nobody wants to be sick or compromised. Nobody has a fear of healing.

What people fear is being ill, and that's what causes people who haven't been sidelined by symptoms yet to utter insensitive remarks. What they're really saying is, "I'll never have to go through what you're going through, right?"

What you need the people surrounding you to say is, "I hear you, I see you, I believe you, and I believe *in* you. What you're going through is real, *and* there must be some way to overcome and triumph over it. I'll hang in there with you for the long haul."

In the process of healing, knowing the cause of your symptoms and conditions (and knowing what *isn't* the cause) is half the battle won. The next step is knowing what tools to use to make them better. If you follow the

guidelines for how to use the chapters ahead that I laid out in the Introduction, this book will help you do both. So will the rest of the Medical Medium book series.

Spirit of Compassion has the answers. He wants you to learn the truth about mystery illness. He wants you and your loved ones to get better, to have a clear sense of direction on how to move forward, to have control over your life and heal.

Spirit understands, with the utmost compassion, what people suffer on this earth.

God granted me the ability to access vast, highly advanced healing information through Spirit of Compassion. Because of this, countless people of all ages—including doctors themselves—who've come to this information have found the solutions to their chronic mystery illnesses and regained control over their health, achieving complete recovery. In the chapters that follow, you can find solutions, too.

CASE HISTORY:
The Real Heal
2004

Lila* was a 34-year-old real estate agent when she started to experience mental fogginess, weakness, fatigue, pressure in her ears, and numbness in her extremities. Her symptoms soon got in the way of her job. She could tell that her fellow agents had noticed she was dropping the ball with some of her clients—forgetting appointments and staging second-rate open houses. Lila frequently failed to recall addresses and names and found herself so fatigued after a day at work that the next morning, she would sleep through her alarm. At property closings, she was on edge, unable to think through the mortgage details coherently, and fuzzy on the numbers, which had once been her strength.

* Names and other select client details throughout have been changed to protect client privacy.

Finally, Lila had to admit to herself and her employer that she was sick. She sat down with her supervisor, who recommended a doctor. At her first appointment, Lila listed her symptoms, but after an exam, the physician couldn't pinpoint a physical cause and declared her perfectly healthy. Depression, he said, was probably behind her ailments.

Lila tried to work with this. Determined to ward off her tiredness, mental fog, and other complaints with a sunny disposition, she returned to her job. Anything that felt like a symptom, she told herself, was a manifestation of her frame of mind. Maybe she'd just been craving attention.

But she started missing more house showings because she was unable to rise from bed, her hands felt too numb to drive, or she was embarrassed that she'd been too weak to bathe. It soon became apparent to Lila and those at her office that no matter her outlook, she was unable to do her job and needed to take a leave of absence. She dragged herself back to the doctor and reiterated her plight. He examined her again and once more concluded that she was perfectly fine. "I'm not going to be the doctor who lets you collect disability," he said.

Devastated and now in survival mode, Lila sought out a second opinion. She submitted to a battery of tests, only to have her new M.D. play it safe and back up the first doctor's ruling. He, too, refused to provide the documentation she needed to receive disability benefits.

This was just the beginning of Lila's years-long journey through the conventional and alternative medical worlds, searching for explanations of her mystery illness. Along the way, she had a few glimpses of hope, but every time she thought she'd found a name for her condition or a shot at getting better, she found herself right back where she'd started—or worse.

That is, until she came to me. Spirit of Compassion provided the long-awaited insights that Lila knew existed, including the underlying cause of her downward spiral and instructions to regain her health. Before long, Lila felt better than she had since she could remember. Her renewed energy brought her renewed trust and delight in life, and she was able to devote herself to her job once more—as well as explore passions she'd neglected for years.

In this book, you'll read about many cases such as Lila's. You might notice a pattern, and you may identify with it: the years of being ill with no validation, the doctor-shopping journey, the isolation, confusion, and frustration. You may resonate with the stories where someone *does* get validation for her or his illness—but it's a misleading validation, either in the form of a misdiagnosis or a prescribed path of healing that leads nowhere fast.

None of the stories end there. You don't have to get stuck in the endless cycle of guesswork. Just like Lila, you can solve the mystery—and real healing can happen.

"Because there's no rule book for mystery illness, there are also no limits to recovery—if you plug in to the truths I reveal in the pages to come.
Healing is one of the greatest freedoms God offers us. Healing is the law of the universe, the light, or whatever you choose to call the higher source—not the law of humans—and so it grants true justice. Untethered by statute, healing from mystery illness can exceed imagination."

— Anthony William, Medical Medium

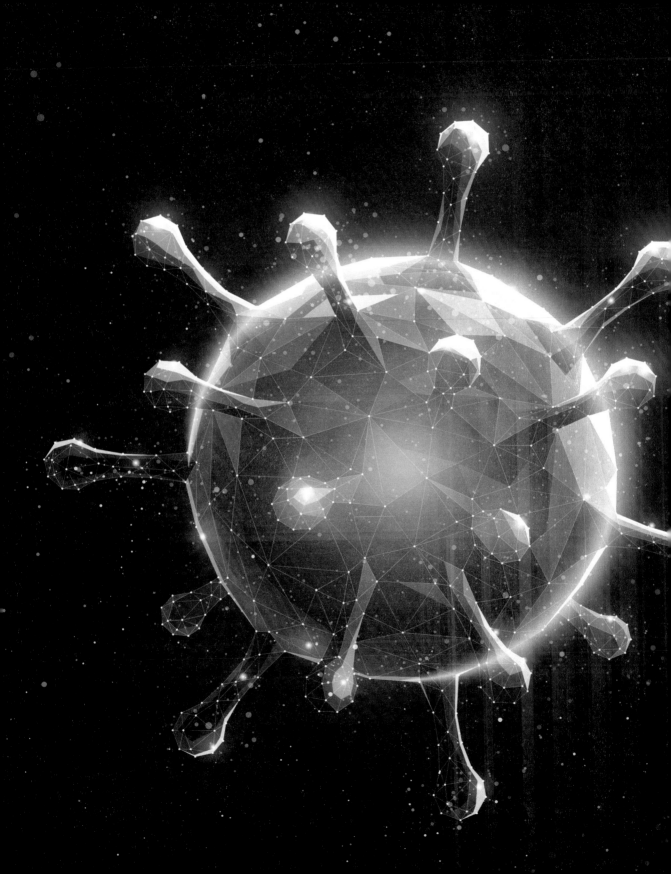

PART II

THE HIDDEN
EPIDEMIC

"Readers continue to introduce more and more health-care providers to this book, and it has prompted a new movement to look for the deeper causes of chronic illness—and to take EBV seriously. Prior to the publication of *Medical Medium*, EBV was practically a non-concern. Medical communities didn't understand what the virus could do—because, for example, medical research and science were unaware that EBV creates symptoms that lead to neurological problems. Now EBV testing and awareness are becoming everyday at the doctor's office. Research and science are finally starting to find a link between Epstein-Barr virus and dozens of conditions."

— Anthony William, Medical Medium

CHAPTER 3

Epstein-Barr Virus, Chronic Fatigue Syndrome, and Fibromyalgia

The *Epstein-Barr virus* (EBV) has created a secret epidemic. We're at a place in time where the majority of the world's population is living with one or more of the many mutations of Epstein-Barr virus.

Epstein-Barr is responsible for symptoms, conditions, diseases, disorders, and illnesses of every category: For some people, it creates fatigue and pain that get tagged as Lyme disease or go unnamed. For others, EBV symptoms prompt doctors to prescribe ineffective treatments, such as hormone replacement. And for so many people walking around with EBV, it gets misdiagnosed.

Among the reasons EBV is thriving: so little is understood about it. Medical research and science are aware of only one version of EBV, when there are actually over 60 varieties and growing. Epstein-Barr is behind several of the debilitating illnesses that stump doctors. As I said in the Introduction, it's the mystery illness of mystery illnesses.

Medical research and science have no idea how the virus operates long term and how problematic it can be. The truth is, EBV is the source of numerous health problems that are currently considered autoimmune, such as fibromyalgia and chronic fatigue syndrome. EBV is also the cause of some major maladies that medical communities think they understand but really don't—including thyroid disease, lupus, vertigo, and tinnitus.

This chapter explains when the Epstein-Barr virus arose, how it's transmitted, how it operates to create untold havoc in strategic stages no one knows about, and the steps (never revealed before) that can destroy the virus and restore health.

EPSTEIN-BARR ORIGINS AND TRANSMISSION

Though Epstein-Barr was discovered by two brilliant physicians in 1964, it had actually begun taking hold in the early 1900s—over half a century before. EBV's initial versions—which are still with us—are relatively slow to act, and might not even create notable symptoms until late in life. Even then, they're only mildly harmful, if at all. There are still some people who have these early EBV strains.

Unfortunately, EBV has evolved over the decades, and each new generation of our population is up against versions of the virus that have grown more challenging than the ones before. The virus is evolving every five years at this point, outpacing the 20 to 30 years it takes us as humans to move from generation to generation.

Until the publication of this book, those with EBV would typically be stuck with it for the rest of their lives. Doctors are starting to accept and learn from the information released here: that EBV is the root cause of myriad problems. In the past, they believed the most trouble EBV caused for a patient was malaise and mild fatigue, with possible fever, all of it temporary. Now some doctors are in the infancy stage of recognizing and addressing the Epstein-Barr virus due to the Medical Medium information published in this book and the rest of the series, as well as the years I spent lecturing before publication.

There are many ways to catch EBV. For example, you can get it as a baby if your parent has the virus. You can also get it through infected blood. Hospitals don't screen for the virus, so any blood transfusion puts you at risk. You can even get it from eating out! That's because chefs are under tremendous pressure to get dishes prepared quickly. They often end up cutting a finger or hand, slapping on a Band-Aid, and continuing to work. Their blood can get into the food . . . and if they happen to have EBV during a contagious phase, that can be enough to infect you.

Transmission can also happen through other bodily fluids, such as those exchanged during sex. Under some circumstances, even a kiss can be enough to transmit EBV. Keep this in mind if you're on the journey of seeking a partner to spend your life with. It's not unusual to pick up multiple varieties of pathogens such as EBV along the way.

Even if you already have EBV, you can pick up new strains of it. You can even heal and overcome the EBV you already have, then pick up another EBV variety, develop symptoms, and think it's the original problem that's come back again. Should this happen to you, the information in this book will still be here for you to access and return to as you go through life. Everybody's got bugs. One way or another, the people you come into contact with have one bug or more. As careful as we can be to safeguard ourselves and our families—and we should take care—we don't always have full control over the transmission of bugs. It's a natural way of life here. That's why having the tools to protect yourself and move yourself forward is key.

Someone with the Epstein-Barr virus isn't contagious all the time. It's most likely to spread during its Stage Two. Which brings up something else that until now hasn't been revealed: EBV goes through four stages.

EPSTEIN-BARR STAGE ONE

If you catch EBV, it goes through an initial dormant period of floating around in your bloodstream doing little more than slowly replicating itself to build its numbers—and waiting for an opportunity to launch a more direct infection.

For example, if circumstances push you to physically exhaust yourself for weeks and you don't get a chance to fully recover, or your body becomes deprived of essential nutrients such as zinc or vitamin B$_{12}$, or you undergo a traumatic emotional experience such as a breakup, betrayal, or the death of a loved one, the virus can detect your intense stress-released adrenaline, which can lower your immune system, allowing the virus to choose that time to take advantage.

EBV can also often awaken when you're naturally going through an immune system shift related to your reproductive system. During menstruation, 80 percent of the immune system watches over the reproductive system, leaving 20 percent of the immune system to watch over the rest of the body. During ovulation, 40 percent of the immune system watches over the reproductive system, leaving only 60 percent to watch over the rest of the body. And during pregnancy, 50 percent of the immune system watches over the reproductive system and baby while the other 50 percent watches over the rest of the body. These times of shift can lead to opportunity for EBV to take root in Stage One.

During childbirth, over 90 percent of a woman's immune system rushes to the reproductive system, which leaves less than 10 percent of her immune system throughout the rest of her body over that course of time. (After giving birth, that ratio changes over the next three days, as the woman's immune system moves on to concentrate around the breast milk and starts to balance out throughout the body.) After childbirth, someone may feel various symptoms, including fatigue, brain fog, aches

and pains, and depression. The symptoms can go on for months and often lead to the umbrella label *postpartum depression*. It's tremendous progress that women now have this recognition, and that postpartum challenges are being spoken about more widely and openly. We also need to be aware that more is going on beneath the surface. Awakened EBV is the frequent reason for postpartum symptoms. On top of the immune system shift at childbirth, there's also the exhausting level of adrenaline output. That large spurt of adrenaline can be a food source for EBV, if giving birth was particularly difficult.

EBV is inhumanly patient. This Stage One period of fortifying itself and waiting for an ideal opportunity can take weeks, months, or even a decade or longer, depending on a variety of factors. Keep in mind, any of the triggers we just covered can also prompt EBV that's already established in the body to travel into its other stages, which you'll read about further in this chapter.

The virus is especially vulnerable during Stage One. However, it's also undetectable through tests and causes no symptoms, so you normally wouldn't know to fight it, because you wouldn't be aware it was there.

EPSTEIN-BARR STAGE TWO

At the end of Stage One, the Epstein-Barr virus becomes willing to challenge your immune system in a battle. That's when EBV first makes its presence known . . . by turning into what doctors call *mononucleosis*. This is the infamous mono that we all grow up hearing about as the "kissing disease." It's what hundreds of thousands of university students worldwide contract every year when they run themselves down with all-night partying and studying.

Medical communities are unaware that every case of mononucleosis is only Stage Two of EBV.

This is one of the periods when the virus is most contagious. It's therefore advisable to avoid getting exposed to blood, saliva, or other bodily fluids from someone who is known to have mono . . . or to avoid exposing anyone to your fluids if *you* have mono. (EBV transmission is still possible through blood, saliva, and other bodily fluids outside of this mono stage; it's just less likely.)

During this Stage Two, your body's immune system goes to war with the virus. It sends identifier cells to "tag" virus cells, i.e., place a hormone on or around them that is released from your adrenal glands and processed and activated by your liver to mark virus cells as invaders. It then sends soldier cells to seek out and kill the tagged virus cells. This is the power of your immune system coming to your defense.

How severely this battle rages will vary from person to person, because everyone is different in what they're up against. One person may be deficient in zinc while someone else may be *severely* deficient in zinc. This difference matters. Someone may already have a weakened immune system from other pathogens it's already facing or keeping in control. (Examples include *H. pylori*, *Streptococcus*, *Staphylococcus*, shingles virus, *E. coli*, HPV, and many other different pathogens.) Someone could be facing emotional hardship, which can prompt fight or flight and the release of lots of corrosive adrenaline, pushing the nervous system and immune system to the edge.

Someone's caffeine addiction, which puts a lot of stress on the immune system, could be weakening immune responses. The range in viral activity from person to person can also be as simple as foods in the diet. For example, eggs feed viruses, so they're very igniting for EBV. If one person eats eggs regularly and another seldom eats an egg, that can make all the difference.

On top of all this, it will also depend on what EBV strain or variety a person has. You can have mono for just a week or two with a mild scratchy throat and tiredness, in which case you aren't likely to realize what's really happening, so you most likely won't visit a doctor for a blood test.

Then again, you can get hit hard with fatigue, sore throat, fever, headaches, rashes, and more that hang on for several months. If this happens, the chances are you'll go see a doctor who'll test your blood, and the Epstein-Barr virus will show up as a form of mono . . . most of the time.

It's during this stage that EBV seeks a long-term home by making a run for one or more of your major organs—typically your liver, spleen, and/or reproductive organs. EBV loves being in these organs because mercury, dioxins, other toxins, and residues from foods such as eggs, dairy products, and gluten are likely to accumulate there. The virus thrives on these poisons, which could eventually lead to endometriosis, fibroids, PCOS, ovarian cysts, prostate issues, and/or mystery infertility.

One other secret about EBV is that it has a best friend, a bacterium called *Streptococcus*. In such cases your body is dealing with not only a virus, but also bacteria that further distract the immune system and produce their own array of symptoms. Strep is Epstein-Barr's number one *cofactor*. In many situations, someone has more than one strain of strep.

During EBV's Stage Two, *Streptococcus* can travel up to create strep throat and/or infest the sinuses, nose, mouth, or ears. It can also travel down to create infections in the urinary tract, vagina, kidneys, or bladder . . . eventually causing cystitis.

EPSTEIN-BARR STAGE THREE

Once the virus settles into your liver, spleen, and/or reproductive organs, it nests there.

From this point on, when a doctor tests for Epstein-Barr, she or he will most likely find antibodies and take these to indicate a *past* infection, when EBV was in its mono phase. The doctor will not find the EBV presently active in the bloodstream. The confusion here is one of the biggest blunders in medical history—this is how this virus has slipped through the cracks. Unless you have already followed the measures outlined in this book to kill the EBV, the virus *is*, in fact, still alive and causing new symptoms . . . and it's eluding the tests. That's because it's living in the liver, spleen, and/or reproductive system, and the test to detect this has not yet been invented. On top of which, there are so many different and newer mutations of EBV, testing may miss them altogether.

With the virus hiding undetected in your organs, your body assumes it's won the war and the invader has been destroyed. Your immune system returns to its normal state, your mononucleosis ends, and your doctor tells you that you're healthy.

Unfortunately, the Epstein-Barr virus has barely begun its voyage through your body.

If you have a typical variety, EBV could lie dormant in your organs for years—possibly for decades—without your knowing it, especially if your immune system hasn't been weakened by other challenges through life. If you have an especially aggressive variety, though, EBV may create serious problems even while it's nesting.

For example, the virus may burrow deep into your liver, spleen, and/or reproductive system, causing those organs to become inflamed and enlarged. And once again, keep in mind that before this book's initial publication, doctors did not know to connect the dots between *past* EBV and its *present* activity in the organs. Now, with this information, doctors are starting to become mindful that there is post-mononucleosis activity that creates new symptoms.

The virus also creates three types of poison:

- EBV excretes toxic waste matter, or viral *byproduct*. This becomes increasingly significant as the virus grows more cells, and its expanding army keeps eating and excreting poisonous byproduct. This waste matter is often identified as spirochetes, which can trigger false positives on tests such as Lyme titers (screening tests for Lyme disease) and lead to a false diagnosis of Lyme.

- When a cell of the virus dies—which happens often, as the cells have a six-week life cycle—the *corpse* that is left behind is itself toxic and so further poisons your body. As with viral byproduct, this problem becomes more severe as EBV's army grows, creating fatigue and other symptoms

- The poisons EBV creates through these two processes have the ability to generate a *neurotoxin* (i.e., a poison that disrupts nerve function and distracts your immune system) and/or a *dermatoxin* (i.e., a poison that rises up through the skin, causing eczema, psoriasis, lupus, or undiagnosed rashes). EBV will secrete these special toxins at strategic periods during Stage Three, and continuously during Stage Four, to prevent your immune system from zeroing in on the virus and attacking it.

The issues that may result from an aggressive variety of EBV nesting in your organs include:

- Your liver performing so sluggishly that it does a poor job of flushing toxins out of your system, creating hot flashes, heart palpitations, skin rashes, and weight gain.

- *Hepatitis A, B,* and *C.* (EBV is actually the primary cause of hepatitis C. It can also cause acute cases of hepatitis A and B.)

- Your liver's sluggish performance leading to stress upon your stomach's gastric glands, which can cause low hydrochloric acid and cause your intestinal tract to start to become toxic. This in turn can result in some food not being fully digested and instead putrefying in your intestinal tract, resulting in bloating and/ or constipation. The strain on your

liver can also lead to bile reserves diminishing, so that fats in your diet are not being dispersed or broken down, causing them to go rancid.

- The stage being set for endometriosis, PCOS, fibroids, ovarian cysts, or enlarged prostate to start to develop.

- Your developing sensitivities to foods that never caused you problems before. This happens when the virus consumes a food it likes, such as cheese or gluten, then "goes to the bathroom" and eliminates it within your body, which transforms the food residue into something your body doesn't recognize.

The virus bides its time until it senses stress-related hormones indicating you're in an especially vulnerable state—say, as a result of burning the candle at both ends; enduring a severe emotional blow such as divorce, breakup, or betrayal; or suffering a physical jolt such as being in a car accident—or when it senses you're undergoing hormonal immune system shifts, as when the immune system changes gears during times such as pregnancy, childbirth, and even menstruation and ovulation.

When the virus is about to reproduce in numbers, a feeding frenzy starts as the virus goes on the search for various foods it likes. Upon consuming these various foods, it begins to excrete neurotoxins. This adds an extra burden upon your liver, because your liver must then filter and process this extra viral waste matter.

An important point to emphasize here is that for the virus to be able to grow in numbers means that most likely, you encountered a viral trigger recently or even months ago. Examples include the types of challenges we just covered: intensely stressful events, difficult circumstances, emotional struggles such as heartbreak and betrayal, or physical trials such as childbirth. Or maybe you faced a lowering of the immune system from ongoing deficiencies or certain foods in the diet that are virus-promoting rather than antiviral. Even vices such as excessive caffeine from common beverages take a toll on the adrenals and liver. Other triggers can include mold exposure; plug-in air fresheners, scented candles, cologne, or perfume; lawn treatment chemicals; the removal of mercury amalgam dental fillings; pesticide or herbicide exposure; or exposure to additional pathogens such as COVID or the flu. This is not an exhaustive list of the triggers that can occur in one's life to allow for the next phase of EBV to begin, only some of the common ones. All of these triggers have the potential to reduce the immune system temporarily.

Lupus

The lowering of the immune system caused by these various triggers I've just described can allow the virus to increase in numbers, which leads to the virus releasing and expelling more byproduct, neurotoxins, virus corpses, and dermatoxins. This can cause an allergic reaction, which can in turn surface as various mysterious rashes and hives on the skin in different parts of the body, prompting the patient to head to the doctor's office. Most of the time, this will lead to blood testing that indicates an elevation of inflammatory markers or numbers that confuse the doctor. This can end up

eventually leading to a lupus diagnosis, especially if other symptoms such as fatigue, body pain in random places, headaches, and brain fog are combined with skin-related symptoms. Medical communities have no understanding that lupus is just the body reacting to Epstein-Barr's byproduct, neurotoxins, virus corpses, and dermatoxins. In truth, lupus is just a viral infection of Epstein-Barr.

Hypothyroidism and Other Thyroid Disorders

While your immune system is in a weakened state, EBV can take advantage by leaving the organs it's been nesting in and making a run for a different major organ or gland. It's most common for EBV to venture out from the liver—even if EBV is also nesting in the spleen and/or reproductive organs, it's the liver that EBV cells are likeliest to travel from when the immune system is lowered. The normal path for most of the over 60 varieties of EBV is to head straight to the thyroid.

Medical communities aren't yet aware that EBV is the actual cause of most thyroid disorders and diseases—especially Hashimoto's, but also Graves', thyroid cancer, and other thyroid ills. (Thyroid complications are also sometimes caused by radiation; but in over 95 percent of cases, the culprit is Epstein-Barr.) That is, medical communities are unaware of this *unless* they have learned from me over the years, read this book, or seen articles or studies published as a result of this book. Medical research has not yet uncovered the true causes of thyroid disorders, and it's still decades away from discovering and accepting that EBV is the virus that directly causes them. If a doctor gives you a Hashimoto's diagnosis, it really means that she or he doesn't know how this happened. The claim is that your body is attacking your thyroid—a view that arises from misinformation. In truth, it's the EBV—not your body—attacking the thyroid.

Once in your thyroid, EBV begins drilling into its tissues. Another undiscovered part of how EBV works is that when it's in the phase of entering a gland, it shape-shifts and its cells becomes much more oval, with one end of each oval-shaped virus cell in a pointed direction. The virus cells then literally twist and spin like drills to burrow deep into the thyroid (just like beetle larvae do when they enter into trees), killing thyroid cells and scarring the gland as they go, creating hidden hypothyroidism in millions of women and many men, from mild cases to the more extreme. Your immune system notices this direct attack and tries to intervene, because the EBV is causing direct inflammation. Your immune system becomes aware of what's causing the inflammation, yet it's very difficult for your immune system to tag the virus when it's already embedding itself into the gland. The EBV's neurotoxins, dermatoxins, viral byproduct, and poisonous corpses raise a smoke shield, making it hard for immune cells to see every viral cell directly, which allows a chance for the viral cells to escape and embed themselves deeper into the gland tissue.

While the above may sound unnerving, don't let it rattle you; your thyroid has the ability to rejuvenate and heal itself when it's given what it needs. And never underestimate the power of your immune system and what it's capable of when coming to your defense. By the end of this chapter your immune system will become activated just by you learning the truth.

Because the virus is injuring and killing cells as it's burrowing into the thyroid, it can create mild forms of scar tissue. This can lead pockets of scar tissue to form, which can become the beginnings of small growths. To stop these mild growths from expanding and the EBV cells inside them from proliferating, your immune system tries to wall off the virus with calcium. This is the process that creates nodules in your thyroid. These calcium prisons that your immune system forms around scar tissue growths don't always stop EBV. First, most of EBV's cells evade this attack and remain free. Second, a virus cell that your immune system successfully walls off typically remains alive and turns its calcium prison into a comfortable home, still allowing it to access food within your thyroid, draining it of energy. Virus cells might even eventually transform their prison into a living growth, called a *cyst*, depending on what mutation or variety of EBV you have, and that creates further strain on your thyroid.

Eating enough calcium-rich foods and foods that are high in vitamin C helps support your immune system in this attack on EBV. Calcium-rich foods such as dairy products are not the type of calcium needed. Your immune system relies on the calcium from fruits, leafy greens, herbs, wild foods, and some vegetables. Because your immune system is constantly using up any calcium available to battle the bigger fire in the moment (trying to save your thyroid), if you don't have the helpful sources of calcium in your diet and you're instead consuming unproductive calcium, your immune system may opt—out of desperation—to use that unproductive calcium from sources such as milk, cheese, butter, and eggs as it tries to wall off a scar tissue growth. With this "wrong" kind of calcium, the calcium prison (thyroid nodule) will not be functional; instead, the virus will expand this growth. These unproductive sources of calcium end up causing more harm.

Even if you have the helpful kind of calcium in your diet from fruits, leafy greens, herbs, wild foods, and some vegetables, you want to be mindful to get plenty of them in your diet. Your immune system is constantly using up calcium to save your thyroid. Without enough of it, your immune system may resort to drawing out calcium from the calcium storage bins inside your liver. Meanwhile, your bones need productive calcium from somewhere. If your immune system doesn't have access to enough useful calcium to battle the virus in your thyroid, then there isn't any leftover for your bones—which means that your bones are robbed of the calcium that should have been distributed to them.

Simultaneously, the hundreds of virus cells that *aren't* imprisoned in nodules can weaken your thyroid, making it less effective at producing its hormones. The resulting strain on your adrenal glands as they fill in for a lack of adequate thyroid hormones, combined with a liver that has become stagnant from long-term low-grade viral infection and EBV's toxins (not to mention other troublemakers inside the liver), can in turn lead to weight gain, fatigue, mental fogginess, impaired memory, depression, hair loss, insomnia, brittle nails, muscle weakness, and/or dozens of other symptoms.

Some especially rare, aggressive varieties of EBV go even further. They can create *cancer* in the thyroid when they're fueled by the "right" toxic troublemakers in the body. The rate of thyroid cancer around the world has been rising rapidly. Medical communities don't know that the cause is an increase in rare, aggressive forms of EBV. These rarer forms become more common every few years.

The Epstein-Barr virus invades your thyroid for a strategic reason: it's seeking to distract and place stress on your endocrine system. The strain on your thyroid in turn puts a strain on your adrenal glands to produce more adrenaline, which is a favored food of EBV.

Not all blends of adrenaline produced by your adrenals will feed EBV in short spurts. What happens is that the long-term condition of your thyroid can prompt the adrenals to release extra adrenaline to compensate long term. This eventually puts the adrenal glands into a more imbalanced, sensitive state because they are already in demand from the stressful events and emotional upheavals of everyday living. Long-term strain leads the adrenals to extra spurts and bouts and inconsistencies. An emotional disturbance or stressful occurrence, even a small one, can shock the adrenals in their weakened state, prompting them to produce a more corrosive variety of adrenaline usually reserved to help us survive fight-or-flight moments.

Day-to-day, normal, gentler adrenaline ends up intermixed with these little bursts of more intense adrenaline blends, and because of its corrosive nature, this more intense adrenaline can penetrate more deeply into body tissue where EBV happens to be nesting. Everyday, gentler adrenaline doesn't penetrate tissue like this and is unlikely to reach EBV in its nesting spots such as the thyroid. It's the corrosive adrenaline blends that can penetrate throughout the body more easily—even becoming easier for EBV within a thyroid nodule prison to reach. They're also the blends that EBV thrives on the most.

This is not always what's needed for EBV to become stronger. Foods such as eggs act as a superfood for EBV, prompting its expansion and growth even more sometimes than corrosive types of adrenaline. Comfort foods such as cheese and gluten also feed EBV.

Sometimes food and adrenaline together play a role. When consuming foods such as eggs, dairy, and gluten, EBV has a better chance of getting ahold of their residues if emotional circumstances and corrosive adrenaline are picking up the heart rate, driving these food residues (and nutrients from other foods) through the blood—allowing EBV to be fed.

All of this can bring EBV to its ultimate target: your nervous system.

EPSTEIN-BARR STAGE FOUR

The ultimate goal of the Epstein-Barr virus is for some of its virus cells to venture past your thyroid and inflame your central nervous system.

Your immune system normally wouldn't allow this to happen. But if EBV has successfully worn you down in Stage Three by entering your thyroid —and all that comes with that— and if on top of that you are abruptly faced with some physical or severe emotional injury, the virus can take advantage of your immune system's vulnerability and start to cause a multitude of strange symptoms that range from heart palpitations to aches and pains that shift and move around to tingles and numbness to mysterious fatigue to nerve pain.

A common scenario is being in an accident, getting surgery, suffering some other physical damage, or even giving birth, and then feeling awful for much longer than would be expected. A typical reaction is to "feel like a truck hit me."

Blood tests, X-rays, and MRIs will reveal nothing wrong, so doctors won't be aware of the virus inflaming the nerves. Stage Four Epstein-Barr is therefore a major source of mystery illnesses—that is, neurological problems that cause doctors massive confusion.

What's actually happening is that your injured nerves trigger an "alarm" hormone to notify your body that the nerves are exposed and need repair. In Stage Four, EBV detects that hormone coupled with an adrenaline surge and rushes over to latch on to those damaged nerves.

A nerve is similar to a string of yarn with little root hairs hanging off it. When the nerve is injured, the root hairs pop off the sides of the nerve sheath. EBV looks for those openings and grabs on to them. If it succeeds, it can keep the area inflamed for years. As a result, you can have a relatively small injury that remains flared up and causes you continual pain.

You don't need to have physical injury to develop any of these neurological symptoms caused by EBV. The nerves can still get inflamed by the virus. As the virus feeds on toxins that are readily available (such as mercury, aluminum, copper, and other toxic troublemakers, plus foods such as eggs, milk, cheese, butter, and gluten), it can release neurotoxins that cling to nerves—whether exposed root hairs, injured nerves, or even non-damaged nerves. This can create symptoms of different types, and each variety of EBV does something a little different. An EBV variety may have an appetite for a more toxic food such as mercury, or it may produce a more toxic neurotoxin that can inflame nerves just by touching them—without the nerves even being injured or frayed.

The issues that result from this viral inflammation can include muscle pain, joint pain, painful tender points, back pain, tingling and/or numbness in the hands and feet, jerking and spasms, tinnitus (ringing, buzzing, humming, or popping sounds in the ears), migraines, ongoing fatigue, dizziness, eye floaters, insomnia, unrestful sleep, and night sweats. Patients with these issues are sometimes diagnosed as having fibromyalgia, chronic fatigue syndrome, or rheumatoid arthritis, all of which are collections of symptoms that medical communities admit they don't understand and for which they have no cure. In such cases the patients are given inappropriate treatments that don't begin to address the real culprit—because these mystery illnesses are really Stage Four Epstein-Barr.

One of the greatest missteps of all time is mistaking women's Epstein-Barr symptoms for perimenopause and menopause. Symptoms such as hot flashes, night sweats, weight gain, heart palpitations, dizziness, depression, hair loss, and anxiety were and are frequently misinterpreted as hormonal change—which is what launched three disastrous movements: the autoimmune theory, the "it's all in your head" theory, and the HRT movement. (To learn more, see Chapter 15, "Premenstrual Syndrome and Menopause.")

Let's take a closer look at some of the chronic illnesses that have puzzled doctors for decades and are the result of Stage Four Epstein-Barr.

Chronic Fatigue Syndrome Also known as Myalgic Encephalomyelitis/Chronic Fatigue Syndrome (ME/CFS), Chronic Fatigue Immune Dysfunction Syndrome (CFIDS), and Systemic Exertion Intolerance Disease (SEID)

There's a long history of womankind facing denial that there's a physical cause of their suffering. Like those with fibromyalgia (see below), people with chronic fatigue syndrome (CFS) often hear that they are liars, lazy, delusional, and/or crazy. It's an illness that affects women in disproportionately large numbers. It's also starting to take hold of men.

And chronic fatigue syndrome is on the rise.

It's becoming common for young women in college to return home mid-semester with the condition, unable to do anything but lie in bed. Contracting CFS as a person in your late teens or early 20s can be particularly devastating as you watch friends move on with relationships and jobs, meanwhile feeling stuck and unable to live up to your potential.

People who get CFS in their 30s, 40s, or 50s have their own obstacles: while you're old enough at this point to have an established life and support network, you also have established responsibilities. You're likely trying to be everything to everybody, taking care of more than you can handle, and so you feel the pressure to act normal when CFS hits.

Compounding the isolation for both age groups are the feelings of guilt, fear, and shame that accompany their misdiagnoses. I'm sure that if you have CFS, you've been in the depths of physical suffering and had someone say, "But you look perfectly healthy," or "You look okay," or even "You look strong." It is so disheartening to feel unwell and hear from practitioners, friends, or family that there's nothing wrong with you. Or a practitioner may hand you a label for what you're experiencing that you can identify with, and yet because people around you can't grasp what it means, they still don't comprehend what you're going through, or else they forget. All they seem to register is that it wasn't a devastating diagnosis of cancer with three months to live, so you must be okay. With the best of intentions, they tell you, "You look fine," or "You look great." They don't realize the devastation of living day in and day out with symptoms that stand in your way.

Chronic fatigue syndrome is real. It's the Epstein-Barr virus.

As we've seen, those with CFS have an elevated viral load of EBV, whether doctors see that elevated viral load on blood tests or not, which systematically afflicts the body by creating a neurotoxin that inflames the central nervous system. This can eventually weaken the adrenals, liver, and digestive system, and create the feeling that you have a low battery.

If you've heard the term *neurological fatigue* before, that originated from Medical Medium information. At this point, the term is in wider use and not cited back to its original source. It's the term I've been using for the last three decades to teach health professionals about viral neurotoxins hampering the central nervous system, leading the nervous system to become sensitive and have an allergic reaction to the neurotoxins, causing mild to severe inflammation of the nerves. Neurological fatigue can be part of many EBV-caused conditions. Often, people will have more than one condition or set of symptoms, with this neurological fatigue in the mix.

Fibromyalgia

We've had over six decades of medical denial that *fibromyalgia* is a legitimate problem. Now, medical communities are finally accepting it as an actual condition. Fibromyalgia is under the autoimmune umbrella, which means that even though they accept it as a condition, it's listed as "cause unknown," with the working theory that the body is attacking the nerves.

One of the theoretical explanations doctors are given by the medical establishment is that fibromyalgia is overactive nerves. What this again really translates to is . . . no one has a clue. It's not the doctors' fault. There's no magic book they receive that tells them what will help their fibromyalgia patients or what is genuinely causing their pain. Alternative medicine doctors play food elimination guessing games and experiment with supplements to see what kind of hit or miss occurs in hopes of getting some relief in their patients. They, too, are unaware of the true cause.

The medical system is still years from discovering the illness's true root—because it's viral, and it takes place at a nerve level that medical tools currently can't detect.

Those suffering from fibromyalgia are facing a very real and what can be a debilitating situation. It's the Epstein-Barr virus that is causing this disorder, inflaming both the central nervous system and nerves throughout the body, which creates ongoing pain that can shift and move around the body (something I call *moving pain*). Discomfort in certain areas one week can shift to other areas of the body a week later. Or someone can live with a constant fluctuation of pain, from mild to more severe, that stays in the same areas.

One of the hard parts of fibromyalgia, out of many, is how everyday accidents and actions can lead to pain that feels insurmountable. Bumping into a doorjamb, for example, or knocking your foot into something as you're walking along, or lifting something too heavy, or pushing your body too far with exercise—these are often experiences of pain that someone would forget about within seconds, if they even registered the pain in the first place. For a fibromyalgia sufferer, the pain these incidents can cause is on a whole other level.

EBV is also behind the common fibromyalgia experiences of sensitivity to touch, severe fatigue (that is, neurological fatigue), and a host of other issues.

Tinnitus

Tinnitus, or ringing in the ear, is usually caused by EBV getting into the inner ear's nerve channel, called the labyrinth. Tinnitus can also be experienced as humming, popping, buzzing, or vibrating in the ear, or for some, what feels almost like a symphony of different instruments at once. These sounds are the result of the virus inflaming and vibrating the labyrinth and the vestibulocochlear nerve. Milder forms of tinnitus can occur from just the neurotoxins themselves that the virus is eliminating—when these neurotoxins gather around the labyrinth, inflaming nerves.

With tinnitus, outside noises such as fans, air-conditioning, and machinery in the distance can change the texture of the ringing or other sound in the ear, making it almost dance around and change tones. It also tends to get worse at the end of the day, going into the evening. Tinnitus can be very hard on people, so it's best to make friends with it while you're working on getting it better. Many notice that the more rest and sleep they get, the more the tinnitus has improved upon waking. That's because the more rest you get, the more time the nerve channel in your inner ear has a chance to strengthen and recover. If you're not sleeping well, this doesn't mean you can't work on healing your tinnitus. Any sleep you get (or, if you can't sleep, any time spent resting with your eyes closed) helps the symptoms of tinnitus stay in check.

Vertigo and Ménière's Disease

Vertigo and *Ménière's disease* are often attributed by doctors to calcium crystals, or *stones*, becoming disrupted in the inner ear. However, most chronic cases are actually caused by EBV's neurotoxin inflaming the vagus nerve.

This can lead to many varieties of vertigo, from feeling like you're standing on a moving boat to the sensation of falling to the left, falling to the right, or even falling forward while you're walking, leading you to try to keep from toppling to the ground. Vertigo can be very mild, where you get dizzy after turning your head really quickly, or have difficulty watching someone or something else moving around you because the movement of anything within your vision can make you slightly nauseous and even partially dizzy. More extreme cases of vertigo can lead to the inability to get out of bed, or the opposite, the inability to lie down in bed, because once you do, your head feels like it's spinning. (I call these the bed spins.) Sometimes the spinning is circular, and sometimes it's a repeated motion that's going across your eyes.

The variety of vertigo you experience hinges on where the neurotoxin or virus itself is touching the vagus nerve. If the bottom of the vagus nerve is more inflamed, then nausea will accompany your dizziness. If the middle of the vagus nerve is more inflamed, then you'll have more of the feeling of being on a boat, or that the earth is moving underneath you as you're standing or walking. If the top of the vagus nerve is inflamed, sometimes this leads to more severe vertigo—the head spins that make it difficult to walk anywhere.

Other Symptoms

Anxiety, dizziness, chest and throat tightness, discomfort in the neck, chest pain, esophageal spasms, some varieties of gastroparesis, panic attacks, asthma, and tingling and numbness in the abdomen, chest, shoulders, and back of neck can also be caused by EBV inflaming the vagus nerve.

Insomnia, tingling and numbness in hands and feet, anxiety, pain in the pinkies, tingling and numbness in the pinkies or other fingers, or even trigger thumb (feeling of loss of control over the use of your thumb at times) can be caused by phrenic nerves becoming perpetually inflamed by EBV.

And heart palpitations can result from buildup of EBV's poisonous virus corpses and byproduct in the liver that lead the organ to become so overburdened that the waste matter escapes the liver and slowly builds up in the heart's mitral valve. This causes a stickiness to occur that can create an ectopic heartbeat or mystery heart palpitations. Certain varieties of EBV can release a neurotoxin that elevates brain inflammation, which can cause more severe heart palpitations or even mysterious

AFib (atrial fibrillation) due to neurotoxins saturating certain neurons, interrupting signals heading from those neurons in the brain to the heart. This can fall under the category of mysterious electrical heart activity, perplexing doctors.

If you have EBV, or suspect you do, you may find the virus in Stage Four beyond frustrating. Take comfort. If you take the right steps with information from the Medical Medium book series—some of which medical communities are starting to glean—you can recover, rebuild your immune system, restore your nervous system, return to a normal state again, and regain control of your life.

TYPES OF EPSTEIN-BARR

As I've noted earlier, there are over 60 varieties of the Epstein-Barr virus. That number is so large because EBV has existed for well over 100 years. It's had generations of people to move through and has even gotten a little help from the industries, mutating and elevating its various hybrids and strains in that time. As the years have gone by, people have become more toxic—meaning their bodies have taken on the burden of increased exposure to toxic troublemakers from our world. EBV has adapted to feeding on this wide variety of toxins, including toxic heavy metals, pesticides, herbicides, fungicides, and pharmaceuticals. Using these troublemakers as fuel sources, EBV has spread and mutated, with different mutations developing different strengths and appetites along the way. Through the decades, EBV has been challenged to adapt by various immune systems, with some of those immune systems much stronger. Because some varieties of EBV have also become stronger, they've been able to spread. The many strains of EBV can be organized into six groups of escalating severity, with roughly 10 types per group.

In a moment, we'll look at those EBV groups in detail. First, it's important to remember that many people have more than one variety of EBV. Someone could have one EBV variety from one group and then 10 years later get another exposure that leads to contracting another EBV variety from another group. Some people have two to three varieties of EBV. What this means is: one person will often experience symptoms from different EBV groups, whether those symptoms are intermixed at the same time or experienced at different times in life. Keep this in mind as you read about the EBV groups.

Also keep in mind that there are different EBV varieties in each group. Those different varieties will have slightly different effects on the body, leading to variations in symptoms within a group. For example, one EBV variety can be a little more aggressive than another in the same group, or have a different appetite for a certain toxin than another. That translates to differences in symptoms.

Any EBV variety from any group can elevate inflammation. The EBV varieties from Groups 3 through 6 have the potential to land somebody a mistaken Lyme diagnosis, if that's what the doctor is looking for. That's because Group 3 through 6 EBV varieties can raise inflammation high enough to trip false positives on Lyme disease tests.

As I always say, just knowing the cause of your suffering can be empowering. Reading through this chapter and recognizing that your mysterious symptoms and conditions match up with how EBV works can give you relief from the fear and worry about what's been happening to you. These EBV group descriptions may help you zero in on a certain variety or varieties of EBV that have been disrupting your life. Even if you can't identify which group or groups of EBV you're dealing with, just the realization that it's EBV at all can help you gain a sense of peace over time. With this knowledge, you can take control and work on ridding the virus, so you can recover instead of staying in the dark about why you're sick.

EBV Group 1 is the oldest and mildest. These versions of the virus typically take years, even decades, to transition from one stage to another. Their effects might not be noticeable until you're in your 70s or 80s, and then result in little more than back pain. They might even remain in your organs and never reach Stage Three or Stage Four. This group is getting rarer every day as the older generations of people pass on and cycle out of the population. This EBV group will most likely disappear in the next 30 years and become extinct as newer mutations in younger people rival these Group 1 varieties.

EBV Group 2 moves from stage to stage a bit quicker than Group 1; you might notice symptoms in your 50s or 60s. These varieties may partially linger in the thyroid and send out only some of their virus cells, which begin to release more neurotoxins that inflame nerves, resulting in relatively mild nerve inflammation. This can in turn lead to mild and/or intermittent versions of a number of different conditions and diagnoses, such as fibromyalgia, neuralgia, joint pain, tendonitis, carpal tunnel syndrome, aches, and pains. The only variety of EBV that medical communities are aware of is in this group.

EBV Group 3 will transition between stages faster than Group 2, so its symptoms might be noticeable around age 40. Also, these viruses fully complete Stage Four—that is, they entirely leave the thyroid to latch on to nerves. This group has an appetite for different toxins, so its neurotoxins are slightly different than the previous group's. Viruses in this group can cause a variety of ills, including joint pain, tingles and numbness, fatigue, heart palpitations, tinnitus, and vertigo. Group 3 varieties of EBV can also create reproductive system conditions. And if high enough levels of copper are present in a person's liver, certain varieties in this group have the potential to feed off that copper and create the dermatoxins behind eczema and psoriasis. If enough aluminum is present in the liver, varieties in this group have the ability to feed off that aluminum and create the dermatoxins responsible for vitiligo.

EBV Group 4 will create noticeable problems as early as age 30. Its more-aggressive neurotoxins can result in symptoms associated with fibromyalgia, chronic fatigue syndrome, brain fog, confusion, anxiety, moodiness, and everything caused by Groups 1 to 3. This group can release the dermatoxins, as well, that are behind skin disorders. This group can also create symptoms of posttraumatic stress disorder, even if a person never underwent any trauma beyond getting inflamed by the virus.

EBV Group 5 will create noticeable issues as early as age 20. This is an especially disruptive form of the virus because it can surface just when a young person is setting out to start an independent life. It can create all the problems of Group 4, and it can feed on the intense blends of excess adrenaline generated from ongoing fear, worry, or other challenging emotions. For this group to cause the most trouble, the toxic heavy metal mercury has to be involved. Younger people these days actually tend to have higher levels of mercury in their organs than older generations; it's easy to think it would be the opposite. EBV varieties in this group tend to have a thirst for eggs, too—mercury and eggs are their top two favorite foods. That means that eliminating eggs from your diet and focusing on removing mercury are two ways to gain some control and work on reversing symptoms and conditions associated with this EBV group. Doctors who can't find anything wrong, and perceive Group 5 EBV patients as young and healthy, have often declared "It's all in your head" and sent patients to psychologists to convince them what's actually happening in their bodies isn't real. As the epidemic of chronic illness has become harder to deny with every passing year, a newer trend has gained footing among younger doctors: "It's all in your head" is being replaced by "Your sickness is real, but you created it." Now some practitioners will tell patients, "You manifested your illness through bad thoughts," or "poor thinking" or "not being positive enough," or they'll imply that you're emotionally faulty and that's why you're sick. Or many doctors, both alternative and conventional, will take your symptoms seriously . . . and still head in the wrong direction of leaky gut, your microbiome, your microflora being "off," your hormones, food sensitivities, or an oversimplified "Maybe it's just your adrenals." As well-meaning as these doctors are, they won't realize there's an underlying low-grade viral infection that's the real problem, unless they're doctors who have learned from Medical Medium information throughout the years. And it's still the case that if a patient happens upon a doctor who's up on the Lyme disease trend, the patient will probably walk away with a Lyme misdiagnosis.

Certain EBV varieties in Group 6 can be very challenging even in young children. In addition to everything Group 5 does, Group 6 can be responsible for leukemia, MS, ALS, some cases of viral meningitis, and severe lupus, if the "right" varieties of EBV are coupled with enough toxic heavy metals such as mercury and aluminum. At the same time, some EBV varieties in this group are responsible for causing symptoms that only *look* like leukemia (or other serious conditions) and therefore lead to misdiagnosis.

This is a subtle difference on the page that will feel anything but subtle to someone living through it. Here's the distinction: an EBV variety in Group 6 can cause a *long-term* viral infection that creates leukemia itself in children and adults. On the other hand, some of the other EBV varieties in Group 6 can cause *acute* viral infections that lead to symptoms that seem very similar to leukemia—without being leukemia itself. Meanwhile, medical research and science don't realize EBV is behind any of it, so diagnostic judgment can be clouded. Well-meaning doctors sometimes misfire, pulling the trigger too fast with the life-changing diagnosis of leukemia. They can accidentally mistake a child's severe case of mono from an aggressive EBV variety (acute viral infection) for leukemia (long-term viral infection), not even realizing that any of it is viral in the first place.

The diagnostic gray area is very similar for neurological conditions such as MS and ALS. Keep in mind that you can get a diagnosis of lupus, ALS, or MS and *not* have one of the

advanced EBV varieties in Group 6. You may be dealing with a milder virus variety; even the mildest of neurological symptoms can land someone a diagnosis these days, depending on the doctor's specialty. For example, while multiple sclerosis—the disease that damages the myelin nerve sheath in the central nervous system—is caused by EBV, so are symptoms that *look* like multiple sclerosis. For myelin sheath damage to occur, it needs to be an advanced variety of EBV. And again, for an EBV variety from Group 6 to accelerate, there needs to be a higher level of toxic heavy metals such as mercury and aluminum present at the same time. There are people with the mildest form of symptoms caused by milder varieties of EBV (not from Group 6) who get misdiagnosed with MS when there is no actual myelin sheath damage, only because of the way some doctors are pulling the trigger. So both *actual* cases of MS and chronic symptoms *mis*diagnosed as MS are caused by EBV, with doctors unaware that EBV is the true cause either way, unless they're familiar with Medical Medium information.

Certain EBV varieties in Group 6 can create a larger amount of more potent types of neurotoxins and dermatoxins, accounting for some of the suffering these varieties can cause. That's due in large part to how certain varieties in this group have an even greater hunger for toxic heavy metals such as mercury, aluminum, and copper. Group 6 varieties also have a greater hunger for eggs, dairy products, and gluten. Their hunger for eggs especially suppresses the immune system, because your immune system is constantly up against the virus, using up its reserves trying to protect you, and anything that fuels EBV the way eggs do makes those battles harder.

Group 6 EBV can lead to a wide variety of symptoms including rashes, weakness in the limbs, and severe nerve pain.

FLU AND COVID COMPLICATIONS

I've always said that when someone gets the flu, it can lower the immune system, allowing other opportunities for viruses such as EBV to take hold. The flu is an Epstein-Barr virus trigger. That's why some people seem to bounce back from a bad flu after a few days and other people need months of recovery. COVID is triggering similar problems, on a larger scale.

There are many different strains of the flu. Some are mild, some are more severe. If the same severe flu hits a group of people, the people with preexisting symptoms or conditions (whether they know about them or not) will likely face more difficult recoveries, unless they have the right understanding of the source of those underlying health issues and the right tools to deal with it all. Again, that's because bad cases of the flu can trigger *other* existing viruses in someone's system. EBV and shingles are the two most common viruses to be triggered by a bad flu. Once they're triggered, viral conditions and symptoms can take hold—ones such as Lyme, CFS, fibromyalgia, brain fog, tingles and numbness throughout the body, weakness of the limbs, depression, and anxiety.

For some people, those symptoms and conditions from EBV or other viruses were preexisting, and the flu trigger either brought them back or brought them on stronger.

For others, these symptoms or conditions from EBV or other viruses were developing inside the body and hadn't yet surfaced—until the flu trigger. These were people on the cusp of low-grade chronic viral infection. An example is if EBV in your system (that you didn't know about) was just on the edge of going into its mono phase. Your immune system was already being challenged by the EBV, and then along came a flu bug—all that was needed to set off the EBV. So after your flu, you could now be dealing with your first bout of mononucleosis. You could be struggling with fatigue, brain fog, body pain, or weakness of the limbs on and off for weeks and weeks, long after the flu. Meanwhile, your friend could have gotten the same flu and after 10 days, been back on track with life, not even thinking about it anymore.

COVID, even more instigative as a trigger, works in a similar way: past symptoms that someone has struggled with can easily come back, or newer symptoms can appear from preexisting viruses (such as EBV) that no one knew were already in their body, awaiting a chance to surface. *COVID is actually quickening people's future symptoms and illness.*

This is a great source of confusion. Many people think that it's all because of COVID; they believe that COVID itself is the reason they're struggling with newfound chronic symptoms. If someone develops breathing issues that become chronic because COVID injured their lungs, then yes, that's a result of COVID. Someone could also have a slow recovery from COVID if the virus created a very high fever for a long period of time. (More on that in a moment.) These scenarios only describe some cases, though. In truth, the majority of lasting problems that people experience post-COVID aren't COVID anymore. They're preexisting or unseen problems that got *triggered*—chronic symptoms and conditions that someone was already going to develop because of viral activity already present in their body. COVID acted as a trigger for the EBV or other viruses that were in the body, undetected. It brought future symptoms and conditions to someone earlier in life, versus waiting 20-plus years to develop them.

Now let's compare this to what it can be like to recover from a COVID-related fever. A high, sustained fever can lead to dehydration and severe electrolyte deficiency crisis, in turn leading someone to experience post-COVID brain fatigue for up to about three to six months before feeling back to normal. Or that fever could put an enormous stress on the adrenal glands, which are highly sensitive to heat, weakening the adrenals to the point that they need a good one to three months of recovery. These effects of high fever don't lead to lots of different symptoms. Someone may just get tired more easily, or feel weaker and have less strength than normal, and it will remedy itself over time. These do not tend to be permanent post-COVID conditions.

In contrast, when COVID triggers an underlying viral condition such as EBV, symptoms can be wider ranging and longer lasting.

Or someone can experience both at once—a slow recovery due to a high, sustained COVID-related fever *at the same time as* the onset or flare-up of chronic symptoms from an underlying viral condition that COVID triggered.

Both the flu and COVID can create confusion in other ways, too. For example, someone may already be struggling with chronic symptoms long term—for example, fatigue, brain fog, aches and pains, sadness—and may have received multiple diagnoses along the way, whether told the suffering is due to gut problems, fibromyalgia, MS, ocular migraines, RA, Lyme disease, anxiety, or depression. Then, that person may contract the flu or COVID and feel worse, not realizing why. Even a milder form of flu can make these symptoms feel so much worse than they already do. While it may be temporary—just two or three weeks of worse symptoms, possibly, depending on what that person is going through—it can be enough to slow the person down.

Mild strains of the flu are especially disorienting. Symptoms could be as simple as little extra body aches, mild fever, scratchy throat, and headache, and when this happens intermixed with the symptoms someone already has, it can confuse the situation. People may think their preexisting chronic conditions are getting worse, or that they're doing something wrong, or that their health is going backward, when what's really happening is that a mild strain of the flu is passing through the body. It's an easy mistake to make. It usually takes mucus forming and maybe a cough developing for people to realize they may have caught something—that it's not a normal condition or symptom they're used to living with intermittently. There are mild flu strains where the mucus and cough never come, so someone never has the realization that it *was* the flu.

The stomach flu confuses people all the time, too. They get hit with it, they're vomiting, they can't eat, and they feel truly lost in that day or two as it's passing through them. They don't know if it's a preexisting condition or if they maybe have food poisoning.

With any flu, you can have the mildest of symptoms, where you just feel a little tired and achy, then it goes away—yet you can pass that flu strain to someone else, and that person can be hit a little harder, especially if the person has preexisting symptoms or conditions.

COVID is very similar. It is not just the one single strain that was started. And COVID is transmissible in the same way the flu is—the same way people pass the flu around in its many strains is how people contract and pass COVID around in its many strains.

COVID is a virus that is alive. It is not an RNA strand that is dead, or fragments of information from the virus itself. That is, COVID is a living virus. The flu is also a living virus. Viruses in the herpetic family are living viruses, including EBV, shingles, cytomegalovirus, simplex, HHV-6, HHV-7, and other known and unknown HHV varieties. These viruses are all alive—and in order for living viruses to stay alive, they need to eat food. Just as EBV feeds on toxic heavy metals such as mercury and other foods, the flu and COVID do the same.

The flu and COVID are manufactured viruses. They've been raised in labs, experimented with, tested with, and fed foods to stay alive. COVID and the flu virus compete with each other (although not with herpetic viruses) inside the body. If someone with COVID also contracts a bad flu strain, COVID will increase its strength to battle the flu for survival. The two viruses attach themselves to each other until one of them slowly breaks down and destroys the other. A preventative measure that may be helpful is to eliminate certain foods that can possibly feed the flu or COVID. The leading food is eggs. Eggs are used to grow and raise viruses in the lab. This is just one helpful preventative measure you can take action with. Having eggs in your body system on a daily or weekly basis can help launch a virus such as COVID or even the flu upon first contracting it.

We're in an age today where viruses don't just appear. They are manipulated, altered, and sometimes even created through purposely mutating original, natural, docile strains of viruses found in our natural environment. The flu virus and COVID do consume toxic heavy metals such as mercury, but only mercury. Both these viruses do not feast on other toxic heavy metals. This is why people with higher mercury levels and higher viral levels from EBV and shingles causing their symptoms and conditions tend to be more sensitive to COVID. We can umbrella it all as "preexisting conditions," but it's more than that—it's preexisting viruses the person has. Which viruses do they have? Are they also high in toxic heavy metals such as mercury? Taking action and removing toxic heavy metals such as mercury out of the body is another step you can take to help your preventative measures with viruses such as flu or COVID.

It's important, too, to be proactive in understanding the preexisting virus you have that's creating the symptoms you live with on a daily basis, because working to overcome your chronic symptoms by killing off viruses such as EBV can make you stronger—more able to take on the flu and COVID we're up against in today's world.

This specific original strain of COVID that found its way into people recently was far more aggressive at the very beginning, because it had never entered human beings before. As it passes through the human population, it becomes less aggressive (unless it's competing with a very aggressive flu strain)—as it goes through millions of people, COVID loses strength because it has to battle the human immune system along the way. Each person's immune system battles and fights COVID, and over time, as it's entering more and more people, the virus itself changes and weakens.

That's the opposite of how viruses such as EBV work. As you read in "Types of Epstein-Barr" earlier in this chapter, as EBV spreads and mutates throughout the years, new groups of EBV develop that become more aggressive. Group 1 was mild and docile. Then as EBV entered more and more people over the decades, it mutated and grew stronger. Newer mutations of EBV are stronger than its past varieties.

COVID, on the other hand, hit the human race hard upon arrival. Over time, it dumbs down as the human immune system shapes it, changes it, and weakens it—meaning that eventually, we aren't going to be contending with the most aggressive strain. As the years go on, we'll be contending with a milder form of this current version of COVID. That doesn't mean that a new variety of COVID won't enter the population through manufacturing, sticking us back in the same position we're in with this variety.

For more than 35 years, I've been teaching people about viruses. Doctors, professionals in health, countless others—I've been teaching them about how viruses work in the body, how we can protect ourselves, and how we can rid viruses to heal and overcome our symptoms and conditions. People tend not to want to know they have viruses until they get sick enough that they have to accept something is wrong. The awareness I've brought to viruses throughout the years has resonated the most with these people—the ones who've already struggled enough with their symptoms to be ready for the awakening that a virus is behind it.

This new global experience of COVID is awakening the wider health movement to the reality that viruses can be an issue in our health. That's not good enough. The focus is always going to be off the mark. Talk such as "COVID is not a living virus" is going to spread more and more, as will the theories "Viruses are not alive," "Viruses don't eat," and "The only virus to be concerned about is COVID, and maybe the flu." We'll also hear, "When you do contract COVID, it can create long-lasting chronic illness," without the understanding that the chronic illness comes from preexisting viruses that people already had that medical communities were unaware of. These are just a few examples of how messaging is always going to be off the mark. There's already been a battle out there where many people didn't even believe COVID was a problem or a concern. That's how antiviral we are as a society today—and not *antiviral* in the helpful way, as in virus protection. We still live in a world where if you can't see it, then it must not be a problem.

To a globe hard hit by COVID, the pandemic *has* brought great awareness around viruses to many. You can use this as an opportunity to spread your knowledge. As I said at the beginning of the book, I've always taught you the tools for dealing with viruses—from the beginning, I've given you information you need to protect yourself and make yourself stronger, so threats like viruses can't take you down.

Since I was a child, Spirit of Compassion has told me that zinc is a fighting weapon against viruses. One reason is because the world is zinc deficient. It's not in our food; we're lacking zinc even in the best organic food we grow. Zinc is an immune system equalizer. It supports it in a way that doesn't allow the immune system to overreact or underreact. With COVID, our immune system tends to overreact because it's such a newly released virus. Our bodies see it as a complete stranger, and COVID can react by waging a war, at the same time your immune system can overreact. That's how it gets truly messy. Zinc can do three things: (1) calm the immune system down, (2) strengthen the immune system, because immune cells feed off zinc, and (3) at the same time, weaken COVID and the flu virus. When zinc weakens COVID, that makes the virus docile and less aggressive. This is a measure that can be very helpful with COVID, the flu, and other viruses that are in the process of being manufactured and will get out of the running gate in future years to come.

Vitamin C is also helpful for viruses such as flu and COVID. It can do two things: (1) feed the immune system and (2) hinder viruses. Vitamin C has an irritating effect upon a virus's membranes. Higher dosages of vitamin C tend to create little pits and divots within a virus membrane—its outer protective cover and shield—and this helps weaken and thwart the virus.

As you read further in this chapter and the chapters that follow, you'll find more tools to strengthen your immune system, free yourself from the troublemakers that feed viruses, and rebuild your body. That's more critical than ever at this time in history.

So is looking after your emotional health. In Chapter 24, "Soul-Healing Meditations and Techniques," you'll find expanded meditations to keep yourself grounded; cope with the many emotions that come with uncertainty, upheaval, and confinement; and access the healing resources within you and right outside your window. In the final chapter of the book, "Keep the Faith," you'll find a powerful technique to keep yourself moving forward.

You carry a special purpose at this point in time. As COVID moves through a lot more people in the coming days and years, it will also continue to act as a trigger for chronic symptoms and conditions. A wave of people who are suffering post-COVID has already begun. People are starting to struggle with the chronic health issues they otherwise would have developed later in life—for example, lasting fatigue, body pain, eye floaters, weakness of the limbs, tingles and numbness, tics and spasms, or migraines. Again, the majority of lasting symptoms are not because of COVID itself. They occur because COVID can act as a trigger, quickening people's future chronic symptoms and conditions.

And yet people won't realize these health issues were already waiting for them. They're going to think their health problems are lasting effects of COVID itself. They're going to feel lost and powerless and think, *I don't have COVID anymore, so I can't do anything about it*. They're in the dark and will continue to be in the dark, unless the information here reaches them.

That's why you play a critical role in history. You understand that when (non-respiratory) symptoms develop and persist long past COVID, the truth is that COVID likely triggered another virus such as EBV or shingles that was already in a person's system—and *that's* usually the real reason for the symptoms. If somebody suffers a Lyme relapse after the flu or COVID, you understand that it's because EBV or another herpetic virus already present got triggered, bringing back the Lyme symptoms. And you understand that there is something you and others can do to put this behind you and move forward. You can not only protect yourself; you can help other people find this information and figure out what's wrong so they can protect themselves and their families.

You hold the knowledge to light the way for others.

HEALING FROM THE EPSTEIN-BARR VIRUS

Because it's very easy to catch and hard to detect, and can cause a number of mysterious symptoms, you might understandably find the Epstein-Barr virus overwhelming and its effects disheartening.

The good news is that if you carefully and patiently follow the steps detailed in this section, and in Part IV of the book, you can heal. You can recover your immune system, free yourself of EBV, rejuvenate your body, gain full control over your health, and move on with your life.

Everyone's healing process is different. There are over 60 varieties of EBV, and that doesn't count the varieties of *other* viruses (such as shingles) that can be present in someone's system at the same time as EBV. Some people may have one variety of EBV; some people may have two. Some people may have EBV *plus* shingles or another herpetic family virus. Some people may have more of the toxic heavy metal mercury causing neurological symptoms; some people may have more toxic copper causing skin conditions.

What this translates to is: Some people may find that just celery juice on its own with no other changes moves the needle with their symptoms. Some people may need to go much further than that, embarking on the 28-Day Healing Cleanse, cleanses from *Cleanse to Heal*, and/or supplement protocols.

The answers are in this book and the rest of the Medical Medium series.

Everyone is different. Everyone has a chance to heal.

Remember, Medical Medium is not just one protocol. That's why millions around the world have already gotten their lives back. There's no such thing as "I tried Medical Medium, and it didn't work for me." More people have recovered their health with the Medical Medium book series and information than from anywhere else in our time. So the results are in. There's a track record of this information changing lives. If you're coming into this brand new, please be aware of this track record. If you put the commitment, time, and effort into reading the books and understanding the various protocols, you have the ability to customize your own personal protocol within this information so you can go as far as you need to go.

I try to make it as easy as possible to understand how to go about your own individual protocol for your symptoms, sickness, or disease. You can bring Medical Medium information to your doctor or practitioners for guidance, if need be.

Keep in mind that if somebody says they've "done celery juice," they could have missed a key point—they could have tried only eight ounces and not appropriately on an empty stomach, or not for long enough. Or maybe they used supplements that contained alcohol or were very low quality. Or maybe they didn't take the time to consider which protocol to customize for themselves. Maybe they didn't approach a protocol one step at a time.

I want everyone to heal within the shortest time span possible. Many people do heal quickly. Some people have a long-term chronic viral infection, lots of toxic heavy metals, and might have come from a route of trying many different approaches in the past that weren't helpful and could even have been harmful. For someone in this situation, even when you kill off the EBV and remove the toxic heavy metals, the nervous system could have been compromised from both the virus and the toxic heavy metals along the way, and so the nervous system needs time to heal. Many who do the Medical Medium protocols start feeling some immediate relief as they clean things up in the body, and then long after they've started, the neurological symptoms finally subside—because again, the nervous system needs time to repair within the protocols.

I believe in you. With the knowledge and power, I know you can heal.

Healing Foods

Certain fruits, leafy greens, herbs, wild foods, and vegetables can help your body rid itself of EBV and heal from its effects. The following are the best ones to incorporate into your diet (listed in rough order of importance). Try to eat at least three of these foods per day—the more the better—rotating your consumption so that in a given week or two, you get as many of these foods as you can into your system.

Also take care to avoid the foods in Chapter 19, "What Not to Eat." When dealing with an EBV-caused symptom or condition, it's critical to begin the process of removing at least one or two of the foods that feed the virus. If you need to take your healing even further, try to gravitate toward removing all the foods that feed the virus.

- **Celery juice:** strengthens hydrochloric acid in the gut by helping to restore the stomach's gastric glands. Provides mineral salts (namely, sodium cluster salts, a subgroup of sodium only found in celery juice) to the central nervous system. Sodium cluster salts are also antiviral and antibacterial. Celery juice is the only food or herbal medicine that contains complete electrolytes, not partial. It helps to flush out neurotoxins, dermatoxins, and bacteria such as *Streptococcus*.

- **Wild blueberries:** help restore the central nervous system during and after toxic heavy metal exposure; flush EBV neurotoxins out of the liver. Also helpful for removing toxic heavy metals such as mercury, aluminum, and copper. Wild blueberries are one of the most adaptogenic foods on the planet and have powerful antiviral properties.

- **Potatoes:** create an easy, sustainable form of glucose that helps stabilize adrenals, feeds the nervous system, restores glycogen in the brain, and is antiviral and antibacterial.

- **Spinach:** creates an alkaline environment in the body and provides highly absorbable micronutrients to the nervous system. Contains trace mineral salts that provide critically needed electrolytes to the brain.

- **Bananas:** help rid viruses and bacteria from the intestinal tract;

contain antiviral and antibacterial compounds.

- **Asparagus:** cleanses the liver and spleen; strengthens the pancreas. Helping to detoxify and strengthen the liver like this automatically leads to cleansing the lymphatic system and keeping it healthy.

- **Cilantro:** removes toxic heavy metals such as mercury, aluminum, copper, and lead, which are favored foods of EBV. Also has mild antiviral properties.

- **Papayas:** restore the central nervous system; strengthen and rebuild hydrochloric acid in the gut. Soothing to the intestinal tract linings, papayas also improve peristaltic action.

- **Lettuce:** stimulates peristaltic action in the intestinal tract and helps cleanse EBV byproduct and other viral waste matter from the liver.

- **Brussels sprouts:** detoxifying for the liver; their phytochemical sulfur compounds are antiviral.

- **Parsley:** can help remove easily accessible surface levels of copper and aluminum, which feed EBV, from the intestinal tract, including the colon (but not from deep-seated place such as the bloodstream, organs, and glands).

- **Sweet potatoes:** help cleanse and detox the liver from EBV byproducts and toxins.

- **Kale:** high in specific alkaloids and trace minerals that help keep our immune system strong, protecting us from viruses such as EBV.

- **Sprouts:** high in zinc and selenium to strengthen the immune system against EBV.

- **Ginger:** helps with nutrient assimilation and relieves spasms associated with EBV; contains antiviral, antibacterial compounds.

- **Garlic:** an antiviral and antibacterial that defends against EBV and strep.

- **Cucumbers:** strengthen the adrenals and kidneys and flush neurotoxins and dermatoxins out of the bloodstream.

- **Tomatoes:** gentle on the digestive system, especially when it comes to sensitive nerves caused by EBV; high in a very absorbable, assimilable form of vitamin C. Also hydrating on a deep cellular level—that little bit of fresh juice that you get from eating a tomato goes a long way in hydrating the liver.

- **Red pitaya (dragon fruit):** helpful in cleansing a stagnant, sluggish liver; also supports liver immune function.

- **Fennel:** contains strong antiviral and antibacterial compounds to fight off EBV and strep; also strengthens the immune system.

- **Raspberries:** rich in antioxidants to remove free radicals from the organs and bloodstream.

- **Grapefruit:** rich source of bioflavonoids and calcium to support the immune system and flush toxins out of the body.

- **Pomegranates:** help detox and cleanse the blood as well as the liver, which then allows the lymphatic system to stay cleaner.

- **Apricots:** immune system rebuilders that also strengthen the blood.

Healing Herbs and Supplements

The following herbs and supplements can further strengthen your immune system and aid your body in healing from the virus's effects. **Before applying these, be sure to read Chapter 21, "Critical Guide to Supplement Protocols."**

You're welcome to intermix supplements from the different lists in this chapter. For example, you may decide to base your protocol on the fibromyalgia list and then bring in some supplements from the chronic fatigue syndrome list. Or you may customize your supplement protocol by selecting supplements from both the autoimmune list and the list of supplements for eczema, psoriasis, and lupus-style rashes. You'll read more options for customization as you go.

When I mention tailoring a supplement protocol for yourself, I'm not talking about bringing in supplements outside of what I recommend in this book or its companion, *Cleanse to Heal*. For reasons you'll read about in Chapter 19, "What Not to Eat," supplements other than what I recommend may be contributing to your problems in the first place.

Supplements for Mononucleosis (Mono, an early stage of Epstein-Barr virus, EBV)

You can use this EBV supplements list if you've been to the doctor and had EBV detected in a blood test, whether or not you received a mono diagnosis at the same time. You can also turn to these supplements if you have mystery symptoms that remain undiagnosed and that you've now matched up with the symptoms in this chapter.

You're welcome to customize your supplement protocol between what's in this list and the list that follows for later-stage EBV.

- **Fresh celery juice:** work up to 32 ounces daily

- **Cat's claw:** 3 dropperfuls twice a day

- **Eyebright:** 3 dropperfuls twice a day

- **Ginger:** 1 cup of tea or freshly grated or juiced to taste four times a day

- **Goldenseal:** 4 dropperfuls twice a day (two weeks on, two weeks off)

- **Lemon balm:** 4 dropperfuls twice a day

- **Licorice root:** 1 dropperful twice a day (two weeks on, two weeks off)

- **L-lysine:** 6 500-milligram capsules twice a day

- **Lomatium root:** 3 dropperfuls twice a day

- **Monolaurin:** 2 capsules twice a day

- **Mullein leaf:** 4 dropperfuls twice a day

- **Oregon grape root:** 2 dropperfuls twice a day (two weeks on, two weeks off)

- **Osha:** 3 dropperfuls twice a day

- **Thyme:** 2 sprigs fresh thyme in hot water as tea or 4 sprigs in room temperature water daily

- **Vitamin C (as Micro-C):** after optional Medical Medium Vitamin C Shock Therapy, 10 capsules twice a day

- **Zinc (as liquid zinc sulfate):** after optional Medical Medium Zinc Shock Therapy for two days, 3 dropperfuls twice a day

Supplements for Autoimmune Disorders and Diseases (later-stage EBV, including Lupus and Rheumatoid Arthritis, [RA])

If you have a condition that is not listed in this chapter and yet your symptoms match up to EBV, you can turn to these supplements. Most of the time someone receives an autoimmune diagnosis, it can be later-stage EBV.

You're welcome to customize your supplement protocol between this list and the previous list, for early-stage EBV.

If you're struggling with lupus and its skin-related aspects are bothering you more, you can turn to the "Eczema, Psoriasis & Lupus-Style Rashes" supplements at the end of this chapter. If you're struggling more with other symptoms of lupus, you can start with this list. Or you're welcome to customize a protocol for yourself using the two lists.

- **Fresh celery juice:** work up to 32 ounces twice a day if possible; if not, work up to 32 ounces every morning

- **Celeryforce:** 3 capsules twice a day

- **5-MTHF:** 1 capsule twice a day

- **ALA (alpha lipoic acid):** 1 500-milligram capsule twice a week

- **Aloe vera:** 2 or more inches of fresh gel (skin removed) daily

- **Barley grass juice powder:** 2 teaspoons or 6 capsules twice a day

- **Cat's claw:** 2 dropperfuls twice a day

- **Chaga mushroom:** 2 teaspoons or 6 capsules twice a day

- **Curcumin:** 2 capsules twice a day

- **Glutathione:** 1 capsule daily

- **Hibiscus:** 1 cup of tea daily

- **Lemon balm:** 2 dropperfuls twice a day

- **Licorice root:** 1 dropperful daily (two weeks on, two weeks off)

- **L-lysine:** 4 500-milligram capsules twice a day

- **Lomatium root:** 1 dropperful daily

- **MSM:** 1 capsule twice a day

- **Mullein leaf:** 2 dropperfuls twice a day

- **Nascent iodine:** 3 small drops (not dropperfuls) twice a day

- **Nettle leaf:** 2 dropperfuls twice a day

- **Oregon grape root:** 1 dropperful twice a day (two weeks on, two weeks off)

- **Raw honey:** 1 to 3 teaspoons daily
- **Selenium:** 1 capsule daily
- **Spirulina:** 2 teaspoons or 6 capsules daily
- **Thyme:** 2 sprigs of fresh thyme in hot water as tea or 4 sprigs in room temperature water daily
- **Turmeric:** 1 capsule twice a day
- **Vitamin B$_{12}$ (as adenosylcobalamin with methylcobalamin):** 2 dropperfuls twice a day
- **Vitamin C (as Micro-C):** 6 capsules twice a day
- **Wild blueberry powder:** 1 tablespoon daily
- **Zinc (as liquid zinc sulfate):** up to 2 dropperfuls twice a day

Supplements for Chronic Fatigue Syndrome (CFS) Also known as Myalgic Encephalomyelitis/ Chronic Fatigue Syndrome (ME/ CFS), Chronic Fatigue Immune Dysfunction Syndrome (CFIDS), Systemic Exertion Intolerance Disease (SEID)

- **Fresh celery juice:** work up to 32 ounces daily, then work up to 64 ounces daily if possible
- **Celeryforce:** 2 capsules three times a day
- **5-MTHF:** 1 capsule twice a day
- **Ashwagandha:** 1 dropperful daily

- **Barley grass juice powder:** 4 teaspoons or 12 capsules daily
- **Cat's claw:** 2 dropperfuls twice a day
- **Chaga mushroom:** 2 teaspoons or 6 capsules daily
- **Curcumin:** 2 capsules twice a day
- **EPA and DHA (fish-free):** 1 capsule daily (taken with dinner)
- **Eyebright:** 1 dropperful daily
- **Glutathione:** 1 capsule daily
- **Goldenseal:** 2 dropperfuls twice a day (two weeks on, two weeks off)
- **Lemon balm:** 3 dropperfuls twice a day
- **Licorice root:** 1 dropperful twice day (two weeks on, two weeks off)
- **L-lysine:** 4 500-milligram capsules twice a day
- **Magnesium glycinate:** 1 capsule twice a day
- **Monolaurin:** 2 capsules twice a day
- **Mullein:** 2 dropperfuls twice a day
- **Oregon grape root:** 1 dropperful daily (two weeks on, two weeks off)
- **Spirulina:** 1 tablespoon or 9 capsules daily
- **Vitamin B$_{12}$ (as adenosylcobalamin with methylcobalamin):** 2 dropperfuls twice a day
- **Vitamin C (as Micro-C):** 3 capsules twice a day
- **Zinc (as liquid zinc sulfate):** 2 dropperfuls twice a day

Supplements for Fibromyalgia

- **Fresh celery juice:** work up to 32 ounces daily

- **Celeryforce:** 2 capsules twice a day

- **5-MTHF:** 1 capsule daily

- **Ashwagandha:** 1 dropperful daily

- **Barley grass juice powder:** 2 teaspoons or 6 capsules daily

- **Cat's claw:** 1 dropperful twice a day

- **Curcumin:** 2 capsules twice a day

- **EPA and DHA (fish-free):** 1 capsule daily (taken with dinner)

- **Lemon balm:** 4 dropperfuls twice a day

- **Licorice root:** 1 dropperful daily (two weeks on, two weeks off)

- **L-lysine:** 3 500-milligram capsules twice a day

- **Magnesium glycinate:** 1 capsule twice a day

- **Monolaurin:** 1 capsule daily

- **MSM:** 1 capsule daily

- **Nettle leaf:** 3 dropperfuls twice a day

- **Spirulina:** 2 teaspoons or 6 capsules daily

- **Vitamin B$_{12}$ (as adenosylcobalamin with methylcobalamin):** 2 dropperfuls twice a day

- **Vitamin C (as Micro-C):** 3 capsules twice a day

- **Vitamin D$_3$:** 1,000 IU daily

- **Wild blueberry powder:** 1 tablespoon daily

- **Zinc (as liquid zinc sulfate):** 1 dropperful twice a day

Supplements for Tinnitus (Ringing, Vibrating, Humming, Buzzing, or Popping in the Ears)

- **Fresh celery juice:** work up to 32 ounces daily, then work up to 64 ounces daily if possible

- **Celeryforce:** 1 capsule twice a day

- **5-MTHF:** 1 capsule daily

- **ALA (alpha lipoic acid):** 1 capsule twice a week

- **Barley grass juice powder:** 2 teaspoons or 6 capsules daily

- **Cat's claw:** 2 dropperfuls twice a day

- **Chaga mushroom:** 2 teaspoons or 6 capsules daily

- **Curcumin:** 3 capsules twice a day

- **Lemon balm:** 4 dropperfuls twice a day

- **Licorice root:** 1 dropperful twice a day (two weeks on, two weeks off)

- **L-lysine:** 6 500-milligram capsules twice a day

- **Lomatium root:** 2 dropperfuls twice a day

- **Magnesium glycinate:** 1 capsule twice a day

- **Monolaurin:** 1 capsule daily

- **Mullein leaf:** 3 dropperfuls twice a day
- **Nettle leaf:** 3 dropperfuls twice a day
- **Olive leaf:** 1 dropperful twice a day
- **Oregano oil:** 1 capsule twice a day
- **Spirulina:** 2 teaspoons or 6 capsules daily
- **Vitamin B$_{12}$ (as adenosylcobalamin with methylcobalamin):** 3 dropperfuls twice a day
- **Vitamin C (as Micro-C):** 6 capsules twice a day
- **Wild blueberry powder:** 1 tablespoon daily
- **Zinc (as liquid zinc sulfate):** 2 dropperfuls twice a day

Supplements for Vertigo & Ménière's Disease

- **Fresh celery juice:** work up to 32 ounces daily
- **Celeryforce:** 2 capsules twice a day
- **Barley grass juice powder:** 2 teaspoons or 6 capsules daily
- **B-complex:** 1 capsule daily
- **Cat's claw:** 2 dropperfuls twice a day
- **Chaga mushroom:** 2 teaspoons or 6 capsules daily
- **Curcumin:** 2 capsules twice a day
- **EPA and DHA (fish-free):** 1 capsule daily (taken with dinner)
- **Eyebright:** 1 dropperful daily

- **Lemon balm:** 3 dropperfuls three times a day
- **L-glutamine:** 1 capsule daily
- **Licorice root:** 1 dropperful daily (two weeks on, two weeks off)
- **L-lysine:** 5 500-milligram capsules twice a day
- **Lomatium root:** 2 dropperfuls twice a day
- **Magnesium glycinate:** 1 capsule daily
- **Monolaurin:** 1 capsule daily
- **Mullein leaf:** 3 dropperfuls twice a day
- **Olive leaf:** 1 dropperful twice a day
- **Spirulina:** 2 teaspoons or 6 capsules daily
- **Vitamin B$_{12}$ (as adenosylcobalamin with methylcobalamin):** 2 dropperfuls twice a day
- **Vitamin C (as Micro-C):** 4 capsules twice a day
- **Wild blueberry powder:** 2 teaspoons daily
- **Zinc (as liquid zinc sulfate):** 2 dropperfuls twice a day

Supplements for Eczema, Psoriasis & Lupus-Style Rashes

- **Fresh celery juice:** work up to 32 ounces daily
- **Celeryforce:** 2 capsules twice a day
- **5-MTHF:** 1 capsule daily

- **Aloe vera:** 2 or more inches of fresh gel (skin removed) daily

- **Barley grass juice powder:** 2 teaspoons or 6 capsules daily

- **Cat's claw:** 1 dropperful twice a day

- **Chaga mushroom:** 1 teaspoon or 3 capsules daily

- **Curcumin:** 1 capsule twice a day

- **EPA and DHA (fish-free):** 2 capsules daily (taken with dinner)

- **Lemon balm:** 2 dropperfuls twice a day or 1 cup of tea twice a day

- **Licorice root:** 1 dropperful daily (two weeks on, two weeks off)

- **L-lysine:** 4 500-milligram capsules twice a day

- **Mullein leaf:** 1 dropperful twice a day

- **Nettle leaf:** 1 dropperful or 1 cup of tea twice a day

- **Selenium:** 1 capsule daily

- **Spirulina:** 2 teaspoons or 6 capsules daily

- **Vitamin B$_{12}$ (as adenosylcobalamin with methylcobalamin):** 1 dropperful twice a day

- **Vitamin C (as Micro-C):** 6 capsules twice a day

- **Zinc (as liquid zinc sulfate):** up to 1 dropperful twice a day

CASE HISTORY:
A Career Almost Lost to Epstein-Barr
2001

Michelle and her husband, Matthew, both had high-paying corporate jobs. Michelle was a star at her firm and made a point of going to work throughout her pregnancy, leaving only when she was about to go into labor.

After giving birth, Michelle instantly fell in love with her new son, Jordan. She couldn't have been happier. *I have it all now*, she thought, *a career I love, and a family I love even more*.

But Michelle's bright future started to dim when she was struck with a fatigue she couldn't shake. No matter how many vitamins she took or how much she exercised, she felt run-down all the time. So Michelle visited her doctor. After giving her a physical, he dismissed her concerns: "You look fine to me. It's natural for a new baby to be exhausting. Just get more sleep and don't worry about it."

Michelle took care to sleep more. After another week, she felt worse than ever. Suspecting a post-pregnancy issue, Michelle went to see her OB/GYN. This doctor drew her blood for a number of tests, including several for thyroid disease. When the lab results came in, the OB/GYN correctly diagnosed Michelle as having Hashimoto's thyroiditis.

Michelle was put on thyroid medication to get her hormone levels back to normal. This made her feel a little better . . . though not quite as well as she had before her pregnancy. She'd been aiming to return to work a month after having her son, and now she had to postpone those plans.

After about six months, Michelle's fatigue was back—and much more severe. That's when Michelle's troubles really began. Soon she had trouble taking care of Jordan. Matthew agreed to help out until she felt better.

Instead, Michelle grew worse. On top of being tired, she started to feel aches and pains, especially in her joints. Michelle returned to her OB/GYN, who ran another set of tests. The lab results showed nothing wrong. Due to the thyroid medication Michelle was continuing to take, her thyroid levels seemed perfect. So were all her vitamin and mineral levels. The OB/GYN was baffled.

Suspecting that Michelle's symptoms were related to her thyroid condition, the OB/GYN referred Michelle to a top endocrinologist (a doctor who specializes in hormonal issues). The specialist conducted a thorough thyroid profile, and tested Michelle's other hormone levels from a variety of angles. He ended up telling Michelle she had "mild adrenal fatigue."

There was some small truth to that. Michelle's adrenal glands were being strained by the Epstein-Barr virus, which her pregnancy had triggered and which was now inflaming her thyroid.

The endocrinologist told Michelle to take it easy and avoid stress. On his recommendation, Michelle handed off the freelance consulting projects she'd been working on from home.

In reality, Michelle's job had nothing to do with her condition. Her source of stress wasn't her work, but the illness that was eating away at her life . . . and her seeming helplessness to understand it or do anything about it.

Michelle continued to get worse. Her knees flared up and swelled, making it difficult to walk. She bought knee supports . . . and decided to pursue help more aggressively. Michelle's intuition told her an invader was present in her body, so she went to see an infectious disease specialist. This would be precisely the right thing to do—if infectious disease doctors actually knew how to recognize and treat past infections of EBV.

Unfortunately, they didn't have this awareness back at the time this was happening to Michelle. So after running an exhausting battery of tests and noticing that Michelle had an antibody from a past EBV infection, the specialist dismissed it as a problem right away. This doctor told her she was physically fit. He added that she might be depressed, and offered to refer her to a psychiatrist.

Infuriated at being made to feel she was crazy for trying to address what she deeply sensed was a real physical problem, Michelle (painfully) rose and strode out of the room.

With increasing desperation, Michelle now visited doctors across the spectrum. They put her through ultrasounds, X-rays, MRIs, CT scans, and loads of blood tests. She was told she had *Candida*, fibromyalgia, MS, lupus, Lyme disease, and rheumatoid arthritis. None of it was right. She was put on immunosuppressant drugs, antibiotics, and loads of different supplements. None of the treatments helped.

Michelle became an insomniac, suffered heart palpitations, and developed chronic vertigo that caused dizziness and nausea. She dropped from 140 to 115 pounds.

Soon, Michelle was spending most of her days in bed. She was wasting away. Her husband, Matthew, was terrified.

After Michelle had spent four years exploring all other options, and based on the recommendation of the naturopath Michelle visited, Matthew called my office as a last resort. When my assistant answered, Matthew burst into tears. "What's wrong?" she asked.

He replied, "My wife is dying."

For our first appointment Matthew planned to do most of the talking while sitting next to Michelle, who was in bed. Less than a minute after Matthew started telling me Michelle's story, I interrupted him. "It's okay," I said. "Spirit tells me it's an aggressive form of the Epstein-Barr virus."

The virus's neurotoxin was inflaming all of Michelle's joints. Her insomnia and foot pain were the result of her phrenic nerves being perpetually inflamed. Her vertigo stemmed from EBV's neurotoxin inflaming her vagus nerve. And her heart palpitations were being caused by buildup of EBV virus corpses and viral byproduct in her mitral valve.

"Don't worry," I told Michelle and Matthew. "I know how to beat this virus."

Michelle exclaimed, with as much joyful energy as she could muster, "I knew it was a virus!"

It was the first critical step in her recovery.

I recommended a protocol of celery juice and papaya, which is great for boosting someone in Michelle's condition (e.g., low weight, not being able to eat, high number of virus cells). I followed that up with the recommendations for healing in this chapter, including a list of helpful supplements, as well as the recommendations from Part IV, "How to Finally Heal."

The cleanse diet immediately stopped feeding Michelle's EBV. Within a week, there was a noticeable reduction of the swelling in her knees. The L-lysine shut down Michelle's vertigo. And the other supplements started killing virus cells and/or dampening the production of new ones.

In three months, Michelle was regularly up and walking again. In nine months, she was once again working part-time at her challenging corporate job.

And in 18 months, Michelle's pain and suffering were just a memory—she'd taken control over EBV. Today, Michelle has fully recovered her health. She's returned to juggling her job and her family energetically and happily.

CASE HISTORY:
An End to CFS Confinement
2005

Cynthia was a mother of two. Shortly after her youngest, Sophie, was born, Cynthia began experiencing fatigue. It took everything she had to push through the day, and she relied on increasing her coffee intake just to function. Within a few years, she had to quit her part-time job at a clothing store because long naps were taking up her afternoons. She needed the rest so she could be strong enough to meet her kids at the school bus, make dinner, and help them with their homework.

Cynthia noticed herself becoming irritable, and arguments arose often with her husband, Mark, who didn't understand why she was tired all the time. After all, the tests that Cynthia's doctor had run indicated nothing was wrong. The doctor said she was healthy and concluded that maybe she was just unhappy or depressed.

This made Cynthia want to walk out of the doctor's office without another word. Any blue mood she experienced was because she was tired all the time and could barely function—not the other way around. Yet her husband sided with the doctor and became increasingly resentful toward her.

The ongoing stress put Cynthia on overload; life felt impossible to keep up with. She couldn't find the energy to brush her hair, and the mere thought of running the vacuum cleaner or washing the dishes exhausted her. From the outside, it looked like she was giving up on life. Mark got angrier—he was talking separation now. "I work too long and hard at the office all day to worry about taking care of things at home," he said. "This is supposed to be your department."

Cynthia felt more pressure than ever to get better, but the worries about her marriage and what would happen to her children put her fatigue at an all-time high. She could barely drive to the grocery store or make dinner for her family. All she could do was lie in bed or on the couch.

This is what a moderate-to-severe case of undiagnosed chronic fatigue syndrome can look like. When Cynthia called me, she felt her life had fallen apart. Her husband had left her, and her daughter, Sophie, now seven years old, and her son, Ryan, age nine, had lost their family unit. What her doctor had misconstrued as a psychiatric condition was an actual physical problem: Epstein-Barr virus. The same story applies to far too many women.

I set to work informing Cynthia that she had a case of EBV that her doctor had missed. With an emphasis on getting her viral load under control and addressing nutritional deficiencies, I laid out the background on CFS that I described earlier in this chapter, and I explained the protocols outlined here and in Part IV. Like her life depended on it—because it did—Cynthia followed Spirit of Compassion's advice.

Slowly, Cynthia began to get better. Her adrenals recovered normal function, and her stamina returned. Once again, she could tend to her children, run errands, keep the house in shape, and do her hair—all without the gallons of coffee she used to rely on. Cynthia finally had the energy to return to work, too.

After witnessing this change in his wife, Mark called Cynthia and asked her out to dinner—his mother would look after the kids, he said. When they arrived at the fancy restaurant, which had long ago been the deli where they had flirted as college students, Mark told Cynthia he'd called ahead and ordered a special healing-food meal for her—and that he'd ordered the same for himself, out of solidarity. Over sun-dried-tomato hummus and vegetable nori rolls, Mark didn't exactly cry (some things would always stay the same), but he did have to dab at his eyes as he apologized for how he'd behaved.

Cynthia was quiet, then answered with a playful smile: "You can make it up to me."

After a few weeks of testing the waters—Cynthia wanted to make sure Mark didn't just want her back as a security blanket and housekeeper—they moved back in together as a family. Mark now wakes up early every Saturday morning so he can get to the farmers' market before they run out of salad greens.

CASE HISTORY:
Fibro Pain Forgotten
2000

Stacy, a 41-year-old part-time receptionist in a doctors' office, had been married to Rob, who worked at a car dealership, for over 15 years. She never had the energy to keep up with the outings Rob planned with their daughters. In fact, she couldn't remember ever feeling that well. She always felt slightly achy and more tired than her friends seemed to be. And since she'd given birth to her second child, who was now 11, the fatigue and muscle soreness had been more pronounced.

One weekend while Rob and the kids were at a museum, she went for a longer walk than usual—she'd decided to push herself to lose some unwanted weight she'd gained in the last few years. Afterward, she noticed an unusual pain in her left knee. Thinking back to her college basketball coach's advice to "walk it off," she tried to ignore it.

It didn't go away. Two weeks later, she scheduled time for an exam with a doctor at her office. Stacy limped out of the appointment with a prescription for an MRI—which revealed nothing visibly wrong with her knee.

Because Stacy's balance was off from leaning on her "good" leg, she found herself tripping easily—stairs, curbs, and corners of rugs had become major obstacles. Then her right knee started to hurt even though it hadn't gotten injured in any of her falls, and exams showed nothing amiss. Stacy's worry escalated to fear—something was really wrong. The doctors in her office ruled out rheumatoid arthritis, though, and guessed that the extra 30 pounds Stacy was carrying were to blame for her pain.

Soon Stacy started to hurt in other places. Now she couldn't raise her hands over her head without her arms and neck hurting. She was unable to work anymore, and depression set in as she started to spend hours at home on the sofa. At night, Rob would make dinner for the family and send their daughter to serve Stacy her plate of food on the couch.

A specialist concluded that Stacy had fibromyalgia. When Stacy asked what caused it, the doctor responded, "We don't know. It's what we think is oversensitive nerves. This should help, though." She handed Stacy a prescription for a medicine popular for treating depression and fibromyalgia pain. At her next visit to the specialist, when Stacy reported no progress, the doctor referred her to me.

After I explained what her fibromyalgia really was, that the real cause was the Epstein-Barr virus and that it had been in her system since childhood, Stacy recalled having a bout of mononucleosis at age 14. She finally felt she had a real answer. She understood now that poor diet, nutritional deficiencies, and increased stress had triggered the formerly dormant EBV to surface as fibromyalgia. Not knowing what was wrong with her—the powerlessness—had been scarier than knowing the true cause; the mystery of her mystery illness had been the hardest part. Now she had direction and felt confident in her ability to heal.

Within six months of our first call, following the same suggestions I describe in this chapter and Part IV, "How to Finally Heal", she was free from fibromyalgia, back to work, and living life again. She told me she felt happier and healthier than ever, and that she'd planned the next family outing—apple picking at an organic orchard.

KNOWLEDGE IS POWER

The first step of the healing process is to know the cause of your suffering is Epstein-Barr—and to realize it's not your fault.

Your EBV-related health problems aren't the result of anything you did wrong or any moral failing. You didn't make this happen, and you're in no way to blame. You did not manifest this; you did not attract this. You're a vibrant, wonderful human being and you have every God-given right to heal. You *deserve* to heal.

Much of EBV's effectiveness stems from hiding in the shadows so that neither you nor your body's immune system can sense its presence. This not only allows it to commit its mayhem unchecked, it leads to challenging emotions such as guilt, fear, and helplessness if you're living with symptoms and conditions and don't have answers.

Now things are different for you. If you have EBV, you now have a mind-body understanding of what's causing your health problems. From this alone, your immune system will strengthen and the virus will naturally weaken. You can also take action against the virus and give your immune system what it needs. So when it comes to fighting EBV, in a very real sense, *knowledge is power.*

"Your EBV-related health problems aren't the result of anything you did wrong or any moral failing. You didn't make this happen, and you're in no way to blame. You did not manifest this; you did not attract this. You're a vibrant, wonderful human being and you have every God-given right to heal. You deserve to heal."

— Anthony William, Medical Medium

CHAPTER 4

Multiple Sclerosis

Since medical science first identified *multiple sclerosis* (MS), grave confusion has accompanied the condition. Every year, far too many people receive an MS misdiagnosis.

In the 1950s, 1960s, and early 1970s, the prevalence of mystery neurological symptoms in women was escalating, yet doctors interpreted their conditions as menopause, hormonal imbalance, or just plain psychosis. Women had an almost impossible time finding a medical professional who would validate their pain, tremors, fatigue, vertigo, and more as real symptoms. In that time period, the only women who could get doctors to take them seriously on the subject were either wealthy or of advanced age.

It wasn't until enough men presented with the same symptoms in the 1960s and 1970s that the medical establishment began to take all of these mystery neurological symptoms seriously. As with many other illnesses, a man's word was taken over a woman's.

Doctors were overwhelmed by the diagnostic task, though, and turned to the label MS.

Multiple sclerosis is most notable for inflaming and damaging the central nervous system's protective layer and message facilitator, called the *myelin sheath.* Your nerves carry electrical signals that direct all the parts of your body; when any portion of your myelin sheath is injured, the messages from the nerves underneath it can become scrambled, wreaking a wide assortment of havoc (depending on which areas of the nervous system are inflamed).

MS can lead to muscle pain and spasms, weakness and fatigue, mental problems, vision problems, hearing problems, dizziness, depression, digestive issues, and bladder and bowel dysfunction. It can also partially or completely paralyze legs, forcing you to use a cane, crutches, or even a wheelchair.

You can also have these symptoms and *not* have MS.

The number of people facing the onset of MS symptoms is increasing globally every year, at a pace not easily documented. And for roughly *half* of the people who receive an MS diagnosis, it's a *mis*diagnosis—meaning that for every person diagnosed accurately with MS, someone else is told she has MS when she doesn't. In these cases of misdiagnosis, myelin nerve sheath injury is not taking place.

Her symptoms are still very real, and there is a reason for them. (More about this shortly.)

Receiving a diagnosis of MS can turn your world upside down—and it can be devastating whether the diagnosis is accurate or a mistake.

This chapter reveals the truth about MS . . . and how you can move past it and take back your life.

IDENTIFYING MULTIPLE SCLEROSIS

If you have multiple sclerosis, the injury to your central nervous system's myelin nerve sheath—and the resulting nerve inflammation and scarring—is likely to create most of the following symptoms. Still, realize that you can have any of these symptoms but not have multiple sclerosis. Only if you have several of these symptoms in their worst forms might your condition be MS.

- Early on, eye issues such as blurred vision, double vision, diminished perception of color, eye pain, and/or complete loss of vision—usually in one eye at a time

- Chronic weakness and fatigue

- Chronic pain, especially in muscles throughout the body

- Tremors

- Numbness in the arms and/or legs—first on one side of the body and then the other

- Weakness or paralysis in the legs that leads to trouble walking or—in severe cases—becoming confined to a wheelchair

- Mental fogginess, such as difficulty concentrating

- Memory issues

- Slurred speech

Beyond this symptoms checklist, there are no definitive tests to pinpoint MS. That's in part why there are so many medical misdiagnoses of the disease.

If you match at least six of the most critical symptoms above in a serious, pronounced form—and if your doctor has ruled out other possible causes for them—you can try to confirm you have MS by asking a neurologist to perform an MRI looking for lesions (i.e., scarring or other damage) on the myelin sheath in the areas of the brain and spinal cord. If two or more lesions are found, it's evidence that your symptoms could be the result of multiple sclerosis.

That said, lesions are very difficult to spot even with medical science's current 3-D imaging tools (and that's not likely to change until around the year 2030). So if your neurologist can't find any lesions, that doesn't mean they don't exist.

On the other hand, many people are walking around with different varieties of spots on their brains—people walk around with dark lesions, lighter-colored lesions, white spots, and gray areas in their brain tissue, and many of them exhibit no symptoms whatsoever. Someone can get an MRI after a concussion and discover that they have a lesion or two that nobody knew about, because the person hadn't ever had any symptoms of the lesions. In other words, detecting lesions in the brain is not always a definitive answer about the symptoms you're experiencing. The next section will offer insights into why.

Another thing to consider is whether you've had a history of ear infections, throat infections, sinus infections, and/or, if you're a woman, vaginal infections. These all will typically occur in childhood and early adulthood before the development of multiple sclerosis.

One other way to get a sense of what's ailing you is to better understand what MS actually is.

WHAT MULTIPLE SCLEROSIS *REALLY* IS

Medical communities believe multiple sclerosis is an autoimmune disease resulting from your immune system somehow confusing areas of your nerve sheath with invaders and attacking them.

As I say in other chapters, this is a philosophy that will hold back the truth in medical research for decades. The human body does *not* attack itself. Pathogens are to blame.

Medical communities also believe that there's no resolution for MS. They're mistaken here too. The truth is that multiple sclerosis can be healed—and that it is actually a version of the Epstein-Barr virus.

As explained in Chapter 3, EBV is a virus that chronically inflames nerves. Most strains of EBV are mild and less aggressive. Then there are more aggressive varieties of EBV that, when there's also a high level of mercury as food for the virus, can create the distinct set of symptoms associated with multiple sclerosis.

In many cases, the symptoms associated with MS come from EBV neurotoxins, not myelin nerve sheath injury. That is, an aggressive EBV variety feeds on mercury and releases large deposits of neurotoxins that can hamper neurotransmitters, weaken electrical impulses, inflame nerves, and create the symptoms associated with MS—without even injuring or damaging the myelin nerve sheath.

(As I mentioned in Chapter 3, there are also people with the mildest form of symptoms caused by milder varieties of EBV who get misdiagnosed with MS, only because of the way some doctors are pulling the trigger.)

A small proportion of MS diagnoses involve actual injury to the myelin nerve sheath. These cases are caused by rare, particularly aggressive forms of EBV that can sit on the myelin nerve sheath itself. Fueled by mercury very nearby in the brain, the virus tries to enter into weak areas of the nerve sheath, causing it to become inflamed on a deeper level. The virus itself can end up injuring the nerve sheath, and that deterioration can show up as a type of lesion on an imaging test. These EBV varieties can also produce neurotoxins that inflame nerves and create further neurological symptoms at the same time.

Keep in mind that identifying what's causing a lesion—and what (if any) effect that lesion is having on someone's health—is outside the scope of medical testing at this time. Again, the viral strains that lead to direct nerve damage are rare. Usually, when lesions are identified in brain imaging of someone experiencing symptoms associated with MS, the spots actually come from mercury and aluminum deposits oxidizing (essentially rusting) and causing stains made of metal byproduct on the myelin nerve sheath or other brain and nervous system tissue.

This is why lesions should not be the number one focus here. As you read in the previous section, many people walk around with different varieties of spots on their brains and experience no symptoms. Conversely, many people have no spots on their brains and *do* experience symptoms associated with MS—because regardless of whether someone has a stain on the brain or not, that person could live with a strain of EBV feeding on mercury in their system and releasing neurotoxins that inflame the nervous system. Besides which, doctors are not yet in a position to be able to know whether a spot they're seeing on a scan comes from a stain, actual myelin nerve sheath damage, or even another cause.

These subtle details are still out of reach of medical research and science. The specific reasons for various MS symptoms are not distinguishable to medical communities yet, nor are the toxic heavy metals and virus behind MS yet recognized by research and science. They still believe the body's immune system is causing the inflammation and damaging the nerve sheath. (As for your immune system, not only is it innocent of any wrongdoing, it's your primary defense against MS. When your immune system gets what it needs, recovery is possible—and within reach.) Something else that distinguishes MS from other forms of EBV is that it's accompanied by a unique combination of bacteria, funguses, and heavy metals. Specifically, if you have MS, you'll typically have the following EBV cofactors in your system:

- *Streptococcus* bacteria (one or more strains from the over 50 groups)
- *H. pylori* bacteria (or at least a previous case of *H. pylori*)
- *Candida* fungus (often misunderstood; it's a friendly messenger of another problem, not a problem causer itself)
- Cytomegalovirus

- Herpes simplex (HSV-1 and/or HSV-2)
- The toxic heavy metals mercury, aluminum, and copper—these metals feed the virus, which then puts more stress upon the immune system's ability to protect the body from viral nerve damage

While these cofactors help give MS its particular characteristics, at its core multiple sclerosis is just a form of EBV—and knowing this illuminates any dark mysteries surrounding the illness. While EBV *can* be serious in some cases, Chapter 3 lays out in detail what you need to understand it—including the steps you can take to end the damage the virus is causing, and eliminate nearly all of the virus and its cofactors.

HEALING FROM MULTIPLE SCLEROSIS

Doctors typically treat multiple sclerosis using immunosuppressant drugs and steroids in the mistaken belief that your immune system is the problem. However, your immune system is *not* attacking you—a *virus* is. Your only hope of killing your EBV is a strong and vibrant immune system, and these medications are designed to make your immune system docile and sleepy. In crisis situations, it's perfectly understandable that people tend to use these medications. The overall goal is to be proactive in working on the real underlying issue so someone may be free from medications someday in the future.

The best approach is to read Chapter 3 to fully understand EBV. Because the strains of EBV causing multiple sclerosis are aggressive toward your myelin nerve sheath, the following supplements are recommended specifically for MS. They'll help reduce pain and help protect your myelin sheath as you heal from EBV. **Before applying these, be sure to read Chapter 21, "Critical Guide to Supplement Protocols."**

Supplements for Multiple Sclerosis (MS)

- **Fresh celery juice:** work up to 32 ounces daily, then work up to 64 ounces if possible
- **Celeryforce:** 2 capsules three times a day
- **5-MTHF:** 2 capsules twice a day
- **ALA (alpha lipoic acid):** 1 capsule daily
- **Barley grass juice powder:** 2 to 4 teaspoons or 6 to 12 capsules daily
- **B-complex:** 1 capsule daily
- **Cat's claw:** 3 dropperfuls twice a day
- **CoQ10:** 1 capsule daily
- **Curcumin:** 3 capsules twice a day
- **EPA and DHA (fish-free):** 1 capsule daily (taken with dinner)
- **GABA:** 1 250-milligram capsule daily
- **Glutathione:** 1 capsule daily
- **Lemon balm:** 4 dropperfuls twice a day
- **L-glutamine:** 1 capsule twice a day
- **Licorice root:** 1 dropperful twice a day (two weeks on, two weeks off)
- **L-lysine:** 4 500-milligram capsules twice a day
- **Magnesium glycinate:** 2 capsules twice a day
- **Monolaurin:** 1 capsule twice a day
- **MSM:** 1 capsule twice a day
- **Mullein leaf:** 2 dropperfuls twice a day
- **Nettle leaf:** 4 dropperfuls twice a day
- **Spirulina:** 1 tablespoon or 9 capsules daily
- **Vitamin B$_{12}$ (as adenosylcobalamin with methylcobalamin):** 2 dropperfuls twice a day
- **Vitamin C (as Micro-C):** 6 capsules twice a day
- **Zinc (as liquid zinc sulfate):** 2 dropperfuls twice a day

Understand that MS is not a life sentence. If a doctor has given you an accurate diagnosis, it doesn't mean the symptoms you have are fully understood. This illness is still a mystery to research and science, so always know there's hope. There are no rules set in place that can tell you that you can't heal.

There's no reason to fear an MS diagnosis. (And if you've heard you have MS, you may be one of the many handed a misdiagnosis. The real culprit behind your symptoms may be EBV, just not a strain that causes injury to the myelin nerve sheath.)

If you stick to the recommendations in this section, and most importantly comply with all of the pertinent advice in Chapter 3 and Part IV to restore your central nervous and immune systems, you'll get the chance to rid yourself of nearly all of the virus inflaming your nerves and be able to resume a normal and symptom-free life. Refer back to "Healing from the Epstein-Barr Virus" in Chapter 3 for a sense of the various factors that can affect your healing timeline. Remember, even when you kill off EBV and remove toxic heavy metals from the body, the nervous system needs time to repair, so take your healing one step at a time.

I believe in you. The answers are here. Millions around the world have gotten their lives back by putting these tools and protocols to work. If you put the commitment, time, and effort into reading and understanding Medical Medium information, you can take yourself as far as you need to go.

CASE HISTORY:
Nursed Back to Health by the Truth
2006

Rebecca, age 41, was a nurse in a hospital emergency room. One afternoon, at the end of a long shift, another nurse didn't show up for work, and so Rebecca had to work another 12 hours, late into the night.

As she was driving home to relieve her mother of babysitting her 10-year-old son, Nicholas, the right side of Rebecca's face went numb. The numbness began to travel down her arm. She'd never experienced anything like it before, though she'd witnessed it in many patients over the years. Rebecca tried to pass it off as a symptom of overwork, though, and went to bed when she got home, hoping it would be gone by morning.

When she awoke, the numbness was still there—on the right side of her face, her nose, part of her mouth, and her arm and hand. Concerned that it was a stroke, Rebecca's mother drove her to the hospital. A doctor she knew looked at her immediately and ran a series of tests, including an MRI with contrast and an EKG. The tests didn't show any problems, so the doctor didn't think it was a stroke. She suspected anxiety was the culprit. "Give it some time, and we'll see if the symptoms ease up," she said, handing Rebecca a prescription for benzodiazepine.

Over the next few weeks, Rebecca experienced very little change. She tried to get along with her mystery numbness, but it was a distraction. Her right arm began to weaken. Eventually she felt that she couldn't handle her normal nursing duties, which included transporting people from stretchers and lifting various pieces of medical equipment. She decided to take a leave of absence—and ask the hospital's top neurologist for a consult.

After a slew of comprehensive tests, he told her it was the beginning of multiple sclerosis—even though Rebecca's MRI and brain scan showed no evidence of the disease. The neurologist said Rebecca should start to receive regular MRIs. Over time, the MS would appear on the imaging if it progressed. Until then, he prescribed medications used to treat MS, such as immunosuppressant drugs and steroids. Rebecca could barely contain a sob as she went to meet her mother in the waiting room. How was she going to take care of Nicholas?

Over the next six months, her symptoms progressed. Now the numbness was accompanied by dizzy spells, fatigue, and—after the latest MRI with contrast—brain fog. One day a nurse Rebecca had worked with, who was a client of mine, recommended that Rebecca call me and make an appointment.

First thing in the reading, Spirit of Compassion informed me that Rebecca had a viral condition—a specific strain of EBV. "But I've been tested for the Epstein-Barr virus," Rebecca said. "It showed I didn't have a present infection in my blood, only an indication that I had an infection decades ago. That wouldn't be causing my problems now."

I explained that the EBV antibodies in the blood aren't necessarily an indication that the virus has left someone's system—but rather that it's traveled deeper into the body. In Rebecca's case, the Epstein-Barr was alive indeed and now affecting her central nervous system. I assured Rebecca that she didn't have multiple sclerosis.

"I'd give anything to believe that," she said.

"It's the truth," I told her, and went on to describe how in addition to the central nervous system, the EBV was inflaming her phrenic and trigeminal nerves, which accounted for the numbness. The virus was also releasing a neurotoxin that caused the dizziness, fatigue, and brain fog.

Finally, Rebecca was convinced. "It's like a weight has been lifted."

By following the protocols outlined in this chapter and in Part IV, Rebecca made a complete recovery within six months. She was free from her medication and returned to her position at the hospital. She no longer works overtime, because she feels that the stress from the extra shifts depleted her and allowed the EBV to take advantage.

Just understanding how her condition worked—and discovering that it wasn't a life sentence—made every difference to Rebecca's healing. She told me that without the knowledge of what was actually behind her mystery illness, she's sure she would have been carrying around the wrong diagnosis for the rest of her life.

"This book is the guide to truly freeing yourself.
It is in your hands at this particular moment for a reason."

— Anthony William, Medical Medium

CHAPTER 5

Rheumatoid Arthritis

Medical communities use the term *rheumatoid arthritis* (RA) as if it's a diagnosis for the condition that chronically and painfully inflames the joints. A better term would be *swollen joint disease*, or *joint hurting affliction*, or *unexplainable aches and pains disorder*. Because let's be honest here. If medical research hasn't uncovered the explanation for certain sets of symptoms—which it hasn't yet with RA—then it's better to call it what doctors do know. Hiding behind fancy names doesn't help anybody, least of all the patients.

Most typically, RA affects the small joints in the hands and feet. It can also affect knees, elbows, and other large joints. Rheumatoid arthritis may afflict other parts of the body, too, such as the nerves, skin, mouth, eyes, lungs, and/or heart. Joint pain and swelling are the most notable results of this illness—and, over time, joint and bone damage and/or deformity may occur. Medical communities don't know that the actual number of people affected by RA is higher than what's reported globally. Their ages range broadly from 15 to 60. The majority of people who get an RA diagnosis are women.

Medical communities believe rheumatoid arthritis is an autoimmune disease—that is, a condition in which a confused immune system regards parts of your body as invaders and responds by perpetually attacking them. This implies your body is turning against you without your say.

The medical establishment trains doctors to use explanations like this about mystery illnesses across the board. It's a decoy to make patients feel safe, to feel like their health-care providers understand what's happening to them and why it's happening, to feel like there's a measure of control over what's going wrong. This explanation of autoimmune disease is not the help the establishment thinks it is. When a patient gets the mental image of cells turning on one another, it sends the wrong message—that the patient's body has betrayed her or him, that it can't be trusted to heal.

It's critical to know that *our bodies don't attack themselves*. Here is the truth: the inflammation in the joints is there to *protect* you from attack by a particularly common virus. Your body is working hard to stop pathogens from digging deeper into the joints and the tissue around them. When the inflammation becomes long term and chronic, that's when it becomes the problem known as RA—but it is still your body working to ward off viral damage.

Doctors also believe that there's no way to heal from rheumatoid arthritis. They're mistaken about that, too.

This chapter explains what rheumatoid arthritis really is . . . and how you can take control and regain your health.

IDENTIFYING RHEUMATOID ARTHRITIS

If you have rheumatoid arthritis, you're probably experiencing many of the following symptoms—and with good reason. These symptoms are the result of your body using its defenses to ward off the common viral pathogen:

- Joint pain—especially in the wrists and knuckles, the knees, and/or the balls of the feet, but *any* joint can be affected

- Joint inflammation

- Stiffness in the joints, especially in the morning, that may last for hours

- Tingling and/or numbness, especially in the hands and/or feet

- Fluid buildup, especially in the ankles or behind the knees

- Fatigue, fever, and other flu-like symptoms on an intermittent basis

- Heart palpitations

- Skin burning or itching

- A roaming, burning pain

- Nerve pain

Doctors employ certain methods to try to identify RA, but none of them are definitive. Below is a list of specific tests they use. Keep in mind that these are fallible, because they are not designed to look for the true root cause of RA. These tests do not find the viral pathogen that causes RA. Rather, they can serve as benchmarks for how much inflammation is present in the body—and even then, these benchmarks are not always accurate as to how much inflammation is occurring.

- **Rheumatoid Factor blood test:** this checks for antibodies doctors believe are associated with RA. However, this test can produce a positive result in entirely healthy people, or in people who have some unrelated disease, such as lupus. At the same time, it can return negative results for those who actually have rheumatoid arthritis symptoms. Therefore, it's not very useful.

- **Anti-cyclic Citrullinated Peptides (anti-CCP) Antibody blood test:** this newer antibodies test is better at identifying rheumatoid arthritis inflammation cases than the Rheumatoid Factor test, but it's still far from definitive. The question is, what is it really detecting? Because remember, they don't know the cause of RA.

- **Erythrocyte Sedimentation Rate blood test:** this tests for a high degree of inflammation. There are many causes for inflammation, so this test doesn't pinpoint rheumatoid arthritis. That said, it can be used to get a sense of how much inflammation is occurring; so if you have RA, this can help you gauge its aggressiveness. On the other hand, someone can exhibit higher levels of inflammation with no symptoms.

- **C-Reactive Protein blood test:** this tests for high levels of a protein associated with active inflammation. Other factors also create this protein, though, including obesity. And again, inflammation alone doesn't pinpoint the cause as being rheumatoid arthritis.

- **Ultrasounds and MRIs:** these can be used to track inflammatory activity that has caused bone damage over time.

- **MTHFR Gene Mutation test:** this is being used as though it identifies a gene mutation issue that could be causing a number of symptoms for any kind of illness where inflammation seems to be the culprit. This test is far from definitive. It gives false positives for gene mutations when really, it is simply acting as a test for inflammation—just like the other ones in this list. Practically anyone with inflammation will test positive on an MTHFR gene mutation. It's a glorified inflammatory test with gene terminology attached to it. (The upside of this test is that it shows there's still a search for answers out there. While MTHFR gene mutations are not the *correct* answers—they're not why people are sick—I commend

medical communities for the ongoing drive to uncover the reasons why people are struggling.)

One other way to determine whether you have rheumatoid arthritis is to learn the truth about what the condition actually is.

WHAT RHEUMATOID ARTHRITIS *REALLY* IS

Medical communities believe rheumatoid arthritis is an autoimmune disease that results from your immune system somehow mistaking your joints and other body parts for invaders and attacking them. As I've said before, *our bodies do not attack themselves.* Our bodies only react to being attacked by *pathogens.*

Rheumatoid arthritis is a version of the Epstein-Barr virus (EBV).

EBV chronically afflicts various parts of the body, including joints, bones, and nerves. It's this virus that's creating the pain and inflammation in your joints. (As for your immune system, not only is it innocent of wrongdoing, it's your primary defense against EBV.)

As mentioned earlier, there are over 60 varieties of the Epstein-Barr virus. It will take decades for medical research to shed light on the conditions and viral mutations of EBV that create RA. When the time, energy, and resources finally go into the cause—hopefully in the coming decades—researchers will easily discover the EBV variants that have wreaked havoc on people's joints and nerves for over a century. And when doctors dig a little deeper, they'll clue in to the real solutions for this virus that are here in this book.

Knowing that rheumatoid arthritis is a form of EBV eliminates any dark mysteries surrounding the illness. While EBV is compromising, it's described in great detail in Chapter 3—including the steps you can take to end the virus's damage and destroy nearly all the EBV in your system.

HEALING FROM RHEUMATOID ARTHRITIS

Doctors typically treat rheumatoid arthritis using a variety of prescription anti-inflammatory and immunosuppressant medications for crisis management, because that's all they have to offer. Given the degree of pain and inflammation caused by RA, this is understandable. However, there are two problems with this strategy.

First, medications don't address the root cause of RA—which is the Epstein-Barr virus. Because these drugs do nothing to curtail EBV, they allow the illness to continue thriving inside of you. They keep your body from reacting to the virus, as if it were not there.

Second, your main defense against EBV is your immune system—and these types of prescription medications actually make your immune system sleepy and docile. So not only are these medications failing to help you defeat EBV, they could potentially aid the virus.

The best approach is to read all of Chapter 3 to fully understand EBV. I hope you'll find it liberating—and I believe you'll benefit from the recommendations you find there.

For supplements to help with RA, refer to the Supplements for Autoimmune Disorders and Diseases list at the end of Chapter 3. Because the EBV that causes rheumatoid arthritis can be especially uncomfortable and difficult to manage, you'll find *natural* anti-inflammatories (i.e., that won't weaken your immune system) recommended in that list. They'll help alleviate pain and promote healing from EBV. And remember, because EBV is the underlying reason for RA inflammation, working to rid yourself of the virus and its fuel is working to rid yourself of the inflammation at its source. Before applying the recommended supplements, be sure to read Chapter 21, "Critical Guide to Supplement Protocols."

Finally, use cold and hot packs. Place a cold pack on painful areas for about 5 to 10 minutes at a time (based on how it feels) for a total of about half an hour a day to reduce inflammation and speed healing. Place a hot pack on the same areas for about 10 minutes a day to loosen up any muscle tension that might be developing around the damaged joints.

If you follow these recommendations, and most importantly follow all the pertinent advice in Chapter 3 and Part IV, "How to Finally Heal," then you can rid yourself of both EBV and RA and take back control of your health and your life. Refer back to "Healing from the Epstein-Barr Virus" in Chapter 3 for a sense of the various factors that can affect your healing timeline. I believe in you. The answers are here. Millions around the world have gotten their lives back by putting these tools and protocols to work.

CASE HISTORY:
Taking Matters into Her Own Swollen Hands
1998

Janet loved her work as an aesthetician. Making people feel good about themselves with in-home spa treatments and makeup application was what got Janet out of bed in the morning. At age 48, Janet had a lot of responsibility, though. As a single mom with two children in their late teens, she was constantly worried about keeping up with rent payments for their home, managing her team of traveling aestheticians, and getting her older son through college. On top of all this, her mother had been sick with cancer for the last year. Janet had needed to spend every weekend and all her spare hours in service to her mom—supervising doctor appointments, paying bills, shopping for groceries, helping with household chores, and getting her mom's affairs in order.

Janet had occasionally experienced aches and pains over the years, but she always passed them off as natural, something that happened to everyone. One night in the midst of this stressful time, after staying up late to complete paperwork for her mother following a day of booked-solid client appointments, Janet noticed a stronger pain than usual in her elbows, wrists, and hands. She told herself it would be gone by morning—but when she woke up, it was even worse.

Feeling like she was unable to perform the hands-on tasks she needed to for her job, Janet booked an immediate appointment with her doctor. After blood work and a complete examination, the doctor told her, "I think you have rheumatoid arthritis." He referred Janet to a rheumatologist, who performed another exam and additional blood tests and concluded that Janet had inflammation from certain proteins and antibodies that were associated with inflammation of the joints.

This circular reasoning didn't fly for Janet. "But what does that *mean*?" she asked.

"It means you have RA," the rheumatologist said.

"But what's causing the inflammation in the first place?"

The rheumatologist answered that her body's immune system was attacking her joints and inflaming them. He handed her a prescription for an anti-inflammatory and immuno-suppressant medication.

The whole thing still made no sense to Janet. Up until now, she'd felt she could trust herself. She might not be able to trust others, like her ex-husband, or like Mrs. Ferguson, who never paid for her facials, but Janet had always trusted her body to be on her side. She didn't understand why her body had decided to start attacking itself. It felt like a betrayal.

She feared the condition would get worse over time. If this had started out of the blue, then what, she wondered, was to stop her body from continuing to hurt her? She looked at her 82-year-old mother, battling cancer, and wondered how much worse off she'd be at that age. At 48, Janet's mother had been in fine health. She'd never had to deal with this RA business. Could Janet's body even make it to 70?

Janet decided to take matters into her own swollen hands and booked an appointment with a functional medicine doctor, who looked at Janet's previous blood work, ordered additional tests, and then came up with the same diagnosis of RA. Janet asked Dr. Tanaka what was causing the rheumatoid arthritis. The doctor told Janet it was autoimmune, that is, that the body was attacking itself. Janet pressed Dr. Tanaka for a better explanation, but she didn't seem to have one. Instead the doctor instructed Janet to eliminate wheat gluten and processed sugar from her diet and to take a pile of supplements, which included fish oil, vitamin D, and B-complex.

On this regimen, Janet felt a little better. The pain wasn't as aggressive in her elbow, but her hands and wrists were still far from normal. She could only perform her job on what she called "good" days, and she only got so many of those a month. Not only was she losing income, she'd also had to hire a helper for her mother, and that was draining her bank account.

One day a special client, Olivia—the woman who'd encouraged Janet to start her own business years earlier—called to book Janet to do the bridal party makeup for her daughter's wedding. When Janet told Olivia she'd have to send one of her team members in her place and explained the reason, Olivia told Janet, "You're calling Anthony."

My initial scan of Janet showed inflammation in her nerves and joints. It wasn't because her body was attacking itself, though. Spirit of Compassion recognized it instead as the viral condition known as Epstein-Barr. Janet's immune system was trying to fight a battle and was working in her favor to fend off the virus. It was doing everything it could to prevent the virus from entering her connective joint tissue. Meanwhile, the immunosuppressant medications she'd been taking were suppressing her immune system so that her body couldn't defend itself against the virus.

When I explained to Janet that EBV takes the form of mononucleosis in one of its early stages, Janet recalled having a case of mono in college, and how all her joints had hurt in a similar manner. Finally, an explanation clicked. She understood that the virus had morphed from its original mono form and burrowed deeper into her body, remaining more or less dormant until the strain of the last year, along with stress-eating certain foods that contained hidden triggers, had brought it to the surface. It all made perfect sense. And learning this truth allowed her to trust her body. She felt her fighting spirit come back, ready to help her heal.

To bring Janet back to health, we focused on the power of fruits, leafy greens, herbs, wild foods, and vegetables, concentrating on the specific antiviral ones as listed in the protocols in Chapter 3, "Epstein-Barr Virus, Chronic Fatigue Syndrome, and Fibromyalgia." After the 28-Day Healing Cleanse I describe in Chapter 22, Janet was back to working almost full-time.

Within three months, she was back to her normal workload and schedule.

Janet kept her mother's aide on part-time and started taking grocery bags of healing foods to her mom's place, showing the helper how to prepare fruit smoothies, mango salsa, spinach soup, and other dishes that would keep her mother's immune system strong.

A year after our first talk, Janet was still following the EBV protocols and staying away from trigger foods—and she didn't have one ache or pain. In fact, she felt better than she had in years. She now owned the truth that she didn't have RA, and she reveled in the fact that she'd finally conquered that little mono virus from college.

When the holidays came and Janet was twice as busy as usual, she didn't flinch when she looked at her jam-packed calendar. Instead, she said, "Bring it on."

"From the beginning, I've given you the information you need to protect yourself and your family, to make yourself stronger, so threats like viruses can't take you down. This has always been one of the foundations of Medical Medium information."

— Anthony William, Medical Medium

CHAPTER 6

Hypothyroidism and Hashimoto's Thyroiditis

To truly understand thyroid disorder and disease, we have to go back in history. Stories get lost through the generations, and it's human nature to forget how things first started as the busyness of daily life distracts us. These days, many stories are purposely hidden or lost. If I don't put this out there, the truth of thyroid issues' origins could be gone forever.

Thyroid disease is in fact a fairly new affliction. It wasn't until the turn of the 19th century, when the Industrial Revolution had started to change the way the world worked, that people started to have real problems with their thyroids. Until this time, goiters had been uncommon. They were a result of nutritional deficiencies in minerals such as iodine and zinc, or toxicity from heavy metals such as copper and mercury.

Then, as newly developed industries started dumping toxic heavy metals into rivers, streams, and lakes, and as factories started to release poisonous emissions of newly born chemicals that our human bodies had never encountered, people's thyroids started to bear the brunt. They were exposed to more toxicity than ever before, and more and more cases of goiters appeared.

Then around the turn of the 20th century, industries began to strip nutrients from our grains, vegetables, and fruit—all in the name of progress—and pack our foods into lead cans. Lead was the perfect heavy metal to help give someone a goiter. And without the proper nutrition in their food, people were doubly vulnerable.

At the same time, medical science made what seemed to be a huge breakthrough. It was based on a philosophy that had been popular in the Middle Ages: the practice of eating an animal's body part to help heal a person's corresponding part. In those days, if someone had heart disease, they'd be instructed to eat heart. Kidney disease was treated by eating kidney, brain disease by eating brain, and eye disease by eating desiccated animal eyeballs. It was a form of quackery that was not effective, yet it was respected as the most sensible trend of its time.

Ages later, at the tail end of the 1800s, medical researchers stumbled upon an instance in which the theory actually worked—for the first time in human history. They found that the thyroid glands of pigs, when dried and ground up, created a medicine that helped relieve the symptoms of human thyroid disorder, specifically goiters.

One reason it actually worked was that the desiccated thyroid provided people with a nutrient that they were critically lacking: iodine. Another reason it gave patients relief was that the medical establishment had accidentally discovered its first steroid compound—that is, a concentrated hormone compound that suppresses inflammation and the immune system. When the thyroid is in trouble, the body will often overreact, resulting in fluid gathering around the gland; this is part of what causes a goiter. The hormone concentration in desiccated thyroid medication acted as an immunosuppressant, slowing down the body's ability to react to the troubled thyroid.

For the first time, it seemed like a cure had emerged from the eating-matching-body-parts philosophy. In altered concentrations, desiccated bovine or porcine thyroid is still the ingredient used in thyroid medications today—which makes them antiquated at best. They still don't address the underlying health issues. So let's not start handing out posthumous medals for this fluke discovery.

We have to realize this wasn't high-minded scientific thought on display. It was a doctor who woke up one morning and thought, *Let's try that old chestnut of a theory*, then visited the butcher shop for some discarded animal parts and started riffing in his lab. *An eye for an eye, a kidney for a kidney, a thyroid gland for a thyroid gland—hey, that last one works!* He'd taken the thyroid from a pig, cured and dehydrated it, then fed it to his patients with

goiters—and they'd happened to see results. It was in no way a grand epiphany based on sophisticated science.

In the 20th century, the viral upsurge began, and women started to present with thyroid-related symptoms very different from the goiters seen years before. Now, years later, this new condition has gotten tagged as thyroiditis, which just means an inflamed thyroid. Often these days, patients get the specific labels Hashimoto's and hypothyroidism—yet these remain mystery illnesses.

Now another wave of this thyroid illness is upon us. Hundreds of millions of people, mostly women, don't even realize they have a thyroid condition, yet are leading diminished lives because of thyroid problems' underlying cause. Patients who do get attention for their thyroids still receive medications made from synthetic or desiccated animal thyroid, and when that doesn't suppress their symptoms enough, they are offered radioactive iodine treatment to try and destroy the thyroid gland.

This isn't progress. Answers have still not surfaced from medical research and science about what actually causes these mystery thyroid conditions, so people aren't learning how to heal, either.

In the sections that follow, I'll uncover the true reason why so many people are struggling with thyroid-related symptoms, and what you can do if you're one of them. If you're suffering, there's a reason—and a way to get better.

UNDERSTANDING HYPOTHYROIDISM AND HASHIMOTO'S

Hypothyroidism is the name for the underproduction of thyroid hormones, which medical research and science are unaware is just a mild, early-stage case of thyroiditis. Whether thyroid hormone underproduction reaches that early stage of thyroiditis depends on how strong the underlying viral cause is, which variety of the virus it is, and how weakened the immune system is. Hypothyroidism and Hashimoto's thyroiditis aren't the goiter conditions of the past, brought on by iodine deficiency and toxin accumulation in the thyroid. And these names—hypothyroidism and Hashimoto's—don't explain what's really going on to cause people's fatigue, heart palpitations, hot flashes, brain fog, weight gain, anxiety, depression, and many other associated issues.

Medical communities believe Hashimoto's is the result of the immune system somehow going haywire, mistaking thyroid cells for invaders, and declaring war on them.

That's not correct. I've said this before, and I'll say it again: The body does not attack itself. Our immune systems do not become confused and go after our own organs. This is as true for the thyroid as it is for any other gland or organ.

The mistaken theory of autoimmune disease is merely a blame game. It points a finger of fault at the patient's own body to distract from the truth that medical research has not yet scratched the surface of what causes thyroid conditions.

Truth is, over 95 percent of today's thyroid disorders, including Hashimoto's, stem from a *viral* infection. (The other 5 percent come from radiation.) That virus is Epstein-Barr (EBV).

As Chapter 3 explains, after a long incubation period—typically in the liver—EBV begins its journey to the thyroid, and then enters into the tissue there. Over time, the viral load will weaken the thyroid, making it less effective at producing the hormones the body relies upon. As time passes, in many people the EBV will also slowly inflame the thyroid, leading from a case of hypothyroidism to a case of Hashimoto's thyroiditis. This is not your body betraying you. Rather, your immune system is going after a real intruder and working hard to protect you.

Your body is working hard to protect you in other ways, too: as the thyroid weakens from being infected by EBV, the liver is capable of releasing storage bins of thyroid hormones to help compensate. The adrenals also start to produce tailor-made hormones similar to the hormones the thyroid would normally produce. With a well-functioning liver and strong adrenals, this becomes a backup for low thyroid hormone production—and remains undiscovered by medical research and science.

One major confusion is that patients think thyroid medications go after the root cause of their illness. In fact, these drugs do not treat the thyroid itself. They just add hormones to the bloodstream in hopes that the body will use them to replace the hormones the thyroid isn't producing. It's a secret that thyroid drugs are mild steroids, and that they slow the immune system down from reacting to your symptoms. It's a secret that unseasoned doctors often don't even know; they just haven't been told. And typically, doctors don't explain to patients that they don't truly understand hypothyroidism or Hashimoto's or that the medications will not alleviate the conditions themselves.

If you're on thyroid medication and feel a positive difference, that's fine. It can act as a mostly harmless Band-Aid to a thyroid condition that comes from a viral load. If you've tried thyroid medications and couldn't find relief, though, now you understand your frustration was valid.

I have heard stories from hundreds of women who started on medication for their thyroid disorders and 10 to 15 years later, when they were in their 50s or 60s, went to get a thyroid exam. The nurse practitioner or doctor took a look at the results and said, "What the heck happened to your thyroid? It looks terrible." All this time, the women thought they were being responsible and proactive. They thought the drugs had been caring for their thyroids.

You don't have to be stuck with this fate. By following the program in Chapter 3, you can rid yourself of the Epstein-Barr virus. And with the advice in the sections below, you can help heal and protect your injured thyroid, as well as fortify supporting glands. You will finally be empowered to reverse your thyroid condition, instead of being told you're addressing and treating it when you're only managing the symptoms temporarily. With the truth about what's causing your condition and how to get better, you can reclaim control over your health.

THYROID BLOOD TESTS

If you suspect you have a thyroid issue or disorder but aren't sure, have your doctor conduct blood tests for your thyroid hormone levels.

Specifically, ask to be tested for TSH, free T4, free T3, and thyroid antibodies. While they're far from perfect, these lab tests have been the gold standards.

One fad that's developed among the alternative medicine community is reverse T3 testing. Its advocates claim that it's an accurate indicator of thyroid problems, while its detractors claim it's just noise.

In a sense, they're both right. Your reverse T3 level *does* reflect genuine thyroid problems—but it's impossible to know what any result means, since the symptoms someone is experiencing are a mystery to begin with to the doctors trying to interpret these test results. It is still okay to have your doctor order the test.

Even though medical communities point to the thyroid as the source of the symptoms in this chapter, there is no evidence, study, or proof that lines up a thyroid problem to these symptoms. People without thyroid problems can have the same symptoms as people with thyroid problems. People on thyroid medication whose doctors claim the thyroid is functioning just fine now can still have these symptoms, too. You know from reading this book that it's because EBV is the true cause, not the thyroid itself. For hypothyroidism and Hashimoto's thyroiditis, they haven't traced the majority of symptoms they claim are thyroid-related to the thyroid.

Finally, it's important to be aware that even if all your thyroid test results are in the normal range, you could still have a thyroid problem. Many people, mostly women, feel low-grade viral symptoms that doctors associate with hypothyroidism regardless of normal test results. One reason: the symptoms are from the virus itself, whether or not the thyroid has begun to show on tests that it's "going hypo." Sometimes it takes months or even years before a thyroid condition develops to the point where blood tests pick up on it. (Plus most lab ranges are too broad, so a mild condition can, and normally does, slip through their cracks.)

Some doctors now prescribe thyroid medications even if a patient's thyroid test results are in the normal range. It's an awareness meant to nip problems in the bud, and it's progress for women because they're finally being taken seriously and heard. However, it's just the medications' mild steroid effect that gives patients partial relief from their low-grade viral infection symptoms, essentially masking the virus's effects. Research is still a long distance away from discovering the underlying cause of thyroid disorder and what will truly help these patients.

If you're feeling viral symptoms regardless of what your lab tests say, make use of the programs in Chapter 3, Part IV, and in the next section below. You'll be working to end your thyroid disorder, recover from the virus that causes it, and spare yourself from future frustrating EBV issues.

ADDRESSING THYROID CONDITIONS

This section offers foods, herbs, and supplements that heal your injured thyroid, strengthen all its fellow glands in your endocrine system (adrenal glands, pituitary gland, pancreas, and so on)—and lower the viral load specifically within your thyroid.

"Goitrogenic" Foods

There's a trend that's making people fearful of vegetables such as cauliflower, kale, broccoli, cabbage, collard greens, and broccoli rabe. Rumor has it that these contain goitrogens, that is, substances that cause goiters.

Don't pay this fad any mind! These so-called "goitrogenic" foods do not contain enough goitrogens to inhibit the thyroid on any level. You'd have to eat a 100-pound barrel's worth of broccoli daily to reach any level of concern.

So please consume and enjoy your favorite cruciferous vegetables. They actually help promote thyroid health.

Healing Foods

Among the most healing foods for thyroid conditions are wild blueberries, cilantro, spinach, artichokes, asparagus, garlic, sprouts, potatoes, butter leaf lettuce, apples, tomatoes, cranberries, hemp seeds (in small amounts), and Atlantic dulse. Variously, they can starve or kill EBV cells, provide micronutrients, repair thyroid tissue, reduce nodule growth, flush toxic heavy metals and viral waste, and eventually halt thyroid hormone decline and boost production of thyroid hormones. Incorporate as many of these foods into your diet as you can.

Also take care to avoid the foods in Chapter 19, "What Not to Eat." When dealing with an EBV-caused symptom or condition, it's critical to begin the process of removing at least one or two of the foods that feed the virus. If you need to take your healing even further, try to gravitate toward removing all the foods that feed the virus.

Healing Herbs and Supplements

Before applying these, be sure to read Chapter 21, "Critical Guide to Supplement Protocols."

(If you're looking for healing insights into hyperthyroidism and Graves' disease, see the Medical Medium book *Cleanse to Heal*.)

Supplements for Hypothyroidism; Hashimoto's Thyroiditis; Goiters; Thyroid Nodules, Cysts, and Tumors

- **Fresh celery juice:** work up to 32 ounces daily, then work up to 64 ounces daily if possible

- **Celeryforce:** 1 capsule twice a day

- **5-MTHF:** 1 capsule daily

- **Barley grass juice powder:** 2 teaspoons or 6 capsules daily

- **B-complex:** 1 capsule daily

- **Cat's claw:** 2 dropperfuls twice a day

- **Chaga mushroom:** 2 teaspoons or 6 capsules daily

- **Curcumin:** 2 capsules twice a day

- **EPA and DHA (fish-free):** 1 capsule daily (taken with dinner)

- **Lemon balm:** 4 dropperfuls twice a day

- **Licorice root:** 1 dropperful twice a day (two weeks on, two weeks off)

- **L-lysine:** 5 500-milligram capsules twice a day

- **Lomatium root:** 1 dropperful twice a day

- **Magnesium glycinate:** 1 capsule twice a day

- **Melatonin:** 5 milligrams at bedtime daily

- **Monolaurin:** 1 capsule twice a day

- **Mullein leaf:** 2 dropperfuls twice a day

- **Nascent iodine:** 2 small drops (not dropperfuls) daily (or 1 capsule of bladderwrack daily)

- **Nettle leaf:** 2 dropperfuls twice a day

- **Spirulina:** 2 teaspoons or 6 capsules daily

- **Thyme:** 2 sprigs of fresh thyme in hot water as tea or 4 sprigs in room temperature water daily

- **Vitamin B$_{12}$ (as adenosylcobalamin with methylcobalamin):** 1 dropperful twice a day

- **Vitamin C (as Micro-C):** 6 capsules twice a day

- **Vitamin D$_3$:** 1,000 IU daily

- **Wild blueberry powder:** 2 tablespoons daily

- **Zinc (as liquid zinc sulfate):** 1 dropperful twice a day

CASE HISTORY:
Stronger Than Ever
1999

Sarah's friends lived in awe (and a little jealousy) of her ability to take on the world with energy that never flagged. On weekends, she and her boyfriend, Rob, would head to the mountains to hike, and then she'd still want to go out with her girlfriends when she got home. She could eat whatever she wanted and never gain a pound. Rob, who worked as a trainer, loved to show her off at the gym where he worked.

When Sarah was 36, she noticed that she'd put on an extra seven pounds between Thanksgiving and New Year's. She could barely fit into her good jeans. At first it seemed like it might just be bloating from her menstrual cycle. But when her period passed, she was still struggling to button her waistband.

She decided she'd go full-throttle at the gym and burn off the extra weight. She also cut out all carbohydrates from her diet.

Sarah's girlfriend Jessica told her she was happy to see her weight go up a little. "You look much healthier," she said. Still, Sarah had been more comfortable at her lower weight and knew it wasn't normal to get heavier out of nowhere. She also knew that Jessica had other reasons for being happy to see Sarah fill out—namely, a history of envy.

In the second week of Sarah's extra workout and no carb regimen, she noticed that the number on the scale hadn't gone down, but her energy had dropped. Rob, who'd never had a problem keeping weight off, told Sarah she just wasn't applying herself enough at the gym. He also put her on protein shakes to try and build her muscle mass.

Yet Sarah's weight was going up at a rate of a pound every two weeks, and her energy just kept dropping. She'd once been 115 pounds. The day the scale hit 130, she called her doctor.

After a full workup, Dr. Kiernan explained that Sarah's thyroid hormone level tests showed that her thyroid levels were elevated, indicating hypothyroidism. Sarah asked what was making that happen. She'd always been healthy, she said, she ate a healthy diet, and she exercised all the time. Dr. Kiernan answered that it was just something that could happen as people aged.

This didn't compute for Sarah. "Aging" wasn't part of her vocabulary. She was still in her 30s, she wasn't even married yet, she didn't have children—and already she was getting the ailments of an older person?

Still, she took the thyroid medication that Dr. Kiernan prescribed, continued her frequent workouts, and kept avoiding carbs. Yet her weight continued to increase by two pounds every month. When she reached 140 pounds, she called her mother to vent about how disappointed Rob was in her weight gain. He no longer liked to be seen at the gym with her, because he said her body reflected poorly on his skills as a trainer. Rob had stopped inviting her out with his friends and colleagues. The one time she'd been out with them in recent weeks, he'd said a defensive, "Don't worry about Sarah. She's just been eating too many carbs," at the beginning of the evening.

Her mom groaned over Rob's behavior and said to Sarah, "I know I've told you about Anthony before and you haven't called him. I really think now's the time."

In the initial scan, Spirit helped me confirm that Sarah did have a thyroid problem—hypothyroidism, just on the edge of early thyroiditis. She wasn't yet at the point of full inflammation of the thyroid, but she was headed there. I hurried to explain that the condition wasn't a symptom of getting older. A virus—specifically Epstein-Barr—was causing Sarah's problem.

Right away, we altered Sarah's diet. We took out hormone-disrupting foods such as eggs and dairy, and minimized her animal protein to once daily. We also increased her consumption of antiviral fruits, leafy greens, herbs, wild foods, and vegetables, including papayas, berries, apples, mâche, mangoes, spinach, kale, sprouts, Atlantic dulse, cilantro, and garlic. For supplements, we concentrated on lemon balm, chromium, zinc, and bladderwrack. With this protocol, we were able to reduce the viral load on Sarah's thyroid, and it returned to producing its normal level of hormones.

At the beginning, Rob was suspicious of this new diet. He thought fruit smoothies (with no protein powder) for breakfast, a spinach salad with orange and avocado for lunch, salmon with vegetables for dinner, and fruit for snacks in between was too much sugar and not enough protein.

Within the first two weeks, though, Sarah had lost four pounds. And within the first month, a total of eight pounds.

The second month, the weight loss was more gradual, but her energy was increasing. Sarah's metabolism had bounced back. As an added benefit, she felt like she was building muscles she'd never even felt before.

After three and a half months, she was back to 115 pounds—with more muscle than the last time she'd been that weight.

Meanwhile, Sarah told Dr. Kiernan she wanted to wean off the thyroid medication. Though it went against what he'd been taught, Dr. Kiernan couldn't deny that Sarah's thyroid was restoring its normal function, and Sarah was coming back to life before his eyes. Soon, Sarah was off the medication entirely.

Now when Rob had gym clients who were having trouble losing weight, he told them all about his girlfriend's weight-loss story (implying he'd been the one to help her), and put those clients on high-fruit, low-fat cleanse diets.

Rob apologized to Sarah for his past behavior and hinted that he might be popping the question soon. Sarah told me that while Rob is easy on the eyes, she's not so quick to commit to him after seeing the way he treated her when times got hard. They remain unmarried.

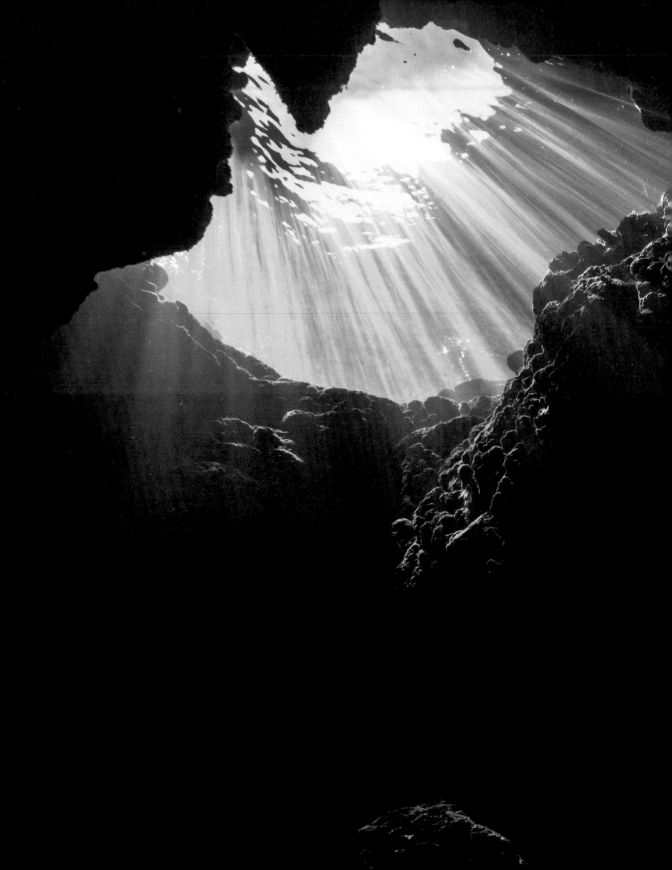

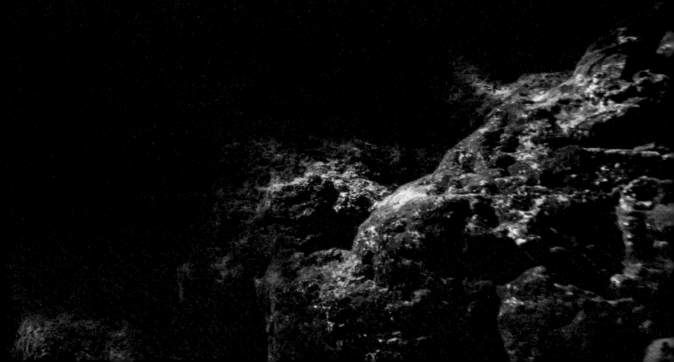

PART III

SECRETS BEHIND OTHER MYSTERY ILLNESSES

"Truth is, millions of people suffer from mystery illness. A mystery illness is any condition or symptom that leaves anyone perplexed for any reason. It can be a mystery because there isn't a name for a given set of symptoms—and so it's written off. A mystery illness can also be an established, chronic condition for which there's no effective treatment of the root cause (because medical communities don't yet understand it), or a condition that's frequently misdiagnosed.

Conditions such as type 2 diabetes, hypoglycemia, TMJ, menopause complications, ADHD, acne, eczema, psoriasis, Bell's palsy, neuropathy, leaky gut syndrome, heart palpitations, autoimmune disease, lupus, fibromyalgia, Lyme disease, multiple sclerosis (MS), chronic fatigue syndrome, migraines, thyroid disorder, rheumatoid arthritis, colitis, irritable bowel syndrome, celiac disease, insomnia, anxiety, depression, and more are merely labels, with no meaning behind them besides confusion and suffering. That makes them mystery illnesses."

— Anthony William, Medical Medium

CHAPTER 7

Type 2 Diabetes and Hypoglycemia

The fundamental fuel for your body is *glucose*, a simple sugar that provides all your cells with the energy they need to function, heal, grow, and thrive.

Glucose keeps us going—and keeps us alive. The central nervous system runs on it, as does every organ in the body, including the heart. Glucose is what we use to build and sustain muscle, and it performs vital functions such as repairing damaged tissue and cells.

When you eat food, your body breaks down the sugars in that food into glucose and places it in your bloodstream so it can travel to all your cells. However, your cells can't access all the glucose directly. They need some help from your *pancreas,* which is a large endocrine gland located behind your stomach. How much help your cells need all depends on the combinations of your food.

Your pancreas is constantly monitoring your bloodstream. When it detects a rise in glucose levels, it responds by producing a hormone called *insulin.* Insulin attaches to your cells and signals them to open up and absorb the glucose from your blood. Insulin therefore both allows your cells to get the energy they need and ensures your blood glucose levels remain stable.

If your bloodstream has more glucose than your cells can consume—for example, if you've eaten a particularly heavy meal (maybe pork ribs slathered in syrupy barbecue sauce; in other words, a lot of fat combined with sugar)—your insulin directs the extra glucose to be stored in your liver. At some later point when your glucose levels run low—for example, in between meals, or during periods of intense physical activity—your liver will release stored glucose for use by your cells. That is, if your liver is strong and functions well.

This is normally an effective system for optimal glucose use. However, it starts to go wrong if your pancreas can't produce enough insulin when it's needed. It also goes wrong if some of your cells start refusing to let the insulin attach and open the cells up to receive glucose because there is too much fat in the bloodstream interfering with this process; this is a true cause of *insulin resistance.* Yet another element that can go wrong is if the liver gets stagnant, sluggish, and dysfunctional, which means it can no longer store glucose or release glucose properly.

When any or all of these problems occur, not enough glucose is removed from your blood by your cells. Your body will expel some of the excess glucose in your urine, which may cause you to urinate more frequently, and also dehydrate you and make you feel thirsty. This is not the fault of the sugar (your glucose). This is the result of how much fat is inside your bloodstream. Even though sugar is being discarded and pushed out through the urine, technically the thirst is because fats inside the bloodstream are causing dehydration. Plus, in most cases where fats are consumed with sugars, excess salt accompanies them in the diet, and salt plays a role in the dehydration process as well.

If your pancreas isn't creating enough insulin when your body needs it, and/or if you're experiencing insulin resistance, and if these issues lead to exceptionally high blood glucose levels, you're at risk for *type 2 diabetes*. While medical research and science are aware of *prediabetes*, the precursor to type 2 diabetes, they are unaware that there are even earlier stages: pre-prediabetes, pre-pre-prediabetes, and even pre-pre-pre-prediabetes. These earlier versions of prediabetes occur as the liver is starting to get stagnant and sluggish from a high-fat diet and not able to store glucose as it should. At the same time, you could have the onset of pre-fatty liver. Precursor stages to both diabetes and fatty liver can go undetected.

Medical professionals don't know why type 2 diabetes happens. This is evident in the diets that physicians and dieticians recommend to diabetics; if they knew what was really happening in these patients' bodies, they'd offer completely different food advice. While doctors get some elements of treatment right,

they aren't able to offer an understanding of how or why this disease starts.

This chapter will tell you precisely what causes type 2 diabetes. It'll also truly explain how insulin resistance occurs, as well as what hypoglycemia is and how to get your system back in balance enough so your body can have the chance to heal.

TYPE 2 DIABETES SYMPTOMS

If you have type 2 diabetes, you may experience one or more of the following symptoms. (Note that it's possible to be in the early stages of diabetes and not experience any symptoms.)

- **Unusual thirst, dry mouth, frequent urination:** this is because of a system that's being overburdened by fats. The liver, lymphatic system, and bloodstream are harboring too much free-floating fat from a long-term diet high in fat. Fat in the bloodstream does not allow water to easily absorb into the bloodstream and become useful. Another reason is because, due to insulin resistance not allowing sugar to enter cells, your body is using up water to expel excess glucose via your urine. These effects of a high-fat diet can create thirst, dry mouth, and frequent urination. (Excess salt consumption usually accompanies high fat consumption, too, although these symptoms can also occur without the salt.)

- **Blurry vision:** the central nervous system requires glucose in order to function optimally. If insulin resistance persists because of a high-fat diet, blurry vision can occur intermittently or continually. It doesn't help that as you become dehydrated, water may be pulled away from the lenses of your eyes to help flush out the excess glucose.

- **Unusual hunger:** this is because your cells aren't getting all the glucose they need to feed themselves, because fat is getting in the way of glucose entering cells.

- **Fatigue and irritability:** as you're not getting the energy you normally do when your cells are fully fueled with glucose. Keep in mind, there could be another condition, such as low-grade viral infection, causing fatigue on top of your insulin resistance, prediabetes, or type 2 diabetes.

- **Digestive problems:** your pancreas doesn't just make insulin; it makes enzymes to help your body break down foods. If your pancreas is underperforming, this creates not only an insulin deficiency but also an enzyme deficiency, making it harder for your body to digest anything. Enzyme deficiency isn't normally the worst thing. What makes it more difficult is when the liver is weak, stagnant, or sluggish, not producing enough bile to break down fats. This puts a strain on the stomach's gastric glands, prompting them to overproduce hydrochloric acid, which can weaken the glands. When your liver is stronger and healthier, it leads to less burden on the pancreas.

- **Hypoglycemia:** these energy lows—blood sugar drops that occur as often as every other hour—are the result of weakness of the liver and underactive adrenals. When the liver is stagnant and sluggish, it can reach the point where it can't store glucose anymore, which means it can't release glucose into the bloodstream when your blood sugar gets low. Instead, the adrenals have to overcompensate for blood sugar drops—when blood sugar gets low, adrenaline surges to fill in as fuel, which over time causes the adrenals to weaken. People who intermittent fast improperly eventually break down and weaken their adrenals because they're running on adrenaline instead of glucose. (Read more about intermittent fasting in *Cleanse to Heal*.)

WHAT *REALLY* CAUSES TYPE 2 DIABETES AND HYPOGLYCEMIA

While medical communities are unaware of this, the causes of both type 2 diabetes and hypoglycemia typically begin with the liver and adrenal glands.

When you're up against continual stress and experiencing difficult and unavoidable trials in life, it sets your adrenal glands to flood your body with *adrenaline*, a hormone that charges you with emergency energy. While this is a helpful response for dire straits, if you're continually operating in crisis mode and aren't able to physically burn off the corrosive adrenaline saturating the tissues of your organs and glands, then the adrenaline, coupled with high-fat diet, can saturate your liver, making it more stagnant and sluggish.

Your pancreas is normally as smooth as a baby's bottom. But chronic scorching by fear-based or other challenging-emotion-based adrenaline, plus adrenaline to fill in for glucose, will wear away at the pancreas, creating calluses that turn it thick and hard.

It's like this: When you're born, your pancreas is like a brand-new credit card. Some come into the world with a sweet deal—a high spending limit, a generous cash credit line, and a cache of frequent flyer miles just for signing up. Others come into the world with lower credit limits, higher interest rates, and fewer bonuses, due to the variety or level of toxins they're born with. Either way, you can use that thing up if you're not careful. When people go through life getting worn down and taming the stress with fried or high-fat foods, ice cream, cookies . . . they run up the balance on the pancreas and use up those frequent flyer miles. (When this happens, it usually means the liver is spent and has become too stagnant and sluggish to act as a protective older sibling to the pancreas, like it usually would.)

Over time, this strain on the pancreas hinders its ability to produce enough insulin to deliver glucose from your bloodstream to the organs and glands that need it. And this underperformance alone is enough to create prediabetes and type 2 diabetes.

That's not the end of it. Your entire body is up against chronic floods of challenging-emotion-based adrenaline. Especially if you eat fat-based food when you're emotional because you're going through a stressful time, your pancreas will produce insulin that mixes with the adrenaline in your bloodstream, and

these hormones clash when they mix together. Over time, this can make many of your cells throughout your body "allergic" to your adrenaline/insulin blend and cause them to shun both hormones. Medical research hasn't yet uncovered this "Franken-sulin" hybrid (as I call it), nor has it understood that the physical body gets affected in this way. It's one of the primary causes of pancreatic weakness, which leads to lowered insulin production and nonacceptance of glucose in the body's cells (insulin resistance).

Heavy, rich meals alone can trigger excess adrenaline production, too. That's because the adrenals are like a fire station, and fat triggers the alarm bell. When the adrenals get the signal that high levels of fat are in the bloodstream—and therefore have the potential to put the pancreas, liver, and heart in immediate danger—the firehouse (the adrenals) sends out the fire trucks (adrenaline) to address the situation by acting as a blood thinner while also slightly increasing heart rate to pull the fat throughout the arteries and veins so the blood doesn't become stagnant from high fat content. That rush of adrenaline increases digestive strength to help move the fat through your intestinal tract, too, in hopes of activating quick peristaltic action so you'll go to the bathroom earlier than you normally would—to get most of the fat out through your bowel movement instead of staying in the digestive tract and getting absorbed into the bloodstream and liver. While these functions of adrenaline protect you from crisis, you also pay a price, as this process can weaken the liver, pancreas, adrenals, and heart over time.

On the flip side, your adrenal glands may be underperforming—that is, producing too *little* adrenaline. This makes your pancreas work overtime to try to compensate. If this condition is chronic and you happen to have any low-grade viral infection, your pancreas will become inflamed or enlarged, and may eventually start underperforming as well. A strong liver and strong immune system can keep pathogens at bay so that neurotoxins or pathogens aren't reaching the pancreas, therefore keeping it from being inflamed.

Then again, you can have *adrenal fatigue,* in which your unstable adrenals are sometimes producing too little adrenaline and sometimes producing way too much. This can play a role in the amount of insulin your pancreas releases. Inconsistency with the pancreas releasing insulin can occur when the adrenals are inconsistent—that is, unstable adrenals that shift between underactive to overactive can lead the pancreas to similar variability. Fight-or-flight can be like a flip switch for insulin production. Caffeine users manually flip the fight-or-flight switch daily, eventually draining the pancreas of energy.

A precursor to type 2 diabetes is a fluctuating but low glucose level—called *hypoglycemia*—which indicates a major issue with your liver's ability to manage glucose properly. This can occur if your liver becomes impaired in its ability to store and release glucose because it is stagnant and sluggish. It can also happen if you're not eating at least a light, balanced snack—e.g., a fruit (for sugar and potassium) and an herb, leafy green, or vegetable (for sodium)—every two hours. Regularly skipping meals forces your body to use up the liver's precious glucose storage, driving the body to run on adrenaline, and as previously mentioned, this can strain your pancreas, create insulin resistance, and lead to adrenal fatigue and weight gain over time.

(If you have a strong liver and you're not dealing with a high pathogen level from viruses and/or bacteria, you can eat inconsistently for more than a few years and not see the effects until down the road. If you're someone dealing with any kind of health compromise, it's critical to snack or graze or at least have some form of mineral salt and carbohydrate—for example, celery juice, coconut water, lemon water, or a balanced snack—regularly throughout the day. Someone dealing with hypoglycemia should not be intermittent fasting.)

One other major factor is the *type* of food you eat. There's a common misconception that diabetes is caused by eating a lot of foods with sugar in them. However, it's not actually the sugar that's the problem. It's sugar and fat combined—mainly fat. For example, you could eat fruit all day and every day for the rest of your life and never get diabetes. (In fact, eating a lot of fruit is the most effective way to add years to your life, as I'll explain in Chapter 20, "Fruit Fear.")

The problem is *fat.* Most people who consume processed foods and junk foods such as cakes, cookies, doughnuts, ice cream, and so on—or people who have a seemingly healthy main dish like chicken but follow it up with dessert—typically eat a lot of fat *and* a lot of sugar at the same time. While sugar that's not attached to nutrients (i.e., that isn't coming from sources such as fruits, leafy greens, herbs, wild food, vegetables, raw honey, pure maple syrup, or coconut water) is definitely unhealthy, it's the *fat* that strains your liver and pancreas.

The first thing that will happen is that instant insulin resistance from the high levels of blood fat that result from an animal protein meal (whether lean versions of pork, steak, or chicken, or fast food battered and fried in oil)—or even a plant-based meal of gluten-free cakes and cookies filled with nuts, seeds, and oils—will stop the body's ability to allow the insulin produced by your pancreas to drive sugar into your cells. This will mean there's a whole lot of sugar floating around the bloodstream that can't go anywhere. A strong liver will help gather up as much glucose as it can to store for a rainy day. Over time, though, a diet high in fat, protein, and processed oils—whether they're healthier fats and oils or not—can burden the liver. Your liver can reach a vulnerable state from the constant responsibility to clean up the excess glucose in the bloodstream while getting bombarded and overloaded by fat, and then having to wait too many hours between meals to be refueled. When the liver becomes overburdened in this way, it dumps all of its glucose storage back into the bloodstream. This can prompt the birthing stage of hypoglycemia into prediabetes.

Since your liver has to take the burden of processing the fat you eat, a diet high in fat (which hides in even the lean protein people tend to think of as healthy) can make the organ sluggish and unable to store and release glucose the way it should. Large, heavy meals plus glucose dry spells caused by not eating in between can eventually result in type 2 diabetes.

At the same time, your pancreas has to produce enzymes to help digest the fat. A lot of fat makes your pancreas work extra hard, and if you've already got other factors straining your pancreas, such as severe emotions leading the adrenal glands to flood it with corrosive adrenaline, a diet high in fat may be all that's needed to push your pancreas over the edge and create type 2 diabetes.

The good news is that all the compromises described above are absolutely reversible. Next we'll cover how to heal your pancreas and your liver, and correct your insulin resistance so you can bring your hypoglycemia or type 2 diabetes to an end.

ADDRESSING TYPE 2 DIABETES AND HYPOGLYCEMIA

Since medical communities don't know the real story of what causes type 2 diabetes and hypoglycemia, they don't provide the proper diet guidance. Typically, they recommend a diet with little to no sugar in it, advising patients to avoid fruit altogether and focus on eating protein (whether plant based, animal, or both) and vegetables. Medical communities usually consider this advice to fall under the umbrella of a "balanced diet," a term that isn't as rational as it sounds, since it isn't based on an understanding of what truly causes these conditions.

Heeding this advice may seemingly give you some improvements. At the same time, it will probably keep you diabetic forever—and not just diabetic and functional, but diabetic and ailing—since too much fat is only going to make your condition worse, while eating fruit is critical for healing diabetes. It's imperative to understand that a diet always high in fat is a leading contributor to what weakened the pancreas and liver to begin with.

Sugar was just the messenger. And in this case, health professionals shoot the messenger. That sugar was showcasing the insulin resistance that had cropped up from a pancreas and liver overburdened by fat.

It's easy to eat a diet high in animal fat and/or plant fat without realizing it. Even a lean-cut 4-ounce piece of meat will contain a tablespoon of concentrated fat that can burden the pancreas and liver. So when a person is insulin resistant (even from a diet that seems traditionally "healthy") and puts sugar into her or his system, that sugar is going to prompt insulin problems—and suddenly sugar is going to get all the attention, when it's not the real instigator.

Now of course table sugar and many other sweeteners aren't good for you—I'm not recommending you eat these. Yet to address type 2 diabetes and hypoglycemia, it is *critical* to lower fat consumption and increase consumption of fresh fruits, leafy greens, herbs, wild foods, and vegetables. I recommend the cleanse in Chapter 22 to help heal the liver, pancreas, and adrenal glands and stabilize blood sugar levels.

Your doctor may prescribe insulin. While insulin lowers your blood glucose level, it does nothing to address core problems such as injured adrenal glands, an injured pancreas, a dysfunctional liver, chronic challenging emotions, and/or insulin resistance.

What follows is a more targeted daily approach that focuses on healing every likely cause of your type 2 diabetes or hypoglycemia. You'll also find guidance in Part IV, "How to Finally Heal." How long you'll need to stick with this program depends on how much damage has to be undone. If you commit to learning the Medical Medium information and customizing these tools to create a protocol that works for you, you will see results.

Since this book was first published, so many people have healed their conditions and symptoms. Some heal in a very short time; some may take longer. It all depends on whether they're putting the information to work correctly and what state they were in when they started.

Take it all in stride. Do what you can for now. A little bit does count—it does go a long way. If you can only try one or two tools here, by all means, stick with them so that you can at least make some improvements or stave off your condition from getting worse. If you ever find that you need to take yourself further, this information will be here waiting for you—so you can take yourself as far as you need to go.

Bolster Your Adrenal Glands

The fact that you have type 2 diabetes means it's likely you have an issue with your adrenal glands. Therefore, one step toward healing is to read Chapter 8, "Adrenal Fatigue." You can follow its advice to make your adrenal glands stable and strong.

Healing Foods

Wild blueberries, spinach, celery, papayas, sprouts, kale, raspberries, blackberries, potatoes, winter squash, cilantro, bananas, melons, lettuce, tomatoes, apples, cucumbers, and asparagus are top foods to eat if you have type 2 diabetes or hypoglycemia. These perform functions such as detoxing the liver, strengthening glucose levels, supporting the pancreas, boosting the adrenal glands, and stabilizing insulin. Incorporate as many of these foods into your diet as you can.

Take care to avoid certain foods as well, most specifically cheese, milk, cream, butter, eggs, and processed oils. Try to keep your overall fat consumption low. Also avoid all processed sugar. The natural sugars in fruit, raw honey, coconut water, and pure maple syrup are acceptable.

Healing Herbs and Supplements

Before applying these, be sure to read Chapter 21, "Critical Guide to Supplement Protocols."

(For insights into the true causes of type 1 and type 1.5 diabetes, see the Medical Medium book *Cleanse to Heal*.)

Supplements for Diabetes (Type 1, Type 1.5 [LADA], and Type 2), Prediabetes, Hypoglycemia, and Blood Sugar Imbalance

- **Fresh celery juice:** work up to 32 ounces daily

- **5-MTHF:** 1 capsule twice a day

- **Amla berry:** 2 teaspoons twice a day

- **Ashwagandha:** 1 dropperful twice a day

- **Barley grass juice powder:** 2 teaspoons or 6 capsules daily

- **Chaga mushroom:** 2 teaspoons or 6 capsules daily

- **Glutathione:** 1 capsule daily

- **Hibiscus:** 1 cup of tea twice a day

- **Lemon balm:** 2 dropperfuls or 1 cup of tea twice a day

- **L-lysine:** 2 500-milligram capsules twice a day

- **Nascent iodine:** 6 small drops (not dropperfuls) daily

- **Nettle leaf:** 2 dropperfuls or 1 cup of tea twice a day

- **Rose hips:** 1 cup of tea twice a day

- **Schisandra berry:** 1 cup of tea twice a day

- **Turmeric:** 2 capsules twice a day

- **Spirulina:** 2 teaspoons or 6 capsules daily

- **Vitamin B$_{12}$ (as adenosylcobalamin with methylcobalamin):** 1 dropperful twice a day

- **Vitamin C (as Micro-C):** 4 capsules twice a day

- **Wild blueberry powder:** 1 tablespoon daily

- **Zinc (as liquid zinc sulfate):** up to 1 dropperful twice a day

CASE HISTORY:
Getting a New Perspective on Sugar
2003

Starting in her teens, Morgan battled what she called emotional highs and lows. Her mother, Kim, learned that if Morgan went too long without eating, she'd start to act out with a burst of frustration or fall into tears out of nowhere.

Kim repeatedly took Morgan to the family doctor to have her blood sugar levels evaluated, but Morgan's A1C and other tests would always come back normal. The doctor passed off Morgan's inconsistent behavior as an aspect of being a sensitive—or maybe even bipolar—girl.

When Morgan was in her early 20s, Kim found an alternative doctor who said Morgan was hypoglycemic. The practitioner instructed Morgan to stay away completely from sugars and other carbohydrates, and to eat a diet of strictly protein and vegetables, with small meals every few hours to stabilize her blood sugar.

At first, Morgan felt an improvement. She and Kim took this as an indication that the diet was helpful, so all through her early adult life, Morgan stayed clear of most carbs and all processed sugars. She focused on eating doctor-recommended proteins such as eggs, chicken, turkey, cheese, fish, and nuts every few hours, as well as salads with tomatoes and cucumbers, which were allowed because they were low carb. This gave Morgan the blood sugar and energy stability to function.

As she got into her late 20s, though, her energy levels became inconsistent again. She started to develop digestive gas and bloating, along with weight gain and fatigue. After exercising, she'd get a huge energy crash and intensely crave sugar.

Morgan had her blood drawn at the alternative doctor's office, and the A1C test showed evidence that she now had type 2 diabetes. She could barely process the information. She'd hardly eaten any sugar over the last seven years. She read every food package, every label, and she studiously sought out protein and avoided carbohydrates. This had once seemed to be saving her.

Kim vented about the predicament to her hairdresser, who was a client of mine. She told Kim I'd be able to get to the bottom of Morgan's health problem.

Within the first minute of my phone call with Morgan and Kim, Spirit confirmed that Morgan was hypoglycemic and now technically had type 2 diabetes.

"How could this happen?" Morgan asked. "I strictly avoid sugar and carbs, and I eat protein every three hours."

"Sugar isn't the issue," I said. "It's fat. Unfortunately, Morgan, you were prescribed a high-fat diet under the guise of a high-protein one."

"I was told this was all protein I've been eating," Morgan said. "Where was the fat?"

"It was in the animal protein," I told her. "For seven years, fat has been your main calorie source, since you weren't living off sugar or carbohydrate calories."

"And why don't doctors know about this?"

"They haven't learned yet," I said. "They're wrapped up in the high-protein trend."

Kim cut in. "Why are these foods just called high protein? Why isn't the fat mentioned?"

"Because that's how it was first marketed back in the 1930s. If all these animal products were marketed as high fat, they wouldn't have been as appealing."

I explained that the animal fat had burdened Morgan's liver and pancreas. "You felt stabilized for the first few years because you weren't going so long between meals, and because the high-protein/high-fat combo had forced your adrenal glands to work harder, pumping out their energy hormones." Now, as she was getting older, she was exhibiting all the symptoms of adrenal fatigue and digestive distress, because her liver and pancreas had become sluggish. This was behind the weight gain, too.

"Your liver can't store glucose anymore to provide you with energy, and your adrenals are running low on adrenaline. We need to change your diet—lower your animal proteins to one serving at dinnertime, eliminate all dairy and eggs, and start bringing in natural sugars from fruit. And you need to let go of the carbohydrate fear that's been drilled into you. Bananas, apples, dates, grapes, melons, mangoes, pears, and berries are going to make every difference in your health. You can keep some nuts and seeds in rotation, just don't eat more than a handful once or twice daily."

Kim hesitated. "You're telling a diabetic that what she needs in her life is more sugar?"

I hear this all the time. "Only the natural sugar in fruit," I said. I assured them both that if Morgan used the grazing technique and ate every two hours, using food combining to balance potassium, sodium, and sugar (as I describe in Chapter 8, "Adrenal Fatigue"), she would do great. Fruits, leafy greens, herbs, wild foods, and vegetables were wonderful components of those snacks and meals. Suggested healing food combos for Morgan were celery or cucumbers with dates, apples, walnuts, or seeds.

Within the first month, Morgan felt more energy and emotional stability than she had in the last 10 years. Her weight was going down, and she could finally exercise without collapsing afterward. Smoothies with dates, bananas, and celery became her favorite post-workout meal. And even though it seemed counterintuitive to all advice on the diabetes front, she decided she was feeling so great with the change in diet that she only wanted one serving of animal protein a week.

Within four months, Morgan had reversed her type 2 diabetes. Her doctor was baffled as he presented the results of her A1C test—that it was back to normal. In the months that followed, Morgan continued to restore her pancreas, liver, and adrenal glands—and get her life back on track.

CHAPTER 8

Adrenal Fatigue

Key components of your endocrine system are your *adrenal glands,* which are small lumps of tissue located directly above your kidneys. Your adrenal glands produce hormones critical for your health, including a number of undiscovered hormones as well as adrenaline, cortisol, and hormones that in turn regulate the production of sex hormones such as estrogen and testosterone. Medical research and science are only at the beginning stages of understanding what role the adrenal glands really play in our bodies and how they affect our health.

The primary trigger for your adrenal glands is stress, which causes them to produce extra amounts of hormones such as adrenaline. This is an excellent survival mechanism built into your body for short-term emergencies, as the additional hormones are likely to help you get through whatever crisis is occurring.

If the stress continues over a long period, however—for example, if you're going through a bankruptcy, a divorce, breakup, betrayal, the death of a loved one, or some other cause of severe emotional turmoil—your adrenal glands may eventually become weakened from being on continual "hyperdrive." Undergoing a very

substantial amount of stress in even a relatively short period can also overstrain the adrenals; a common example is childbirth, which requires an enormous amount of adrenaline.

In fact, medical communities are unaware that overstrained adrenals are one reason for postpartum fatigue and depression—these struggles are often the result of adrenal glands becoming so exhausted after the process of childbirth that they lose the strength to produce enough of the right hormones at the right times to keep the mother strong, vibrant, and happy.

When your adrenal glands become overextended, they have the equivalent of a nervous breakdown and behave erratically.

Some alternative medicine doctors believe that when the adrenals partially "burn out," they simply stop producing the full amount of hormones needed. That's an oversimplification of the complex role these glands play in reacting to moment-by-moment emotional and environmental changes. What really happens is that instead of operating in a rock-steady manner that creates precisely the right amount of hormones for each new situation, exhausted adrenals may produce *too little* or *too much* hormone—something like the massive mood swings in someone with bipolar disorder.

For example, a temporary bout of depression can result when out-of-control adrenals wildly overreact to a situation and flood you with *too much* adrenaline. The excess adrenaline may in turn burn away your brain's neurotransmitter chemicals. One of those neurotransmitters, out of many, is *dopamine*. All neurotransmitter chemical compounds are vital to your feeling stable and happy, so a lack of them can leave you feeling depressed. It's this variable behavior producing adrenal extremes on either the low or the high side at any moment that characterizes genuine *adrenal fatigue.*

While alternative doctors don't grasp all the nuances of adrenal fatigue, they're way ahead of some mainstream doctors who don't even recognize that this illness *exists.*

The truth is that adrenal fatigue has been with us since the start of the human race.

What's changed is how pervasive it's become—thanks to our fast-paced and stress-filled times, as well as the explosion of pathogens that started in the 20th century, plus toxic heavy metal exposure, which is rampant. Because of the Quickening, over *95 percent* of us will undergo adrenal fatigue multiple times in our lives.

ADRENAL FATIGUE SYMPTOMS

If you have adrenal fatigue, you may experience one or more of the following symptoms: weakness, lack of energy, trouble concentrating, becoming easily confused, forgetfulness, trouble completing basic tasks you could once

handle easily, hoarse voice, poor digestion, constipation, depression, insomnia, not feeling rested after waking from sleep, and relying on naps during the day. Keep in mind, this can accompany a low-grade viral infection such as EBV—that is, both adrenal fatigue and viral symptoms can be combined.

Adrenaline plays a vital role in dreams (when you're running in a dream, for example, your adrenals become stimulated and release the hormone), so in extreme cases of adrenal fatigue, some people are unable to dream enough for the needs of the mind, soul, and spirit. In very extreme cases, some people are so weak that they can't get out of bed for more than a couple of hours a day.

Fatigued adrenals will often also have effects on other glands and organs. For example, your pancreas can become stressed from working overtime to compensate for adrenal underperformance. Your heart may need to work harder as it tries to regulate unusual levels of adrenaline, cortisol, and blood sugar. If excess adrenaline-cortisol blends abruptly race through your body and empty your liver's reserves of glucose, glycogen, and iron, your liver will have to work extra hard to create more. And your central nervous system and brain can go off-kilter from sudden floods of adrenaline-cortisol blends, and lack of glucose.

Too little cortisol can wreak its own havoc. Cortisol plays a key role in converting the thyroid storage hormone T4 into the usable hormone T3, and in allowing the T3 to penetrate and "charge up" your cells. When your adrenals underperform, they can create a thyroid hormone shortage on the cellular level. In this case, even if you have a healthy thyroid that's testing as normal, you can experience what doctors believe are hypothyroid symptoms such as weight gain, depression, hair loss, brittle nails, rough or thinning skin, feeling cold, fluctuating blood sugar, and a myriad of other issues that are really from underperforming adrenals in combination with a low-grade viral infection and a stagnant, sluggish liver.

You can also have some of these symptoms with perfectly healthy adrenal glands but a malfunctioning thyroid (see Chapter 6, "Hypothyroidism and Hashimoto's Thyroiditis"). Then again, you can have *neurological fatigue,* which is caused by the swelling of the central nervous system as a result of neurotoxins produced by such viruses as Epstein-Barr and shingles. Because there are myriad causes for energy loss, it's difficult to know whether you have adrenal fatigue based on a list of symptoms alone. Fortunately, there are some additional clues you can look for.

MORE SIGNS YOU HAVE ADRENAL FATIGUE

If you have several of the symptoms described in the previous section, and your condition also matches two or more of the scenarios that follow, then it's very possible you have adrenal fatigue.

(If the distressing or demanding circumstances that led to your adrenal fatigue reduce and your symptoms still persist and become chronic, consider the information in Chapter 3, "Epstein-Barr Virus, Chronic Fatigue Syndrome, and Fibromyalgia." You could be dealing with an underlying viral infection coupled with toxic heavy metals.)

You "crash" in the early part of your day and/or throughout your day. Again, even if you've had a normal amount of sleep the night before, you may feel the need to lie down and close your eyes before lunchtime if you lack adequate adrenal hormones.

You feel tired all day at work, but feel more energetic at home in the evening. This happens when your exhausted adrenal glands hold back their limited reserve of hormones during your stress-filled day in case an emergency arises, then let go of the reserves when you're back home in a relaxed environment where you're much less likely to encounter a crisis.

You're exceptionally exhausted at night but have trouble falling asleep. The act of sleeping, and especially falling into REM sleep, requires adrenal hormones. If you're short on these hormones, you may experience insomnia, unsatisfyingly light sleep, and/or dreamless sleep.

You feel unrested even after a full night's sleep. Again, if you lack enough adrenal hormones to fuel REM sleep and dreaming, you won't have a satisfying night. On top of that, low hormones can rob you of so much energy that you'll feel weak no matter how much sleep you get.

You experience continual sweating under your armpits after performing even light tasks. This is the result of your entire endocrine system working overtime to compensate for the lack of adequate adrenaline.

You're continually thirsty and can't seem to quench your thirst; or you have a continually dry mouth; or you're frequently craving salt. This is caused by a substantial number of electrolytes in your bloodstream and nervous system getting destroyed by an abrupt flood of an adrenaline-cortisol blend. Water, soda, coffee, alcohol, and most other beverages won't solve this problem. You need to replenish the electrolytes by drinking something that has the right balance of sodium, potassium, and glucose—e.g., coconut water, freshly pressed apple juice, freshly pressed celery juice, or a juice blend of cucumber and apple.

Blurry vision or difficulty focusing eyesight. This is caused by a flood of excess cortisol—which tends to dehydrate any area—affecting one or more sensitive spots near the eyes, which require a great deal of constant hydration. Other symptoms are dark circles around the eyes and/or sunken eyes.

Continual craving for stimulants. If you frequently feel the need for stimulants to keep you going—such as cigarettes, coffee, caffeine-infused soda, sugary snacks such as cookies or doughnuts, or even prescription-drug "uppers" such as amphetamines—you may instinctively be seeking a substitute for your missing adrenal hormones. While stimulants will give you a quick energy boost, you'll soon "crash" after their effects fade away. Plus, by forcing your adrenals to regularly over-perform and then become exhausted, these stimulants create an up-and-down cycle that makes their already poor functioning even worse over time.

AVOIDING ADRENAL FATIGUE

Daily stress is not easy to avoid. We all have responsibilities and obligations, some that can't be avoided in any way. Not all of us have a choice in the way we live our lives, due to financial needs, taking care of others, or other responsibilities. Little things go a long way when helping to support and even recover your adrenal glands. If it's out of reach

to do the big things like getting a lot of sleep, toning down your schedule, creating a more manageable workload, or focusing on the best options to eat, know that every bit of support you do give your adrenals means a great deal for helping out these glands. So let's explore options for small steps to help you feel more in control of your health.

One step you can take is to avoid caffeine, which is designed to give you an adrenaline "rush." While caffeine may make you feel good temporarily, in the long term, it risks burning out your adrenal glands. Relying on coffee drinks, matcha tea, chocolate, and cacao—even when they seem medicinal—is a sure path to not allowing your adrenals to heal. It's understandable if caffeine is the only way that you can power through something at this moment in your life. If that's not the case, consider reducing the amount of caffeine you consume. Small dietary shifts can make this easier. Bringing glucose into your diet (fruit is a great source of glucose), especially in the morning, can be really helpful to give you the strength and energy you need. And when you lower the amount of fats you consume (again, especially in the morning), you can get the most energy out of that glucose—plus your adrenals can start to restore. Glucose is like a cutoff switch to unwanted adrenaline production; it prevents your body from running on adrenaline every minute. Instead, the glucose itself gives you energy, especially when lower fats in the bloodstream mean that glucose can be delivered to your cells most efficiently.

Another strain on your adrenals is strong emotion. That doesn't mean you should avoid *all* powerful emotions. For example, if you're feeling extreme joy, your adrenals will generate a hormone that's *good* for your body and won't overtax the glands. If you're feeling fear, however, your adrenals will produce a form of adrenaline that can over time wear down both the glands and other vital parts of your body.

You might ask, "How is it possible that some emotions are better for the body than others? Don't my adrenal glands excrete the same adrenaline in response to *any* emotion?" That's what medical communities believe—and they're mistaken. The truth is your adrenal glands produce 56 different blends in response to different emotions and situations. More specifically, they produce 36 varieties of adrenaline that address everyday situations (e.g., feeling afraid, conversing with a stranger, walking briskly, moving your bowels, bathing/swimming in water, dreaming), and 20 for less common scenarios (e.g., going through a breakup, childbirth, fighting off a physical attack, getting into a car accident, mourning a death).

As a rule of thumb, if something makes you feel bad emotionally, it's probably compromising your body and can act as a trigger to some symptoms you're already experiencing. If you're someone who deals with migraines, for example, intense emotional stress can act as a trigger. While it's not the *cause* of your migraines, it can prematurely bring one on. If the emotional strain persists, it's also putting a strain on your adrenal glands. So you ideally want to let challenging or difficult feelings such as fear, anxiety, anger, hatred, guilt, and shame arise and pass by instead of suppressing or engaging with them.

Turning away from painful emotions and toward joyful ones is much easier said than done. For emotional support, you'll find a number of suggestions in Chapter 24, "Soul-Healing Meditations and Techniques," and

Chapter 25, "Essential Angels." These chapters also include spiritual balance exercises you can tap into when life seems to be throwing everything at you at once.

ADDRESSING ADRENAL FATIGUE

If considering the symptoms and scenarios described earlier in this chapter leads you to believe you have adrenal fatigue, don't despair. In addition to the suggestions above, you can take a number of concrete steps, as described below and in Part IV, to heal your adrenals and return them to their optimal strength.

If you commit to learning the Medical Medium information and customizing these tools to create a protocol that works for you, you will see results. Countless people have used the information in this book to heal. Some heal in a very short time; some may take longer. Your individual timeline depends in part on how much of this information you're able to put to use right now and what state you were in when you started. Other factors that can affect this time span include your overall health and what's going on in your life—e.g., if you're in a state of crisis that's continuing to strain your adrenals, you'll require a lot more time to heal. And again, if your adrenal fatigue persists, consider the information in Chapter 3, "Epstein-Barr Virus, Chronic Fatigue Syndrome, and Fibromyalgia," because you could be dealing with a low-grade viral infection that causes fatigue and other symptoms.

Take it all in stride. Do what you can for now. A little bit does count—it does go a long way. If you can only try one or two tools here, by all means, stick with them so that you can at least make some improvements or stave off your condition from getting worse. If you ever find that you need to take yourself further, this information will be here waiting for you—so you can take yourself as far as you need to go.

However long it takes, the sooner you get started on the road to recovery, the sooner you'll start feeling better and restoring your adrenals to full health.

Your Body Is on Your Side

Your adrenal glands support each other. They lean on one another. That's because your adrenal glands never weaken exactly equally. One adrenal is always a little more compromised or sensitive than the other. That means one is always a little stronger.

When one adrenal gland is lacking, the other picks up the slack. For example, if one adrenal gland is weakening faster, the stronger one will compensate so the weaker gland has a chance to recover—in the hopes that if the stronger gland starts to flag one day, the other gland will be in a position to help save it in its moment of need. This is a built-in mechanism of our endocrine system that is undiscovered by medical research and science.

Whenever we get emotionally challenged, for example by a betrayal or tragedy, the area of the soul that resides in a certain location in the emotional center of the brain will signal one adrenal gland to release more adrenaline than the other. That's what determines whether your left or right adrenal is used more during a challenging situation. This is a natural defense mechanism of our body that prevents both adrenals from being summoned to

discharge adrenaline in large amounts at the same time.

(Caffeine works around this defense mechanism. It stimulates both adrenals glands at the same time.)

As you're working to heal, it can be very helpful to remember that your body is on your side. You're not battling against some innate weakness or failing of your body. You're working *with* your body's natural, restorative mechanisms that have always been looking out for you. Even when we're up against emotional trials, we have a system put in place that's supporting and protecting us.

External Cortisol: For Emergencies Only

If you're in a state of crisis, a quick fix is taking cortisol replacement medication. This will provide your body with extra hormones to take the place of the ones not being generated by your underactive adrenal glands.

While this is the treatment of choice by doctors, it isn't an ideal solution, because your body needs a variety of types and amounts of hormones from your adrenal glands throughout the day to address different situations. Taking one pill in the morning isn't comparable to adrenal glands that are actively reacting to your body's needs every moment.

Also, cortisol medication is an immunosuppressant that makes your immune system sleepy and docile, making you more sensitive to a host of other issues.

So medication is, at best, a temporary fix to get you functional again . . . and buy you time to heal your adrenal glands properly using the techniques that follow.

Graze Every One and a Half to Two Hours

Most of us eat three relatively heavy meals a day with long stretches in between. This is tough on the adrenal glands, because one and a half to two hours after a meal your bloodstream runs low in glucose, which means you've run out of the sugars you've consumed. Once your blood sugar drops, your adrenal glands are forced to produce hormone blends to keep you "running." This means that if you frequently go without eating for long stretches, you're putting your adrenals under a steady strain and not giving them a chance to recuperate.

Therefore, the best way to heal your adrenal glands is to eat a light, balanced meal every 90 minutes to two hours. (This is especially helpful if you're struggling from other conditions or neurological symptoms, such as those mentioned in Chapter 3, "Epstein-Barr Virus, Chronic Fatigue Syndrome, and Fibromyalgia.")

In other words, use a *grazing* approach to food. This is critical to know—because diet trends right now are sending people in the opposite direction. Following the fashion on skipping meals will rob you of the opportunity to heal your adrenal fatigue.

For example, the intermittent fasting trend leads people to avoid meals for half the day or even longer. Intermittent fasters claim it gives them more energy. The reality is that most intermittent fasters consume caffeine beverages to replace the energy from meals. If you take away the caffeine, you'll feel the true effects of having low blood sugar, and that's the opposite of having energy. If someone has energy while intermittent fasting without

caffeine, that's because when you hold off mineral salts and glucose for too long, your adrenals take over and release adrenaline to fill in for blood sugar as your body's defense mechanism to power you through your day. That momentary feeling of energy comes at the price of strain on your adrenal glands that can affect you down the road. The real reason that intermittent fasting can provide temporary benefits is because by default, it has people avoiding foods high in fat (what I call *radical fats*) for the morning or even most of the day. Avoiding these foods, such as eggs, bacon, cheese, butter, milk, meat, avocado, nut butters, and oil, in the morning can be very helpful. That doesn't mean it's done properly. Find more about intermittent fasting in *Cleanse to Heal*.

The grazing technique works because the frequent meals keep your blood sugar steady throughout the day, and as long as your glucose isn't dropping, your adrenal glands don't have to interfere. Giving your adrenal glands lots of rest allows them to devote energy to healing and restoring themselves.

Each of your meals should ideally contain a balance of potassium, sodium, and sugar. Understand that we're talking about natural sugars from fruit here, the type that contains critical trace minerals and nutrients, unlike table sugar or lactose, the sugar present in dairy. Some examples of great meals for healing your adrenals include:

- A date (potassium), two celery sticks (sodium), and an apple (sugar)

- A banana (potassium), spinach (sodium), and an orange (sugar)

- A sweet potato (potassium), parsley (sodium), and tomato (sugar)

To be clear, you're welcome to have larger meals. The examples above needn't be substitutes for your breakfast, lunch, and dinner; rather, they can serve to keep your blood sugar levels steady in between those bigger meals. Or if you can't have a snack, you can turn to coconut water (that's not pink or red) or lemon water with raw honey to keep yourself going between meals.

You're also welcome to focus on any of these options and not eat larger meals, especially in the morning. Starting your day with lemon water (16 to 32 ounces) followed 15 to 30 minutes later by celery juice (16 to 32 ounces) is a very helpful technique, because both the lemon and celery provide a large dosage of mineral salts to support your adrenals from the get-go. (Remember not to squeeze lemon *into* the celery juice. Drink the lemon water and celery juice separately.)

The fruit smoothie options in Chapter 23 are also supportive. The Heavy Metal Detox Smoothie, for example, provides a helpful combination of potassium, sodium, natural sugar, and trace minerals to support your adrenals.

Beyond eating frequent light meals, there are specific foods you can eat to restore your adrenal glands.

Healing Foods

Certain fruits, leafy greens, herbs, wild foods, and vegetables either help protect your adrenal glands or speed their recovery by strengthening the nervous system, reducing inflammation because of their antiviral and antibacterial compounds, easing stress, and providing critical nutrients for adrenal function. The following are among the top foods to eat to bounce back from adrenal fatigue:

sprouts, asparagus, wild blueberries, bananas, potatoes, papayas, tomatoes, mangoes, cilantro, spinach, garlic, broccoli, kale, raspberries, blackberries, romaine lettuce, and red-skinned apples. Incorporate as many of these foods into your diet as you can.

What *Not* to Eat

If you have mild adrenal fatigue, you might be set with following the other advice in this chapter. If you have a moderate to severe case, however, then until you get stronger, you'll probably need to take the temporary extra step of cutting out foods that put a strain on your adrenal glands and slow them from healing. Please note that many diet experts recommend eating foods that are high in fat, whether plant based, animal based, or both. This is either because they don't realize how much fat can hide in even lean protein or because they think that fat content is a good thing. This protein advice can seem very convincing, so beware; it's bad for *anyone,* and especially unhealthy if you have adrenal fatigue. The high fat strains your pancreas and liver and eventually creates insulin resistance, making it difficult for your body to maintain a stable level of glucose . . . which in turn creates a massive strain on your adrenal glands as they struggle to produce hormone blends to compensate. If you're plant based or vegan, this does not grant you immunity. If your diet is mostly composed of foods high in fat such as avocados, almond butter, peanut butter, nuts, seeds, soy, coconut oil, and other healthier oils, it still creates a strain on your pancreas and liver.

Diet experts also often counsel people to cut out carbohydrates from their diets. Again, this is not good and can result in strain, because your body needs carbs for energy. Following these diet trends will slow you down and keep you from healing your adrenal fatigue.

For more background on the effects certain foods can have on our health, see Chapter 19, "What Not to Eat." Especially if you're dealing with a low-grade viral infection that's contributing to your fatigue and other symptoms, you may feel ready to gravitate toward removing foods that feed viruses from your diet.

Healing Herbs and Supplements

Before applying these, be sure to read Chapter 21, "Critical Guide to Supplement Protocols."

Supplements for Adrenal Problems

- **Fresh celery juice:** work up to 16 ounces twice a day or 32 ounces every morning
- **Celeryforce:** 3 capsules twice a day
- **Amla berry:** 1 teaspoon twice a day

- **Ashwagandha:** 1 dropperful twice a day
- **B-complex:** 1 capsule daily
- **Chicory root:** 1 cup of tea daily
- **Hibiscus:** 1 cup of tea daily
- **Lemon balm:** 2 dropperfuls twice a day
- **Licorice root:** 10 small drops (not dropperfuls) twice a day (two weeks on, two weeks off)
- **Magnesium glycinate:** 2 capsules twice a day
- **Nettle leaf:** 1 dropperful twice a day
- **Schisandra berry:** 1 cup of tea daily
- **Spirulina:** 2 teaspoons or 6 capsules daily
- **Vitamin B$_{12}$ (as adenosylcobalamin with methylcobalamin):** 1 dropperful twice a day
- **Vitamin C (as Micro-C):** 4 capsules twice a day
- **Zinc (as liquid zinc sulfate):** up to 1 dropperful twice a day

CASE HISTORY:
Fatigued from Radical Fat, Fixed by Fruit
2001

Mary, age 35, went to the doctor with the complaint that she was tired all the time. No matter how much rest she got, she couldn't seem to shake her fatigue. On the job at the shipping company where she worked, she never felt fully awake or alert. Mary's doctor performed a number of tests and called when he received the results. "Nothing is wrong," he said. "You're just a little overworked. You'll bounce back when the holidays have passed."

But the fatigue persisted and steadily worsened in the new year. This time, Mary visited an integrative medical doctor, who diagnosed her with adrenal fatigue. He was correct. However, along with a huge list of supplements to take, he instructed Mary to remove all carbohydrates and sugars from her diet, except for one green apple a day and occasional berries. She was to stick to three meals per day, with animal protein at each, plus various vegetables.

At first, Mary felt a burst of energy and thought she was healing. Here's what was really going on: to compensate for the loss of sugars in her diet that had resulted in reduction of glucose in her bloodstream, her already exhausted adrenals were now in overdrive and flooding her system with adrenaline. Further, eating animal protein—which naturally included fat—three times a day was burdening Mary's liver and pancreas and forcing her adrenals to pump more of their hormones to keep everything in balance. This is an example of the risk associated with a fad diet that's not backed up by true understanding of what the body needs and how it operates.

After 30 days of eating this way, Mary felt a noticeable decrease in energy. The fatigue was now even worse, and it was harder than ever to drag herself to work each day. On top of this, she had an irresistible hunger for sugar; she started reaching for processed carbs and sweets from the vending machine to feed the cravings. In her bloodstream, the sugars combined with the very high fat levels and triggered insulin resistance. Now her adrenals started releasing even more adrenaline and reached a point of near-total exhaustion.

At this point, an intern at Mary's company told her about how I'd helped his mom, so Mary gave me a call. Right off the bat, we removed the animal fats from her diet and switched her over from three meals a day to the every-two-hour grazing technique. This kept her glucose levels active and stable and put an end to her insulin resistance. We also brought balance into her diet with sodium-rich herbs and vegetables, potassium-rich fruits, and protein-rich leafy greens.

Very soon, Mary was back to where she'd started when she went to see the first doctor. Within a month, she was feeling functional again.

And within a year, she was full of energy.

When I checked in with her recently, she said she'd noticed blood sugar–related fatigue in others at her company, so she and the intern had started making their coworkers afternoon smoothies—which were very popular. She said she still liked to graze and felt so much better eating the way Spirit had recommended that she only ventured off her healing diet for very special occasions.

CHAPTER 9

Candida

The popularity of the *Candida* diagnosis was born out of a time when conventional medicine was in complete denial. It was the mid-1980s—practically the Dark Ages in chronic illness—and the medical model was not validating women's health concerns, except by offering hormone replacement therapy or antidepressants. Hundreds of thousands of women globally felt unheard and fed up.

Meanwhile, the alternative medicine movement had reached a turning point. An increasing number of alternative doctors and healers were rolling out practices or joining established ones. This was a time when conventional and alternative doctors were starkly divided. You wouldn't find a naturopath or a holistic doctor working in a conventional practice. This was also a time when alternative medicine wasn't owned by conventional. Alternative was on its own; conventional medicine hadn't infiltrated alternative yet. Now we're in an age where Trojan-horse approaches have introduced conventional thinking into alternative medicine. Conventional and alternative medicine are almost one and the same now, with much of alternative medicine doing the bidding of conventional medicine. This has taken

away much of alternative medicine's ability to think outside the box. Back in the 1980s, alternative doctors were still independent and felt primed to trump conventional medicine—they just needed something to sink their teeth into so they could prove their knowledge.

A surge of women frustrated with their regular physicians began filling the waiting rooms of alternative practices. Problem was, the practitioners didn't know what was wrong—though they did believe the women were suffering from *something*. This was the great awakening of the early-to-mid-1980s through the early 1990s. Women and their health complaints were finally being taken seriously. It was an important time, one that should be celebrated, as women's suffrage is. Yet this historic shift in women's lives didn't make it into any history books.

By this point, the hormone movement had already made a major impact. It was a well-established practice in the conventional medical community to blame anything and everything on menopause and perimenopause. As alternative doctors attempted to diagnose the flood of patients with mystery symptoms, though, they weren't yet on the hormone train. They suspected something else was in play.

The alternative medical community landed on the fungus *Candida*. The label was a breath of fresh air to women who'd gone through decades of conventional medical care and couldn't find answers. *Candida* became synonymous with, *We finally know why everyone isn't feeling well.* It was wrong, but it was still an amazing breakthrough.

Sitting in the office of her naturopath, chiropractor, acupuncturist, or herbalist and hearing that she had *Candida,* a woman would feel the blessing of validation: "You *are* sick with something." (Keep in mind, it was still a rare occurrence to find these practitioners. There wasn't one around every corner, and they weren't usually covered by insurance.) She was still getting a side order of blame as the doctor pointed to lifestyle as the culprit, but it all seemed to make perfect sense. And she might even feel some improvement in her health as she followed the doctor's instructions to cut out fried and processed foods and rich desserts. The concern at that time wasn't gluten. Instead, the focus was more on "white foods"—foods stripped of their nutrients and often battered and fried in grease.

By the late 1990s, the popularity of the *Candida* diagnosis had spread from the alternative to the conventional medical world, in part because conventional medicine was losing patients and its reputation was starting to wane. Now the diagnosis is mainstream, and it's one of the easiest ways to tell someone, "This is why you're sick."

Do women actually recover when they're treated for *Candida*? No. And the drastic recommended diet of no sugar but high fat and protein only provides temporary relief . . . and later backfires.

In truth, *Candida* is the most inappropriately maligned yeast of our time. We *all* have *Candida,* which is a beneficial fungus residing in the intestinal tract that aids food digestion and absorption. It's possible to be virtually riddled with *Candida* and yet be perfectly healthy. There are people with extremely high levels of it who eat and drink whatever they want without a hint of fatigue or stomach upset. *Candida* by itself is typically harmless.

What isn't yet fully understood by medical communities is that *Candida* is a frequent companion, or harmless cofactor, of diseases and organisms such as viruses and bacteria that are causing the real problem. These include Lyme disease, shingles, EBV, herpes, *C. difficile, Streptococcus, H. pylori,* diabetes, MS, HHV-6, cytomegalovirus, and many more.

For example, if you have Lyme disease symptoms (see Chapter 16), the conditions that triggered them (e.g., antibiotics, troublemaker foods, lack of sleep, intense stress, fear)—plus the viral infection responsible for the symptoms—are likely to result in a higher reproductive rate for *Candida*. Any type of viral and/or bacterial infection makes it more probable that a test for *Candida* will turn up positive. And *Candida* is often suggested to be the problem regardless of whether it shows up on a test. Keep in mind that tests for *Candida* are still fallible and inconclusive. They are part of the guessing game system. Even if the test doesn't show a positive, you can have *Candida*—because we all have *Candida*. What level of *Candida* depends on the factors in this chapter. Still, no matter how much *Candida* you have, what's causing the compromise to your body isn't this beneficial fungus; it's everything else.

Blaming *Candida* is like shooting the messenger. A large buildup of *Candida* can be an indicator that there's something wrong that bears investigation, *not* that the problem is the *Candida* itself.

Yet it's comparatively easy for doctors to employ a handful of tests to detect *Candida*, while it's currently almost impossible for them to detect the true culprits behind fibromyalgia, MS, Alzheimer's, dementia, UTIs, certain types of adrenal fatigue, chronic fatigue syndrome, lupus, rheumatoid arthritis, Lyme disease, thyroid disease, small intestinal bacterial overgrowth (SIBO), eczema, psoriasis, and numerous other illnesses for which medical communities don't yet have answers. *Candida* became a convenient scapegoat, and it still is today.

THE TRUTH ABOUT *CANDIDA*

A number of absurd notions have arisen in medical communities regarding *Candida,* built on misinformation and reinforced by decades of fads. You'll have to read these next sections with an open mind, because they contradict everything you've been told about this innocuous fungus and most likely everything you will be told in the future.

Recognizing the Rare Case

Whenever someone contracts a virus or bacterial strain and develops fatigue and fever, whether severe or mild, the beneficial fungus *Candida* can take the blame for the person's symptoms. In cases where *Candida* is believed to be the cause of a severe condition, what's really going on is that the person who is sick is suffering from an entirely different cause: viral or bacterial infection. *Candida* will often naturally upsurge to try to work in that person's favor—to try to support, not hurt or hinder. In these less than 0.1 percent of cases in which *Candida* seems to be doing notable harm, doctors tend to believe the fungus is out of control, creating a moderate-to-high fever that can become chronic and long term, ranging from weeks to months. In truth, it's the viral or bacterial infection causing the fever, fatigue, and more. Clinical blood work may show high levels of *Candida* in the bloodstream. While this is a true case of *Candida*, it only means that there's a rampant bacterial infection or acute viral infection that's the real reason for the symptoms. That's the only time that *Candida* will "explode" and proliferate to an extreme degree. These true cases of *Candida* are typically due to post-surgical complications, and—again—there's always a rampant bacterial or viral infection at the same time.

When someone is living with the symptoms of a chronic, low-grade bacterial or viral infection (versus a severe, acute bacterial or viral infection), *Candida* can still get the blame, even though testing will show its levels as moderate to mild. Today, what typically happens, especially in alternative medicine, is that your chronic, long-term symptoms of fatigue and digestive issues are blamed on *Candida*—or, more and more often, SIBO. Eventually SIBO will take the lead as the *Candida* diagnosis of the future. As I've said elsewhere, SIBO is the new *Candida*.

Bottom line: if a doctor tells you that your symptoms are from *Candida*, the odds are enormous that she or he is mistaken.

Candida and Leaky Gut Syndrome

Candida has been accused of drilling through the linings of the colon and intestinal tract, resulting in leaky gut syndrome.

This is not true.

The worst that can result from a high level of *Candida* is formation of calluses on irritated portions of the intestinal lining that have been chronically infected by bacteria such as *Streptococcus*. Wherever unproductive bacteria were, *Candida* moved in with them. Calluses and scar tissue inside the intestinal tract are from bacteria and viruses that mildly hinder food absorption. *Candida* tends to make a home in these patches that were created by pathogens. That's as bad as *Candida* can get. (For the true cause of leaky gut syndrome, see Chapter 17, "Gut Health.")

The Canary in the Mine

Candida's home is the gut, but it can also appear in the liver, the spleen, the vagina, and elsewhere. This causes no notable harm beyond some slight extra strain on your immune system. That slight extra strain is compensated for by how hard *Candida* works to defend you from unproductive bacteria and viruses. So it's a give-and-take relationship.

Like a canary in a coal mine, *Candida* is an indicator of something else truly worrisome that's spurring the fungus's growth. For instance, a vaginal *Streptococcus* infection could go unnoticed by doctors, while yeast that's also present could receive the blame for the patient's discomfort. Doctors would do well, instead, to take the *Candida* as a sign to look for the underlying strep bacteria. *Streptococcus* is the cause of UTIs, bladder infections, many vaginal infections (including yeast infections and bacterial vaginosis, or BV), and interstitial cystitis. An elevation of fungus is just a sign that there's another real culprit—in this case, one that's bacterial—causing the problem.

Treat the Root Cause

You almost never need to treat an overabundance of *Candida* directly. Instead, address the root cause of the illness that's creating your symptoms. Once you put an end to the real illness, *Candida* levels will naturally return to normal.

One bright spot in medicine today is that popular treatments for *Candida,* such as healthier eating habits, are helpful components, if done right, of effective treatment for many of the genuine illnesses *Candida* accompanies. When someone changes her diet to eliminate foods such as cake, bread, and, processed foods, her immune system will naturally strengthen because the gluten, dairy products, and eggs in these foods were feeding viruses and bacteria. By eliminating them, she makes her body less hospitable to autoimmune disease and other conditions.

However, other aspects of the diet recommended for *Candida* can be detrimental . . .

Fear of Fruit

One of the greatest misconceptions about *Candida* has to do with what foods feed it. Even though medical communities may use the term *feed*, they don't look at it quite that way; they're merely referencing foods they believe trigger a *Candida* upsurge. For example, while it's known that *Candida* may feed on sugar, they look at sugar as a *cause* of *Candida* proliferation; they don't believe *Candida* literally feeds on it. Besides which, major confusion lies around what *kind* of sugar.

People often think that all sugar is the same. That's like saying all water is the same, from a glass of fresh drinking water to the water in the toilet bowl.

In fact, the fructose that naturally occurs in fruit is actually bonded with compounds and substances—including antiviral compounds, antibacterial compounds, antioxidants, polyphenols, anthocyanin, minerals, phytochemicals, and cancer-killing micronutrients—that annihilate almost all diseases and actually kill off *Candida*. Even when sugar is separated from fruit and concentrated into fructose, it still doesn't have the ability to create or feed *Candida*.

Further, fresh fruit sugar starts to quickly leave your stomach in three to six minutes and doesn't even touch the intestinal tract. So if your fear is that fruit sugar feeds *Candida*, you needn't worry anymore. Fruit's fiber, pulp, skin, and seeds kill not only varieties of bacteria such as *Streptococcus*, *E. coli*, and *Staphylococcus*, along with some viruses; fruit also helps kill off unproductive fungus (that is, not the beneficial *Candida*), plus parasites and worms. These fruits naturally lower *Candida*, because *Candida* doesn't need to thrive when the environment is clear and foods are removed that, unknown to medical research and science, literally do feed *Candida*. Without gluten, dairy products, and eggs in the digestive system, *Candida* doesn't need to gobble up these foods in order to defend and protect you. Fruit is your anti-pathogen secret weapon. And while you now know that *Candida* is a saving grace, you can also look

at fruit as an anti-*Candida* weapon or tool, because *Candida* does naturally reduce when you're using fruit. (For more information, see Chapter 20, "Fruit Fear.")

Sugars that *do* feed *Candida* include table sugar, processed cane sugar, processed beet sugar, sugar from sources like agave nectar, processed grain sugar of any kind, and sugar from corn (such as high fructose corn syrup). What exacerbates the effects of these sugars, making them more problematic, is that they're mixed with fats. So this is where the alternative doctors were helping people—by encouraging them to lay off the chocolate cake.

The Fat and Protein Myth

It's a huge misconception that eating a high-fat, high-protein diet stops *Candida*. Fat and protein actually *feed Candida*.

Certain proteins, which are inflammatory because they feed bugs, are sticky and bind to the intestinal tract. The buildup of undigested proteins in someone with a weakened digestive system can result in a breeding ground for all forms of unproductive bacteria and nonbeneficial funguses. In turn, the beneficial fungus *Candida* starts to proliferate, because it's trying to manage the problem occurring with the unproductive bacteria and nonbeneficial fungus that are breeding due to the undigested proteins.

Relying on fat (whether it's plant fat, animal fat, or both) as your main calorie source will result in the highest *Candida* growth. A patient may follow a doctor's outlined diet to a T and it may *seem* like everything is okay. Silently, though, the *Candida* is multiplying in the patient's system, trying to manage the unproductive bacteria that are gorging themselves on milk, cheese, butter, eggs, oils that become rancid, and poultry that doesn't digest well and becomes putrefied in the gut because of weak digestion due to a weak liver. The day the patient caves to a craving for ice cream (fat, lactose, and processed sugar combined) at her son's birthday party, it may prompt symptoms to return a few days or a week later. The doctor can be concerned the *Candida* is returning and exposing itself due to the sugar in the ice cream, when the truth is that the high fats and undigested proteins were feeding unproductive bacteria in her digestive system all along. After the ice cream, she may be worse off than when she started, with more unproductive bacteria and nonbeneficial fungus causing a return of the beneficial *Candida* to clean it up.

The best approach to creating a friendlier, healthier environment in your gut—which reduces the need for *Candida* to have to clean up the mess—is to keep your fats low in your diet. That means once per day or less, whether it's a plant fat or an animal fat. Remember that if you're on a high-protein diet, it normally correlates with being high fat as well, even if it doesn't seem to be.

Avoiding the troublemaker foods such as gluten, dairy, eggs, processed oils, processed foods, and others in Chapter 19, "What Not to Eat," is a great way to stop feeding the unproductive bacteria and toxic fungus inside your intestinal tract and liver.

Also incorporate plenty of fruits, leafy greens, herbs, wild foods, and vegetables. Consider learning how to use them within the Medical Medium information.

HEALING FROM *CANDIDA*

The best way to heal from a flare-up of *Candida* is to address the illness that's the real cause of your symptoms.

The advice in Chapter 17, "Gut Health," will benefit anyone, including those who just want to address *Candida* as a side issue to an underlying health problem. Your goal in addressing your *Candida* is to increase levels of hydrochloric acid to break down and digest proteins, cleanse the intestinal tract, strengthen and detoxify the liver (so bile production increases and fats can break down and digest), and starve and kill off unproductive viruses and bacteria.

Learning how to address gut problems with these tools can eventually take you to a place of not needing to rely on antifungals and antibiotics being used for guessing games associated with your gut.

Healing Herbs and Supplements

These two supplement lists give you options if you're dealing with symptoms that you've been (mistakenly) told are from *Candida*. If your symptoms are more gut-related, you'll likely resonate with the SIBO list. (SIBO is very often misdiagnosed as *Candida*.) If your symptoms are centered around your reproductive area or urinary tract, you'll likely resonate with the list for UTIs, yeast infections, bladder infections, and BV. If you're dealing with symptoms in both categories, you're welcome to customize your supplement protocol using both lists.

Before applying these, be sure to read Chapter 21, "Critical Guide to Supplement Protocols."

Supplements for SIBO (Small Intestinal Bacterial Overgrowth) (Often misdiagnosed as an overgrowth of *Candida*; also applicable for those with a history of Acne, Sinus Infections, Strep Throat, Bloating, and Acid Reflux)

- **Fresh celery juice:** work up to 32 ounces daily
- **Aloe vera:** 2 or more inches of fresh gel (skin removed) twice a day
- **Barley grass juice powder:** 2 teaspoons or 6 capsules daily
- **Burdock root:** 1 cup of tea or 1 root freshly juiced daily
- **Cat's claw:** 3 dropperfuls twice a day
- **Chaga mushroom:** 2 teaspoons or 6 capsules daily
- **Curcumin:** 1 capsule twice a day
- **Ginger:** 1 cup of tea twice a day or freshly grated or juiced to taste daily
- **Goldenseal:** 4 dropperfuls twice a day (two weeks on, two weeks off)
- **Lemon balm:** 4 dropperfuls twice a day
- **Licorice root:** 1 dropperful twice a day (two weeks on, two weeks off)
- **Mullein leaf:** 4 dropperfuls twice a day
- **Olive leaf:** 3 dropperfuls twice a day
- **Oregano oil:** 1 capsule twice a day
- **Oregon grape root:** 2 dropperfuls twice a day (two weeks on, two weeks off)

- **Spirulina:** 2 teaspoons or 6 capsules daily
- **Turmeric:** 2 capsules daily
- **Vitamin B$_{12}$ (as adenosylcobalamin with methylcobalamin):** 1 dropperful twice a day
- **Vitamin C (as Micro-C):** 4 capsules twice a day
- **Zinc (as liquid zinc sulfate):** up to 1 dropperful twice a day

Supplements for UTIs (Urinary Tract Infections), Bladder Infections, Yeast Infections, and Bacterial Vaginosis (BV)

- **Fresh celery juice:** work up to 32 ounces daily
- **Aloe vera:** 2 or more inches of fresh gel (skin removed) daily
- **Amla berry:** 2 teaspoons twice a day
- **Barley grass juice powder:** 2 teaspoons or 6 capsules daily
- **Cat's claw:** 3 dropperfuls twice a day
- **Chaga mushroom:** 2 teaspoons or 6 capsules daily
- **D-mannose:** 1 tablespoon powder in water four times a day
- **Goldenseal:** 4 dropperfuls twice a day (two weeks on, two weeks off)
- **Hibiscus:** 2 cups of tea daily
- **Lemon balm:** 4 dropperfuls twice a day

- **Lomatium root:** 2 dropperfuls twice a day
- **Mullein leaf:** 3 dropperfuls twice a day
- **Olive leaf:** 2 dropperfuls twice a day
- **Oregon grape root:** 1 dropperful twice a day (two weeks on, two weeks off)
- **Raw honey:** 1 tablespoon daily
- **Rose hips:** 2 cups of tea daily
- **Thyme:** 2 sprigs of fresh thyme in hot water as tea or 4 sprigs in room temperature water twice a day
- **Vitamin C (as Micro-C):** after optional Medical Medium Vitamin C Shock Therapy, 6 capsules twice a day
- **Zinc (as liquid zinc sulfate):** after optional Medical Medium Zinc Shock Therapy for two days, up to 2 dropperfuls twice a day

CASE HISTORY:
Not *Candida* After All
1992

Margaret was a 42-year-old kindergarten teacher when she started to experience extreme fatigue. Even if she got a full night's sleep, she'd wake up unrested and feel tired for the remainder of the day.

Soon her elbows, knees, and ankles began to feel tender and achy, and she had trouble getting up and down from the floor for circle time with her class. Foods that used to give her no problem were now causing gastrointestinal distress, and she constantly felt bloated. On top of all this, Margaret periodically ran hot or cold, and started to dress in layers so she could adjust at a moment's notice to her sweat spells or freezing fingers.

When Margaret returned to school yawning and with dark circles under her eyes after a long weekend of doing nothing, her assistant teacher suggested she get a checkup. At Margaret's visit to her regular M.D., he took a blood sample to test for thyroid issues. After the doctor got the results, he called to say that nothing was wrong. "You're perfectly fine."

Unsatisfied, Margaret asked her sister for the name of the functional medicine doctor she'd raved about. As Margaret sat fanning herself in the doctor's air-conditioned exam room, he smiled knowingly. "The problems you've been experiencing are hormonal," he said, and added that it was possibly a disorder or the initial stages of perimenopause. Either way, the doctor insisted that the issue had coupled with *Candida* to cause her symptoms.

Margaret was so relieved she had to fight the urge to hug the doctor. She finally felt she had an answer. She bounded out of his office with prescriptions for bioidentical hormone replacement therapy (BHRT) and antifungal medication, as well as a printout explaining the need to clean up her diet and eliminate processed sugar, processed oil, and fried food.

After taking the 10-day course of the antifungal drug, she didn't feel better. She returned to the functional medicine doctor to say that, in fact, her gut felt worse. He sold her a probiotic and assured her that it would take care of the discomfort. A week later, even with the probiotics, the BHRT, and her new diet, Margaret was doubling over with stomach cramps during show-and-tell at school.

This time, Margaret decided to go to a naturopath. The naturopath nodded as Margaret recounted her story, then agreed that hormonal imbalances and *Candida* were to blame. To address the *Candida*, the doctor put her on a round of colon cleanse supplements and directed her to remove all carbohydrates from her diet. Margaret was to eat mainly animal protein and vegetables.

School was out for the summer by now, so Margaret devoted herself to applying the naturopath's recommendations, even cutting out her favorite balsamic vinaigrette and nightly glass of wine. Her aches and pains, she estimated, felt about 15 percent better from the changes. It seemed like she was on the right track . . . but she couldn't improve past that initial uptick.

The naturopath put her on another cleanse program, but now Margaret watched her progress dissipate. Her tenderness and achiness were back, she developed extreme gas, and she was more fatigued than ever (which I would later tell her was because she had no carbohydrates to carry her). Margaret longed for berries, grapefruit, and bananas—but the naturopath had scared her away from even going near fruit. Through sheer determination, she kept sugar out of her diet for another 30 days and didn't consume carbs of any kind.

Now, she feared that she was worse than before she'd sought help. She felt hopeless and sequestered from the world, completely unsure how she'd function once school started back up in a few weeks. The *Candida* she'd been diagnosed with, she felt, was destroying her quality of life.

At this stage, Margaret found me. Spirit quickly gave me the reading that *Candida* wasn't the problem at all. In fact, it was nearly nonexistent in Margaret's body. The real reason for her suffering was an undiagnosed case of the stomach bacteria *H. pylori*, coupled with the cytomegalovirus (in the herpes family). Her liver was sluggish, functioning at only 40 percent, versus the 65 percent typical for a woman her age. And she had very low hydrochloric acid in her gastric fluid, as well as a moderate amount of mercury-based toxic heavy metal poisoning.

When I brought this up, Margaret recalled that she'd had her metal dental fillings removed six months prior to the onset of her condition. I explained that during the removal process, mercury had been released into her system, saturating and overloading her liver. This had fed and grown the cytomegalovirus and *H. pylori* and diminished the hydrochloric acid she critically needed.

To address the situation, I made a quick adjustment to Margaret's diet plan. We reduced her animal fat and animal protein intake, and allowed certain fruits back into rotation, including wild blueberries, apricots, and even dates. The rest of her diet consisted of vegetables, herbs, leafy greens, potatoes, avocados, various additional fruits, and wild salmon—with an overall emphasis on low fat. With this change, her body was able to drive out a large amount of mercury from her intestinal tract and liver. It also shut down the growth of *H. pylori* immediately and lowered the cytomegalovirus load.

By September, Margaret had gotten better enough to greet her new class in good spirits. Within three months of our first call, she'd lost all of her symptoms—which were never *Candida* or hormone issues to begin with—and completely recovered her health.

"Today, what typically happens, especially in alternative medicine, is that your chronic, long-term symptoms of fatigue and digestive issues are blamed on Candida —or, more and more often, SIBO. Eventually SIBO will take the lead as the Candida diagnosis of the future. As I've said elsewhere, SIBO is the new Candida."

— Anthony William, Medical Medium

CHAPTER 10

Migraines

A large part of the global population suffers from migraines or recurring headaches of varying types. Some people experience migraines in the back of the head, some on the top of the head, some at the temple, some in the eyes—to name only a few variations. Migraines can also be experienced as intense pulsing or throbbing focused on one side, or a migraine can feel like it takes over the person's entire head and neck. The majority of migraine sufferers are women, although anyone can be struck with migraines, at any age, even children. Migraines can make life very difficult to navigate.

Those familiar with migraines know well that the pain may be accompanied by extreme sensitivity to light, sound, and/or smell; blurry vision; seeing flashes of light; nausea and/or vomiting; difficulty speaking; and lightheadedness that can result in fainting spells. A migraine can last anywhere from a couple of hours to several days and may rob you of the desire to do anything but lie down in a dark, quiet room until it's over.

This mystery illness can be debilitating, making it difficult to maintain a job or enjoy a social life. People with migraines often feel that they have to schedule their lives around their headaches. They're constantly trying to predict whether meetings, appointments, or lunch out with friends will be ruined by a migraine.

For some, it even becomes a superstition—they can't mention the word *migraine* for fear they'll trigger one. Some people have told me it feels like life imprisonment. The sense that migraines rule over you and control your every move—as well as the degrading effects of physical pain—can make sufferers feel extremely vulnerable and emotionally sensitive.

This is a complex mystery illness. The combination of issues that trigger it is different for each person. Doctors try to treat migraines with drug "cocktails" on a trial-and-error basis. If one group of drugs doesn't work, your doctor will put you on another, and another, until you start to experience some symptom relief. However, side effects of the drugs can create entirely new problems; plus they might work only temporarily. In some cases, the body can develop resistance to a drug over time—yet weaning yourself off the medication can trigger migraines, too.

This chapter offers information on migraines that's never been brought to the table. It reveals the secrets behind migraines' many triggers and points you toward recovery.

MIGRAINE TRIGGERS

Medical communities don't know what causes most migraines. That's in part why they have a haphazard approach to treating them. So far, the big theory is that a neuropeptide released in the trigeminal system (cranial nerves) results in head pain for people particularly sensitive to the compound. Other theories include that it's all in your gut—that your microorganisms are out of balance, that maybe you have leaky gut, that your microbiome is "off"—or that in women, migraines are hormonal—because for many women, migraines tend to worsen at certain points in their menstrual cycle. (More on that later.)

In fact, it's often not just one thing but a combination of issues that triggers a migraine. Below, I'll lay out the most common triggers. Read through the descriptions and do your best to identify the ones that apply to you—and fully address each one so you can begin your healing process.

Also be aware that you shouldn't stop looking after you identify a single cause. Migraines often result from a cluster of causes—two, three, four, or more issues that *collectively* act as a trigger. For example, if you're not getting enough sleep, and you're under chronic stress, but otherwise you're healthy, you probably won't get migraines. But if you also have toxic heavy metal exposure (such as to mercury or aluminum) and on top of that you're eating dairy and eggs (foods that can be mucus-forming because they feed pathogens such as EBV, other viruses, and bacteria such as *Streptococcus*, and these pathogens can release poisons that are allergenic), then the lack of sleep, stress, toxic heavy metals, and pathogens could combine to push your system over the edge and trigger a migraine.

The Usual Suspects

There are certain conditions that are well known for creating migraine symptoms. A trustworthy doctor will first go through the following checklist to see if you have any of these issues. If you suffer from migraines, you've no doubt visited multiple doctors and explored a variety of contributing factors and diagnostic tests. Just for reinforcement, here's the list:

- **Concussion:** a traumatic brain injury, usually caused by a blow to the head or violent shaking of the head and upper body. If you've experienced anything that might have resulted in a concussion, tell your doctor about it. Even if you had a concussion a long time ago and the migraines didn't start until much later, it could have triggered the sensitivity.

- **Meningitis:** severe inflammation and swelling of the protective membranes surrounding the brain and spinal cord. This is typically caused by a viral infection. Other causes are bacteria and certain drugs. If you once had meningitis, even a long time ago, chances are it was a trigger for your future migraine sensitivity, especially if it was viral meningitis.

- **Stroke:** a brain injury in which the blood supply to part of the brain is interrupted or greatly reduced, causing brain cells to die from lack of nutrition and oxygen. This is the easily identified, injury-induced type of stroke.

- **Transient ischemic attack (TIA):** this results in a smaller brain injury than a stroke; it can be so subtle that it's not even felt when it happens, but it can have a substantial impact on health.

- **Brain aneurysm:** the ballooning of a blood vessel in the brain.

- **Brain tumor:** an abnormal mass of tissue in the brain. A tumor can be cancerous or benign, but both types can create migraines.

- **Brain cyst or microcyst:** a sac filled with air, fluid, or other material (usually benign) that forms in the brain.

- **Impeded cervical nerves:** the cervical nerves are eight nerves branching off from the spinal cord that help control different areas of the body. The first two cervical nerves (C1 and C2) control the head. If something interferes with them, a variety of issues can result, including migraines.

If you've gone through the battery of tests, reviewed your medical history with your doctors, and ruled out the elements on the list above, then you're in the mystery realm. What follows are explanations of migraine triggers that medical communities don't yet fully understand . . . along with triggers that I'm disclosing here for the first time.

Epstein-Barr Virus and Shingles

Doctors don't know that millions of people suffer from migraines as a result of the Epstein-Barr virus (EBV), or even the shingles virus.

As explained in Chapter 3, EBV continually inflames your central nervous system—which includes your brain. If EBV or its neurotoxins get into or onto your vagus nerve, the inflamed nerve can be a migraine trigger.

Alternatively, shingles can inflame your trigeminal and/or phrenic nerves, which also have the potential to trigger migraines. Herpes simplex 1 (HSV-1), the virus behind the common fever blister, can also nest within the trigeminal and/or phrenic nerves, elevating their inflammation ever so slightly, just enough to be a trigger.

To learn if you're being afflicted by the Epstein-Barr virus, read Chapter 3 and see whether you have other EBV symptoms beyond these headaches. If you do, then follow Chapter 3's instructions to fight the virus. To learn whether the shingles virus may be the culprit, read Chapter 11. Taming your EBV or shingles may be all you need to do to end your migraines.

Micro-Transient Ischemic Attack Trigger

Micro-transient ischemic attack is similar to transient ischemic attack, but on a much smaller scale. Medical communities are not yet aware that this micro-stroke-like activity can occur—and trigger migraines.

Sinus-Related Migraines

Some migraines stem from chronic strep-tococcal infections that sit in the linings of the sinus cavity. In these cases, ear, nose, and throat specialists often recommend sinus surgery to remove scar tissue. Because strep is very difficult to remove once it gets into the sinus linings, if these surgical procedures work at all, then the relief they give patients is only temporary.

A better way to address sinus-related migraines is to strengthen the immune system so that the body can naturally fight infection. The recommendations in this chapter and in Part IV, "How to Finally Heal," will guide you through that. Also check the "Healing Herbs and Supplements" section of Chapter 9, "Candida," for a supplement protocol that's helpful for those with a history of chronic sinus infections and sinusitis.

Ammonia Permeability Trigger

Another major migraine culprit is a burdened gut. Medical communities don't know that when your digestive system isn't working properly, ammonia gas can drift out from your gut to your vagus, phrenic, and/or trigeminal nerves. Ammonia can cross the blood-brain barrier and find its way into all parts of the central nervous system. As the gas deprives the brain of some of its needed oxygen, tension can arise and these nerves can spasm, creating migraines.

To determine whether this is happening to you—and, if so, how to fix the problem—read Chapter 17, "Gut Health."

Electrolyte Deficiency Trigger

To remain healthy, your body must maintain a certain level of *electrolytes*. These electrolytes are used to maintain neurotransmitters, strengthen neurons, and send the electrical nerve impulses that run your body and your brain, which is the center of your body's electrical activity. When you run low on electrolytes, it can severely disrupt the activity of your brain, which puts a load on your central nervous system and sets off migraines, especially if you're someone with toxic heavy metals inside the brain or you're living with a chronic low-grade viral infection like EBV.

The most common cause of electrolyte deficiency is chronic dehydration, often caused by caffeine beverages, foods that are dehydrating, and a lack of fresh juices and good water. Celery juice and coconut water (that's not pink or red) are top sources of electrolytes to replenish your supply. If you can't drink 16 ounces or more of celery juice or bring in coconut water, then try to drink a daily minimum of 12 ounces of cucumber, cucumber-apple, or celery-apple juice (the blends can be half-and-half). Also, 16 to 32 ounces of lemon water is a great way to defeat electrolyte deficiency and chronic dehydration.

Stress Trigger

Everyone feels stress now and then, in both big and small ways. Some of us have been through so much more than others. If you experience chronic stress, then you're up against a lot of fight-or-flight, where adrenaline surges can occur on a daily basis. Adrenaline is extremely stimulating and has an up-and-down pattern of charging us up, then dropping us down. This influx of an adrenaline "up" for someone who's very sensitive, especially if they have chronic illness, can be enough to create a hypertensive reaction that can tighten specific areas such as the trigeminal nerves, resulting in a migraine trigger. This can even trigger migraines on a daily or weekly basis.

For ways to ease your mental tension, read Chapter 24, "Soul-Healing Meditations and Techniques."

Menstrual Cycle Trigger

Many female migraine sufferers notice that their migraines come on right before, during, or after their menstrual cycle. This is because when a woman is menstruating, her reproductive system requires 80 percent of her body's immune system functionality. If your body is fending off other triggers such as stress, heavy metal toxicity, dehydration, or, most often, viruses or bacteria such as EBV or strep, then when menstruation happens, *boom,* you can end up with a migraine, because those reserves and immune system power switch over to helping the reproductive system. This is why such a large proportion of migraine sufferers are women. Men's immune systems don't switch over to the reproductive system once a month, leaving the rest of the body vulnerable to low-grade viral infections and effects from toxic heavy metals.

If this trigger is the case for you, turn your attention to minimizing other possible causes so that your monthly cycle will have less chance of overwhelming your system.

Sleep Disorders

If you aren't getting enough sound sleep, then if you're also dealing with other issues such as toxic heavy metals, other toxic troublemakers, viral symptoms, or other symptoms and conditions, that lack of sleep can be a trigger for your migraine.

If you have a sleep disorder such as insomnia, take comfort: as you lie awake in bed with your eyes closed, half of your brain can actually sleep while the other half is awake. This means that your body is still healing and your central nervous system is still rejuvenating—so if you can, try not to get frustrated or angry when you have a wakeful night. Understanding this secret alone will make you less susceptible to sleep-related migraines.

If it's a physical illness that creates insomnia and is covered by this book—e.g., EBV, shingles, Lyme disease—use the advice in the pertinent chapter and in Part IV, "How to Finally Heal," to help recover from it.

If you're not getting enough sleep because there aren't enough hours in the day with all of your obligations, try to think about where you can cut back. It may feel impossible. Since the alternative is losing hours or days to migraines, though, carving out more hours for sleep is a better trade. You deserve to respect your body's limits.

Heavy Metals and Other Environmental Toxic Triggers

Toxic heavy metals such as mercury, aluminum, lead, copper, arsenic, cadmium, nickel, and barium can settle into the brain and other organs, such as the liver, and affect their ability to function properly. Potential consequences include anxiety, depression, obsessive-compulsive disorder (OCD), attention-deficit/hyperactivity disorder (ADHD), autism spectrum disorder (ASD), bipolar disorder, depersonalization, Alzheimer's, dementia, tics, and spasms. Another possible result is migraines.

There are also thousands of questionable or flat-out toxic chemicals that you're regularly exposed to in your office or other workplace, your home, your food, your water, the air you breathe, and so on. These chemicals can eventually enter your brain and disrupt its electrical impulses. Many of us have no control over our environments—what we breathe, what we're exposed to—but we do have the power to remove these toxins from our bodies. For information on that, see Chapter 18, "Freeing Your Brain and Body of Toxins." In some cases, continual detoxing—coupled with any possible avoidance of new toxins—is enough to eventually stop migraines.

Common Migraine Food Triggers

You're unlikely to get migraines from eating a certain food if you don't have pathogens such as viruses or bacteria.

The chances are that *multiple* issues are contributing to your condition—and the following foods are very likely to be triggers:

- **Dairy:** mucus-forming because it feeds all unproductive bacteria and viruses such as EBV and *Streptococcus* in the gut and the body. This overburdens the liver, ultimately leading to an overburdened lymphatic system. Toxins released from viruses and/or the additional mucus created

by these viruses and bacteria put pressure on the central nervous system.

- **Eggs:** feed all viruses and all unproductive bacteria, allowing them to proliferate and expel neurotoxins and other pathogenic byproducts that can irritate the central nervous system. This can, in turn, inflame the phrenic, vagus, and/or trigeminal nerves, and even areas of the brain itself, leading to a migraine.

- **Gluten (e.g., wheat, rye, barley, spelt):** gluten feeds unproductive bacteria such as *Streptococcus* and viruses, which then release neurotoxins and other byproducts that can result in inflammation. The immune system becomes burdened down as pathogens increase in strength. All of this can trigger existing migraines, making them worse.

- **Meat (e.g., beef, chicken, pork):** when you have a weakened digestive system, including low hydrochloric acid, and a liver that's overburdened and can't produce enough bile, then when these proteins and rancid fats rot, ammonia production can occur, minimizing oxygen levels to the brain, creating a migraine trigger.

- **Fermented foods (e.g., pickles, vinegar [including ACV], sauerkraut, kimchi, ketchup):** fermented or vinegar-based foods lower the pH in the intestinal tract, making your intestinal tract more acidic, which can trigger migraines. Apple cider vinegar (ACV) alone is a trigger for most people with migraines.

- **Salt:** try to avoid excessive salt if possible. Consider bringing celery juice or Medical Medium Spinach Soup (recipe in Chapter 23) into your diet. Add lemon to your water, too. If you're going to use salt, use a high-quality sea salt or rock salt. Do not use table salt.

- **Oils:** canola, corn, cottonseed, and palm oil are fats that burden the liver and thicken the blood. Canola and corn oil, especially when GMO, can feed pathogens, creating inflammation.

- **Additives (e.g., MSG, aspartame):** these are neurotoxic and can be aggressive triggers for migraine sufferers.

- **Alcohol:** extremely dehydrating, and also hard on the liver.

- **Coffee drinks, matcha tea, chocolate, cacao, and other caffeine:** overstimulating and highly aggressive to the central nervous system, caffeine acts as a neurotoxin that can trigger migraines. Some people claim that chocolate and other forms of caffeine can help a migraine—because the truth is these people are in and out of withdrawal. They've experienced that effect because caffeine triggers the adrenals to flood the body with adrenaline, which acts as a steroid for the inflammation that causes migraines. Over time, though, that caffeine has unproductive repercussions.

To facilitate your healing, it's highly recommended that you stop eating all of the above *at least* until your migraines go away. If that's too difficult, start with the choices you think you can handle and take it from there. It's very positive to be proactive in any way.

Allergic Reactions

When you encounter something to which you're allergic, your body makes histamine to protect you from the potentially dangerous substance. Low-grade viral infections such as EBV are constantly releasing neurotoxins, byproduct, and other viral waste matter. This can raise histamines all on its own, making you more sensitive and allergic to different things at different times. In some cases your body may overreact and produce too much histamine—and this can contribute to migraines. The reaction may be delayed, occurring days after eating an allergenic food—a food that may not seem allergenic, yet can feed pathogens, creating toxins that make you more sensitive in a variety of ways.

Think about whether there's anything you're eating, drinking, breathing, touching, or otherwise exposed to that might be giving you a migraine or headache. This can range from secondhand smoke, to pollen, to a new neighbor's pet.

If your migraines began only recently, pay special attention to anything with the potential to be allergenic that was introduced into your life shortly before your first episode. For example, plug-in air fresheners, scented candles, cologne, perfume, aftershave, and incense are all migraine triggers. Once you identify all possible causes for a migraine reaction, try to cut them out and see if that eliminates your migraines. Your intuition about what you're sensitive to is far more accurate than doctor's office testing, which can be flawed, so make a point to listen to your body and stay aware.

Addressing Migraines

As you've just seen, there are a dizzying number of potential triggers for migraines. If you've identified the likely causes for your headaches, then the most helpful thing you can do is eliminate the triggers from your life.

Herbs and supplements, as well as healing foods, are also important. They will help lower your pain and inflammation, mitigate allergic reactions, soothe nerves, help calm you, improve your liver health, starve and kill off pathogens, and provide a mild detox.

Healing Foods

Specific foods can help prevent and/or heal your migraines by killing off pathogens, flushing out toxins, bolstering brain tissue, improving digestion through your liver and stomach glands, soothing nerves, providing critical nutrients, and relaxing muscles. Fresh celery juice, cilantro, hemp seeds (in small amounts), potatoes, bananas, asparagus, oranges, brussels sprouts, tomatoes, broccoli, spinach, papayas, chili peppers, garlic, ginger, kale, cinnamon, and apples are among the top foods to eat for addressing migraines. Incorporate as many of these foods into your diet as you can.

Healing Herbs and Supplements

Before applying these, be sure to read Chapter 21, "Critical Guide to Supplement Protocols."

Supplements for Headaches and Migraines

- **Fresh celery juice:** work up to 32 ounces daily
- **Celeryforce:** 3 capsules three times a day
- **Ashwagandha:** 1 dropperful twice a day
- **Barley grass juice powder:** 2 teaspoons or 6 capsules daily
- **Cat's claw:** 2 dropperfuls twice a day
- **CoQ10:** 1 capsule daily
- **Curcumin:** 3 capsules twice a day
- **Elderflower:** 1 cup of tea daily
- **Feverfew:** 2 dropperfuls or 2 capsules daily
- **Goldenseal:** 1 dropperful twice a day (two weeks on, two weeks off)
- **Kava kava:** 2 dropperfuls or 2 capsules daily
- **Lemon balm:** 4 dropperfuls twice a day
- **L-lysine:** 4 500-milligram capsules twice a day
- **Magnesium glycinate:** 2 capsules twice a day

- **Nettle leaf:** 4 dropperfuls twice a day

- **Oregano oil:** 2 capsules daily

- **Skullcap:** 2 dropperfuls or 2 capsules twice a day

- **Spirulina:** 2 teaspoons or 6 capsules daily

- **Turmeric:** 2 capsules twice a day

- **Vitamin B$_{12}$ (as adenosylcobalamin with methylcobalamin):** 2 dropperfuls twice a day

- **Vitamin C (as Micro-C):** 4 capsules twice a day

- **White willow bark:** 2 dropperfuls or 2 capsules daily

- **Wild blueberry powder:** 1 tablespoon daily

CASE HISTORY:
In the Dark No More
2007

Erica had been suffering from migraines since she was 10 years old. She could remember the first one clearly: she'd been standing under the bright stage lights in a school play when out of nowhere, a pain developed in the back of her head that suddenly intensified and radiated to the side of her head.

After that, Erica learned that the only way to manage a migraine was to lie in a dark, silent room. Sometimes the headache would radiate to the other side of her head. Sometimes the pain would make her vomit. When she got older, migraines often hit before, during, or even shortly after her menstrual cycle. She also noticed that being a passenger in a car could trigger the headaches, as could staying out a little too late with friends. Any kind of emotional conflict could start the pulsing, too.

Now 30 years old, Erica was having problems with her boyfriend of three years.

Derek couldn't understand Erica's need for extra rest and quiet. "I don't appreciate having to tiptoe around my own apartment," he'd say. He also couldn't grasp why his girlfriend didn't join him anymore for a few drinks out on the town. Erica would tell him it was because she'd get a migraine from the late night and cocktails, and Derek would go out without her, sending texts about how noble he was for not hooking up with the cute girls at the bar. This always sent Erica into a tailspin, and they'd exchange angry texts until the familiar pain took hold and she had to go lie down.

Erica never felt relief from the many different medications her doctor prescribed. She tried to change her diet based on articles she came across, but that never seemed to be the answer, either. In search of relief, she visited neurologists, nutritionists who specialized in food allergies, and even a psychotherapist when she'd begun to feel isolated and lost.

An integrative medical doctor diagnosed Erica with an overabundance of *Candida* and told her to remove all sugars from her diet . . . but she didn't get any real results

When Erica called me, her voice was quiet. She said Derek was in the other room, and he'd make fun of her if he knew she was still looking for ways to get better. He'd told her he had a theory that she had a victim mentality, and that her "migraines" were an elaborate scheme to get more attention.

The first thing Spirit instructed me to tell Erica was that this was nonsense. Her pain was all too real.

Then I told Erica that Spirit said she had high levels of mercury in her brain and liver, due in part to heavy metal exposure when she was a child. This wasn't all: she was also chronically dehydrated, as well as allergic to eggs, dairy, and wheat gluten. She'd developed deficiencies in nutrients critical to her nervous system, including vitamin B$_{12}$, zinc, selenium, and molybdenum. These were also essential cofactors to electrolyte preservation.

To help Erica heal, Spirit advocated potassium-rich foods for rehydration, cilantro for heavy metal removal, and straight celery juice as a source of much-needed mineral salt for the central nervous system. Following this protocol, Erica started to balance out quickly. She stayed away from the instigative foods mentioned in this chapter, focused on staying hydrated, got plenty of rest, and started taking several of the supplements from the "Healing Herbs and Supplements" section.

For the first time in 20 years, she was now migraine free.

And for the first time in three years, she was free of Derek. With a clear head, she'd reevaluated their relationship and decided to set her sights higher.

"Never forget the power of your steps toward healing. Whenever you work to take care of yourself, your own pursuit of truth and vitality helps free others."

— Anthony William, Medical Medium

CHAPTER 11

Shingles—True Cause of Colitis, TMJ, Diabetic Neuropathy, and More

In the medical world, *shingles* seems like an open-and-shut case. You've got a patient with the textbook rash, skin pain on the side or back, and that's all, folks.

If that were true, there wouldn't be any need for this chapter.

The truth is that the shingles virus is responsible for millions of people's mystery symptoms, from rashes that confound dermatologists to neurological symptoms like twitching, tingling, burning, spasms, chronic migraines, headaches, and much more. Undiscovered varieties of shingles are responsible for Bell's palsy, frozen shoulder, diabetic nerve pain, colitis, vaginal burning, TMJ, trigeminal neuralgia, sciatica, tooth and gum pain, tooth grinding, jaw pain, burning tongue, many cases of Lyme disease, and even misdiagnosed MS.

Shingles is an illness that can result in fever, headaches, rashes, joint pain, muscle pain, neck pain, sharp nerve pain, burning nerve pain, and other highly unpleasant symptoms. The earliest shingles strains came into existence around the turn of the 20th century. Medical communities believe shingles is caused by the *zoster* virus, which is a species in the herpes family. And that's actually correct—as far as it goes.

What medical research and science don't yet know is that there isn't merely one type of shingles virus, but *31* varieties and counting. This matters because different types of shingles cause different symptoms. It also matters because medical communities don't even recognize the majority of shingles cases as being the result of a virus. For example, any of the more aggressive varieties of shingles can cause Lyme disease (including neurological Lyme) symptoms. (For more on Lyme disease, see Chapter 16.)

This chapter covers the 15 types of shingles virus from which people most commonly suffer, and which are almost always treated improperly, sometimes with immunosuppressant drugs, steroids, and antibiotics that could lessen a patient's quality of life. You'll learn about shingles symptoms, how the virus is transmitted and triggered, the unique qualities of many strains of shingles, and how to most effectively deal with the two major categories of shingles—those that cause rashes and those that don't—so you can identify and overcome whatever version of the virus you have and live a healthy life.

SHINGLES SYMPTOMS

Signs that you could be suffering from the onset of a shingles infection include flu-like fever and chills, headaches or migraines, aches and pains, burning pain, itching, tingling, red rash, and/or pustules (blisters on the skin containing pus).

Medical communities believe that those last two symptoms—red rash and pustules—always accompany shingles. In fact, this is merely the classic presentation of one type of the zoster virus. It's usually on the lower back, upper back, rib cage, shoulder, or neck. If a patient displays pustules and blisters that look different than the barcode-style rash, and the blisters and pustules are in unusual areas, doctors often won't consider it shingles at all. This is a common diagnostic error. Seven of the strains of shingles *do* cause rashes somewhere on the body, just not always in expected areas.

And the other eight strains cause *no* rashes. So if you're experiencing most of the symptoms of shingles but have no signs of it on your skin, and your doctor can't identify a reason for your suffering, there's a good chance you're the victim of a non-rashing shingles virus.

SHINGLES TRANSMISSION AND TRIGGERS

As with any virus in the herpes family, there are numerous ways to catch shingles. You can get it passed down from your parents, through a transfusion of infected blood, via an exchange of bodily fluids, from a public bathroom . . . and even from the blood of a chef's cut finger while eating out!

The Chicken Pox Myth

Contrary to the current beliefs of medical research and science, one way that you *can't* get shingles is through chicken pox. Your doctor may tell you that if you've had chicken pox, sooner or later you'll get shingles. This is not the case. The only thing chicken pox has in common with shingles is that they're both viruses in the herpes family that can cause a rash. Chicken pox is an entirely different species of herpes virus from shingles. They essentially have nothing to do with each other.

Why are we being told shingles is chicken pox–related when it's not? This is a prime example of misinformation that was accepted at one point because it *sounded* like it made sense, then was perpetuated to the point where it's now ingrained. Not to mention that medical research and science don't have a lot of accountability when it comes to viruses. They lack information and know very little in this area. The plague of COVID has shown this to be true.

Dormancy and Triggers

If you're infected by shingles or harboring one of the older varieties of the virus, you probably won't know it for a long time. The chances are you'll carry the virus around for at least 10 years, possibly even 50 years or more, before it strikes. With newer shingles varieties and mutations, the dormancy period can be much shorter, meaning that symptoms could appear just months after becoming infected.

The virus hides in one of your organs—typically your liver—where it can't be detected by your immune system. It bides its time until some traumatic physical or emotional event weakens you and/or provides an environment that makes the virus stronger (for example, feeding the virus the foods it likes to eat). Events such as a betrayal, financial stress, or a broken heart can sometimes be enough to act as a trigger.

If you have an especially strong immune system, and/or if you're spared from shingles triggers, some varieties of shingles virus might remain in their dormant state for your entire life and never cause you notable harm.

Then again, if your immune system is a bit shaky (for example, from a zinc deficiency, toxic exposure to toxic heavy metals or other troublemakers, or other viruses such as EBV or herpes simplex 1), the shingles virus might leave its hiding place and embark on little forays into your body even before a trigger leads to a major outbreak. The virus will typically go into your lower spine, inflaming the sciatic nerve. So if you periodically feel lower back pain that seems to come and go for no apparent reason, it could be a shingles virus shuttling between your liver and spine. In many cases, when shingles gets into the lower spine, it can create debilitating and even crippling back pain. Often if the pain persists, a specialist will recommend surgery. In many cases, surgery does not help, and the pain continues,

sometimes even becoming worse. If you've had a back surgery and the outcome wasn't as beneficial as you'd expected, consider that you could have a simultaneous shingles virus infection creating inflammation and pain.

The best strategy against both minor and major shingles attacks is preventative—that is, to steer clear of situations that might embolden the virus to leave its dormant state. One easier way of doing this is to avoid foods that feed the shingles virus.

SHINGLES WITH RASHES

There are seven strains of shingles that cause rashes. While the resulting pustules are painful, if they're in an easy-to-spot location that the doctor associates with the standard variety of shingles and they look like the classic version doctors are accustomed to from medical school, in a sense they can be a blessing—because the rash makes it more likely that your doctor will at least realize you have shingles and not call the condition idiopathic or a mystery rash. However, most shingles rashes may be unidentifiable to the doctor because of their location or pattern.

These seven strains have very similar symptoms. They're primarily distinguished by the different types and locations of rashes they create.

Classic Shingles

Rash appears anywhere from the chest to the thighs. This might include a rash on the lower back or near the top of the buttocks. It can also include one side of the body or the other, or one leg or the other (but not both).

This is the variety you see on TV commercials about the condition, and it's the type that's (wrongly) associated with chicken pox. This is one of the most common strains of shingles—and what doctors mistakenly believe is the only type.

Upper Body Shingles

Rash appears from the chest up—e.g., on the upper chest, shoulders, or neck—but not on the arms. This rash is the closest in appearance to the most common shingles variety.

Both Arms Shingles

Rash appears exclusively on *both* arms and on *both* hands. Also, the rash has an altered pattern, somewhat spotty, with large and small pustules sometimes spaced apart.

One Arm Shingles

Rash appears on one arm only. It can be either arm, but *not* both arms. This breakout also has an altered pattern, somewhat spotty, with large and small pustules spaced apart.

Head Shingles

Rash appears on the top and sides of the head (including the face). Also, you can have this variety inside the mouth—on the tongue, throat, or anywhere else in the mouth. The resulting pustules are tinier than those of the above strains, and they sometimes have little "horns" on top. Medical communities often misdiagnose this type as a fungus that needs to be treated with antifungal or steroid cream.

Both Legs Shingles

Rash appears on *both* legs, but nowhere else. It has a different appearance than standard shingles, with pustules that look almost like constellations.

Vaginal Area Shingles

Affecting only women, this strain causes a rash that appears outside but near the vagina—e.g., between the rectum and vagina, or on the lower buttocks, or inside the crotch area. This strain is especially notable because doctors often misdiagnose it as sexually transmitted herpes . . . creating unnecessary emotional pain for hundreds of thousands of women globally. The primary way to tell these illnesses apart is that this strain of the shingles virus causes substantial pain, while genital herpes—i.e., herpes simplex virus 2, or HSV-2—is typically less painful. Also, this shingles virus creates pustules that are relatively spread out in the genital area and/or lower buttocks, while HSV-2 pustules tend to cluster within a small area.

Shingles Neurotoxin

One of the misconceptions about shingles is that the virus is lurking directly within the skin rash. That's never the case. The virus lies much deeper under the skin, and even inside the bloodstream and liver at the very same time, positioning itself for the most effective inflammation possible of your nervous system.

However, the virus releases a unique mix of neurotoxin and dermatoxin; and in these seven strains, the viral poison travels outward to your peripheral nerves and your skin.

It's this neurotoxin-dermatoxin that causes the itchy, irritable red rashes and pustules for which shingles is famous.

Toxic heavy metals (such as mercury, aluminum, and copper) are some of the shingles virus's favorite foods. It's these metals that allow shingles to create its neurotoxin and dermatoxin. (Shingles also loves eggs; that's another one of the virus's favorite foods.)

While these seven strains create nerve damage both on the skin and far below it that can be quite painful, they're actually the mildest forms of shingles. If you have a strong immune system, and you do nothing to empower the virus, your body might drive out your shingles by itself.

SHINGLES WITHOUT RASHES

While this is entirely unknown to medical communities, there are eight strains of shingles that typically do *not* cause rashes.

As just explained, the rashes from the first seven strains result from a poison, or neurotoxin-dermatoxin, produced by the virus that travels outward into your peripheral nerves and skin.

The eight non-rashing strains produce a neurotoxin, too. In these cases the poison doesn't usually contain a dermatoxin element that moves outward into the small peripheral nerves and skin. Instead, the neurotoxin produced by non-rashing shingles travels *inward* into larger nerves. These nerves are already aggravated by the virus, but the neurotoxin inflames them even more. (Note that these varieties of shingles can still produce *some* dermatoxin that can create very mild mystery rashes in some cases.)

If you have one of these non-rashing varieties, in many cases you may undergo more internal pain and nerve injury than you would from the strains that cause rashes. Further, you'll feel these symptoms without any outward sign to let your doctor know you're being inflamed by a shingles virus. As a result, if your doctor isn't familiar with Medical Medium information, she or he may not have any idea that your symptoms are related to shingles and could instead recommend a battery of tests heading into an area of guessing games.

For example, your doctor may guess that you're suffering from an immune system that's mistaken a part of your body for an invader and has begun attacking it. As a treatment, your doctor may prescribe one or more immunosuppressant drugs or steroids to lessen the severity of the attack. However, as noted before, your immune system is not only entirely innocent of wrongdoing, it's your primary defense against the real source of harm. The drugs that make your immune system sleepy and docile therefore give the shingles virus the opportunity to further reproduce and become substantially stronger.

Another situation is if your doctor guesses that it's Lyme, decides you're being attacked by bacteria, and gives you antibiotics, which create a double blow to your health, as they weaken your immune system *and* strengthen the shingles virus. When nerves are inflamed by shingles, some antibiotics can have an abrasive effect, causing the nerves to hurt a little bit more. Your doctor may say that this is a "kill-off" of the Lyme bacteria. Meanwhile, it's sensitive nerves from the shingles.

You can help protect yourself against such situations by learning the characteristics of the eight non-rashing varieties of shingles.

Neuralgic Shingles (also known as Diabetic Neuropathy)

Neuralgic shingles—which primarily attacks the lower extremities, creating nerve pain, numbness, and/or burning in the legs and feet—is often called *diabetic neuropathy* and misidentified as a complication of diabetes. This is a huge medical myth that needs to be debunked. Unless there's an obvious injury or impediment to the nerves, the sensations a patient is feeling are *not* neuropathy, which doctors believe means that the nerves in a certain area have died. Rather, the nerves are inflamed, creating neuralgia.

And the truth is, there is no link whatsoever between diabetes and so-called diabetic neuropathy. (In fact, this shingles variety occurs more often in patients *without* diabetes than in patients with diabetes.) Doctors, though, have no idea that they're dealing with two separate problems, and so they either do nothing or attempt to treat the nerve issue with more medications—which makes the virus stronger.

Maddening Itch Shingles

This virus creates a continually moving itch that can't be scratched. That's because the virus is irritating nerves too far beneath the skin to be reached with fingers. There's no burning, so it's not especially painful; but having a perpetually roaming itch that you can't do anything to relieve can be maddening. If the virus is empowered by a weak immune system and/or by triggers, the severe itching can destroy your ability to get a solid night's sleep, hold a job, or otherwise lead a normal life.

Vaginal Shingles

This virus affects only women. It goes deep into the inner vaginal walls and inflames the nerves there. It also travels inside the bladder and rectum to wreak additional havoc, creating a burning so irritating it's akin to torture.

If a doctor doesn't dismiss it as being "all in your head" because she or he can't find the cause, she or he will typically misdiagnose it once again as a hormonal imbalance and prescribe hormones to treat it. This is not an effective treatment and can sometimes make the situation worse. Many women have truly suffered from this variety—and so far the medical industry has ignored it.

Colitis Shingles

Medical communities don't know that this virus is responsible for almost all cases of *colitis*, which is a condition that causes severe inflammation and bleeding in the inner lining of the colon. Colitis symptoms include intestinal pain, blood in the stool, weakness, and weight loss.

Colitis has always been a mystery illness and will continue to be so until medical research reveals that it's a variety of shingles. No one knows this yet! Society is once again three to four decades away from learning the truth.

Medical research and science believe colitis is an autoimmune condition where the immune system is attacking the lining of the colon, causing inflammation. This belief means that doctors typically try to treat colitis with immunosuppressant drugs or, even worse, antibiotics, which make the virus stronger. Steroids can put colitis in remission, but because the drugs don't address the shingles itself, the remission tends not to last.

Arm and Leg Burning Shingles

This virus creates a hot, burning pain in your arms and legs. Unlike the rash-based strains that attack arms or legs, with this strain the nerve inflammation and burning sensations all take place far below the skin, so you can't pinpoint them or relieve them.

And because no rash appears to indicate a shingles virus, doctors are likely to prescribe inappropriate medications that make the situation far worse.

Mouth Shingles, TMJ, and Bell's Palsy

This virus affects the gums and/or the area by the jaw. It's also responsible for Bell's palsy (viral inflammation of critical facial nerves), trigeminal neuralgia, and TMJ disorders (a result of trigeminal nerve inflammation and pain). It's frequently mistaken for a dental issue, leading to unnecessary root canals. Not only does the dental surgery not help, the medications involved weaken the immune system, which allows the virus to grow even stronger.

This viral torture of the mouth can go on for years.

Frozen Shoulder Shingles

This virus aggravates the nerves in the shoulder, causing it to freeze up for anywhere from a month to a year.

This condition is often misdiagnosed as infectious bursitis and treated with antibiotics . . . which only serves to make the virus much

stronger. Sometimes, unnecessary surgeries are even performed, since doctors have no idea that shingles is behind the affliction.

Body on Fire Shingles

This virus makes every part of your body feel like it's on fire, simultaneously and relentlessly. It operates by finding a central location by the ganglia deep in the nervous system and releasing its neurotoxin, which spreads throughout the body and inflames nerves everywhere. Needless to say, it creates a great deal of anxiety and fear . . . and these challenging emotions can prompt the adrenal glands to produce an abundant amount of intense adrenal hormones that can feed the virus and make it even stronger.

This is an especially terrible shingles condition, but thankfully, relatively rare. Keep in mind that the body always has the ability to heal—even from this uncommon variety. I've seen hundreds of people throughout the decades heal this condition with the right tools. There are also milder versions of this variety that can heal more quickly.

Healing Shingles

Being struck with any kind of shingles is painful and stressful. Whether you have a variety that creates a rash or doesn't, it can be maddening.

Fortunately, there are simple yet powerful Medical Medium protocols for this condition. The goal is to knock the virus back into a dormant state, kill off as much of it as possible, or kill it off altogether—to render it virtually harmless.

How long this process takes will depend on a variety of factors, including the amount of time the virus has been in your system, how many toxic heavy metals you have, and what you're doing in your diet (for example, are you eating eggs, dairy products, and gluten?). Also, medications taken throughout life get into our liver, making it stagnant and sluggish, which can lead to nutritional deficiencies because it can't function optimally. The healing timeline with shingles depends, too, on whether your immune system is being used to battle other viruses such as the Epstein-Barr virus, herpes simplex 1, or cytomegalovirus, or *Streptococcus* or other forms of bacteria. People who are living with the symptoms of shingles virus varieties are often dealing with additional symptoms from EBV. That can mean that it takes longer to rebuild your immune system.

Everybody is different in what they're up against. While it may take a little time to customize your protocol with the tools here to get it just right for you, you have all the information necessary to do so. And remember, the results are in. Countless people have already healed their shingles using this book. This information has already proven itself. If you work with these protocols, you have the ability to take yourself as far as you need to go and move past living a life with shingles symptoms. For additional support, read through Part IV, "How to Finally Heal."

Flare-Ups and Post-Shingles Symptoms

As you go through your healing process, keep in mind that you can still experience post-shingles symptoms that have the potential to last a little while. That's because nerves can take time to heal from the shingles neurotoxin and dermatoxin. So after you've battled a shingles infection or flare-up, these leftover neurological symptoms are not unexpected. They just take more time to fade.

Also be mindful that even after healing from shingles, it's critical to stay proactive with your antiviral measures. If you're not staying proactive after recovering from one case of shingles, you're still susceptible to periodic flare-ups of that shingles variety, or you could even contract a whole new case of shingles. Stay aware and continue to take care of yourself.

Healing Foods

Certain fruits, leafy greens, herbs, wild foods, and vegetables can greatly aid the body in healing from shingles with and without rashes. One reason is because certain foods won't feed the shingles virus—plus they have antiviral, antibacterial properties that can ward off, weaken, and even destroy virus cells. These foods can also help by, variously, supporting the body in recovery from neurotoxin and dermatoxin flare-ups, boosting the immune system, healing nerves and stimulating new nerve growth, soothing inflamed skin, and cleansing the body. The ideal foods to concentrate on are wild blueberries, garlic, ginger, celery, cilantro, sprouts, tomatoes, papayas, red-skinned apples, potatoes, artichokes, bananas, sweet potatoes, spinach, asparagus, lettuce (varieties that are leafy and deep green or red), green beans, kiwis, red pitaya (dragon fruit), and rosemary. Incorporate as many of these foods into your diet as you can.

Also take care to avoid the foods in Chapter 19, "What Not to Eat." When dealing with a shingles-caused symptom or condition, it's critical to begin the process of removing at least one or two of the foods that feed the virus. If you need to take your healing even further, try to acclimate yourself to removing all the foods that feed the virus.

Healing Herbs and Supplements

Before applying these, be sure to read Chapter 21, "Critical Guide to Supplement Protocols."

Supplements for Shingles (Trigeminal Neuralgia, TMJ, Frozen Shoulder, Ulcerative Colitis, Bell's Palsy; Many Cases of Neck Pain, Jaw Pain, Gum and Tooth Pain, Tongue Pain, Burning Sensations inside Mouth, Burning Sensations on Skin, Pain in Back of Head, Migraine-Related Pain, Mystery Sciatica, Mystery Lower Back Pain, Neuropathy)

- **Fresh celery juice:** work up to 32 ounces daily

- **Aloe vera:** 2 or more inches of fresh gel (skin removed) daily; also apply fresh gel to shingles rash

- **California poppy:** 3 capsules or 3 dropperfuls twice a day

- **Cat's claw:** 2 dropperfuls twice a day

- **Curcumin:** 3 capsules three times a day

- **Lemon balm:** 4 dropperfuls three times a day

- **Licorice root:** 2 dropperfuls twice a day (two weeks on, two weeks off)

- **L-lysine:** 6 capsules twice a day

- **Mullein leaf:** 4 dropperfuls twice a day

- **Nettle leaf:** 4 dropperfuls twice a day

- **Propolis:** 3 dropperfuls three times a day

- **Spirulina:** 1 teaspoon or 3 capsules daily

- **Vitamin B$_{12}$ (as adenosylcobalamin with methylcobalamin):** 3 dropperfuls twice a day

- **Vitamin C (as Micro-C):** 8 capsules twice a day

- **Zinc (as liquid zinc sulfate):** 2 dropperfuls twice a day

CASE HISTORY:
A Pain in the Jaw
2010

Terrence had always experienced fairly good health. He liked to play tennis, go on adventures with his friends, and work long hours at the consulting business he owned. When Terrence was 51 years old, though, he began to develop some sensitivity in his bottom right jaw. Every time he chewed anything on that side, a pain would radiate from his jaw into his face.

His dentist noticed an old metal amalgam filling in one of his molars and pinpointed it as the potential culprit. "There's a low-grade bacterial infection in your jaw," she said. Her solution was to dig out the filling and perform a root canal.

Following the procedure, Terrence experienced a change for the worse. The pain increased, affecting his entire jaw now and making it impossible to chew. The discomfort was barely manageable with mild pain medications. One morning, Terrence woke up with tension in his jaw. It was there every morning afterward.

At a return visit to the dentist, she concluded that Terrence needed more dental work. It seemed to her that the molar next to the tooth where she had done the root canal now needed attention. She believed the root on this adjacent molar was dying, too, so she performed another root canal. Afterward, Terrence's pain didn't lessen. In fact, he now felt it spreading to his neck and shoulder.

Terrence decided to visit an oral surgeon. At first the surgeon was baffled, but he finally said that the problem must be Terrence's temporomandibular joint (TMJ). While the joint looked okay, his pain could be the beginning of a TMJ issue. In case a bacterial infection was in play, the surgeon prescribed antibiotics. After the two-week course of pills, though, Terrence still hadn't found relief.

It had been eight months since his problems started. Each night, it took hours to fall asleep. On a scale of 1 to 10, he called this level 10 pain. To top it off, Terrence's tennis partner had found a new teammate, and the bills were piling up at work. His friends had stopped inviting him on outings, too.

One day Terrence called one of his friends, Jim, to see if they could meet for coffee, but Jim mistook Terrence's need for sympathy for an apology instead. "Don't worry, man," Jim said. "Only Reggie thinks that you've abandoned us."

When Terrence got angry at this, Jim said, "Just a joke! Calm down and get yourself better so you can come on the next hike."

Terrence felt defeated, alone, lost, and in need of answers.

That's when he found my website and scheduled a call. Right away, in the initial scan and reading, Spirit noticed a non-rashing variety of the shingles virus that was inflaming

Terrence's trigeminal and phrenic nerves, causing the pain in his jaw, face, neck, and shoulder. A mechanical TMJ issue had not been the underlying cause. However, the nerve inflammation had put pressure on his jaw, which is what caused the tension he felt there at night and upon waking.

I explained to Terrence that he'd had the virus before his first root canal—in fact, he'd had the virus his entire life. When the first dentist had removed the metal amalgam filling, it had released mercury toxins, which along with the anesthetics used for the procedure, had fed and strengthened the shingles virus.

We immediately addressed the virus with the appropriate herbs and healing foods. To allow Terrence to reclaim his immune system, we also removed antagonistic foods from his diet—ones that specifically strengthened the virus, such as corn products, canola, and the whey protein powder his trainer had him consuming twice a day.

Learning the real cause of his pain took away the mystery and fear and allowed Terrence to gain back the confidence that he would heal.

Within a month on this new regimen, Terrence's pain had noticeably decreased.

After three months, he was completely out of the woods.

He'd made many new friends at the local food co-op, too, since he'd started going there for cases of organic produce. The next time a group e-mail came from his friends about a day hike, he wasn't so quick to join them. Instead he decided to sign up for a co-op workday, where he spread the gospel of fruit's healing power to anyone who would listen.

"If you are struggling with your health in any way, the game has to change. Eating restorative foods—and eliminating foods that feed problems—is the most critical aspect of healing any illness or health condition."

— Anthony William, Medical Medium

CHAPTER 12

Attention-Deficit/Hyperactivity Disorder and Autism

Listing a dozen or more symptoms to determine if your child struggles from *attention-deficit/hyperactivity disorder* (ADHD) or *autism* is not a productive way to begin our discussion here. There's already so much confusion out there, so many books, websites, and articles about ADHD and autism indicators, that I don't want to add to the mess that you've already had to sort through in your search for answers. Here's what's important to keep in mind: ADHD and autism are mystery conditions to medical research and science.

A mother's intuition is the best tool for identifying ADHD and autism. The bond between mothers and their children, whether biological or adoptive, is a spiritual force that can never be broken. Moms (and other primary caregivers) know their children better than anyone else can or ever will. They know that attention issues don't arise from their children being selfish, stubborn, or insensitive. They know their children are intelligent and sensitive. They know that their children often don't have a choice in their behavior; they know when something deeper is going on.

A primary caregiver's gut instinct overrides all clinical systems set in place to diagnose children—and all informational pamphlets, all teacher assessments, all judgments by playmates' parents. It's a caregiver's sense of her child that will best detect if she or he is struggling with more than just growing pains.

Tens of millions of children have ADHD and autism, and the number is growing at an alarming rate. This chapter is primarily written for parents and caregivers of children who have ADHD and autism—people who know how frustrating it can be to understand their children in the face of certain behaviors, and how challenging it can be not to get the answers and support they need from the outside world.

The chapter can also be useful if you're an adult who has one of these conditions.

Either way, it will help you better understand ADHD and autism by providing information beyond anything that research, science, or medical communities know. It will also offer you options for ways to address both conditions.

THE HIDDEN UPSIDES OF ADHD AND AUTISM

You're probably familiar with the characteristics associated with ADHD and autism. You understand that it goes beyond fidgeting here and there, not paying attention now and then, and occasional difficulty communicating.

The traits of attention difficulty, hyperactivity, and impulsivity are considered ADHD when they're so extreme that a child has difficulty functioning in school, at home, or in other settings. When symptoms go a step beyond ADHD, they fall into the category of autism (also called autism spectrum disorder, or ASD).

It's common for a child to receive a label from a small group of classifications, because the medical industry loves to keep things all snug and cozy with a handful of labels. Allowing for more complication would make the industry uncomfortable, and the medical industry likes to be comfortable. It doesn't like the feeling of so many variables and variations making diagnosis confusing and a mystery—and revealing that it doesn't have a grip on deep-seated causes. The medical industry doesn't like when symptoms leave the box; it likes when they stay inside the box. As a result, the medical industry can try to put children inside that box. It has been trying to do so for years.

In truth, there's a much deeper issue going on—and the labels ADHD and autism shroud the deeper causes and deeper meanings. The labels, and the classifications within them, often serve as boxes that allow the medical industry to package up these complex sets of experiences so that they appear known and understood.

There are upsides to ADHD and autism. Children with these conditions often have a high level of intuition, are exceptionally creative, possess an extraordinary ability to see beneath the surface, and—though this goes against traditional thinking—actually have the ability to "read" people easily. Kids with ADHD and autism often think fast, feel deeply, and are intuitive and artistic, in part because of their limited patience for doing things in the "standard" way. (There are also physiological reasons these traits develop in tandem with the well-known challenges of attention-deficit/hyperactivity disorder and autism; we'll cover that in the next section.)

The truth is, ADHD and autism are producing new generations of children who will grow up, adapt, and be better equipped to solve future problems and chart the best course for humanity.

While being different makes life harder for children struggling with a mystery condition—as well as for their families—learning how to grow and adapt with it also increases their chances of living extraordinary lives.

WHAT CAUSES ADHD AND AUTISM

A popular misconception is that ADHD and autism are the result of a poor intestinal environment. Some current thinking goes that an overproduction of *Candida*, yeast, mold, and non-beneficial bacteria are to blame for children's hyperactive, inattentive, impulsive, or antisocial behavior, and that improving intestinal flora will improve children's brain health and alleviate their symptoms.

This theory is a distraction from what's really in play. Anybody can benefit from cleaning up their gut health, even if they're unaware of how or why. In the case of ADHD and autism, trying to improve the intestinal environment with probiotics and probiotic-rich foods is a good intention—that's peripheral. It doesn't address the true underlying cause of ADHD and autism: toxic heavy metals.

Specifically, ADHD and autism are born from (primarily) mercury, plus aluminum, that settles in the brain's midline cerebral canal, which divides the left cerebral hemisphere from the right. The mercury and aluminum can also be in other areas of the brain, "sprinkled" about in smaller deposits, some even inside the emotional center of the brain.

It might occur to you that it's hard to build up significant exposure to toxic heavy metals in just a few years of a young life. Mercury, however, is a neurotoxin that slips under doctors' noses. Most doctors are oblivious to which medical treatments they offer that contain mercury, and if they are aware of it, they're either in denial, afraid to break traditional protocol, or they believe in the treatment, and that belief overrides their common sense about the nature of the toxic heavy metals. Medical communities are due for a massive wake-up call about obvious mercury contamination.

Mercury is a great instigator of ADHD and autism in children in the 21st century. (Mercury is also responsible for most seizure disorders.) Until mercury and aluminum are addressed, the conditions will continue to affect millions of new kids each year.

It's very easy for a baby to take in toxic heavy metals from her or his mother while in the womb, and for a father to pass along toxic heavy metals at conception. That's because the parents have likely accumulated mercury over decades, and so did their mothers and fathers before them—and mercury tends to stay in the family bloodline generation after generation, in some cases for centuries, unless specific steps are taken to remove it.

Genetics are not behind ADHD and autism. Do you remember reading in other chapters about how the theory of autoimmune disease—the theory that the body attacks itself—is false and merely a way of blaming the person who's sick? The genetics theory is a similar scapegoat. Blaming DNA blames the very essence of the child who struggles with ADHD and/or autism, and that's a shame. The reason that ADHD and autism sometimes run in a family is a generation-to-generation transfer of mercury, as well as family patterns of exposure to toxic heavy metals.

It's easy to transfer aluminum, the other toxic heavy metal typically involved in ADHD and autism, from generation to generation, too, and to get aluminum from medical treatments. Also, other outside sources lead to aluminum exposure: most soda cans are made of aluminum, aluminum foil is a popular item in the kitchen, and aluminum siding is common on homes. Aluminum and mercury show up in pesticides, fungicides, and herbicides, too. This list represents only a fraction of the places where you can get aluminum and other toxic heavy metals.

(Copper is another common toxic heavy metal that gets passed from generation to generation and is also very easy to be exposed to in daily life. Many children with ADHD or autism have elevations of toxic copper deposits inside the liver, resulting in eczema, psoriasis, or other skin conditions either in childhood or adult life. While copper doesn't play a role in the symptoms of ADHD or autism themselves, it doesn't help—because when you have an uncomfortable skin condition while struggling with ADHD and autism, it becomes even more of a strain emotionally.)

Also critical in the story behind ADHD and autism is the physical location in which the toxic heavy metals mercury and aluminum settle.

The Cerebral Midline Canal

The brain's midline is located directly between the right and left cerebral hemispheres of the brain. This midline looks like an open canal, but instead of water running through it, a channel of electrical energy does. It's not yet documented in medical research that this canal forms an electrical charge that makes an energetic connection between the two cerebral hemispheres and allows information to be exchanged between them. This exchange of information is powered by neurons, and the true nature of this connection may never be discovered by medical research and science.

Children have free-flowing midline canals. It's what allows them to learn how to communicate with other people and with the metaphysical realm, and to see things adults don't see anymore, such as angels.

When toxic heavy metals enter this midline canal—which is supposed to be open and free—they block the electrical and metaphysical energetic transmissions between the cerebral hemispheres. This challenges the child's brain to develop alternative ways to make that exchange happen. Adaptations set in, and the child unconsciously begins accessing areas of her or his brain that most of us never use (at least not until we're older). Metaphysical and electrical energy struggles to find its way into

uncharted territory. Electrical nerve impulses begin igniting neurons and firing off neurotransmitters onto brain pathways that aren't supposed to be explored until after a person reaches early adulthood.

Autism is essentially a more advanced and complicated form of ADHD. Toxic heavy metals are present at higher levels in the midline cerebral canal, and gathered in uneven layers. This helps explain why there's an autism spectrum, with the syndrome displaying in different intensities depending on the child. It all has to do with the amount of heavy metals in the canal, and in what positions they have accumulated. With autism (versus ADHD), the additional layers of mercury interfere even more greatly with the metaphysical and electrical energy communications trying to cross the canal. The small amounts of toxic heavy metals "sprinkled" throughout the brain also have an effect here.

To understand ADHD and autism, imagine the Grand Canyon. There's a symbiotic relationship taking place in and around it, between physical and metaphysical elements. There's the water running through the canyon, the wind rising up out of it, the electrical fields from storms and the earth, and the light and heat of the sun. All of it combines just so to make the canyon a visible, energetic, and spiritual force. The brain's midline canal is like the Grand Canyon in this way—so many elements interacting at once to make it work just so.

Now what if something altered the pristine environment of the Grand Canyon? What if someone started dropping cars into it, and metal barrels? Everything would change. Wind patterns would redirect themselves. The sun would refract at different angles, no longer reaching certain areas but lighting up nooks and crannies that hadn't seen sunshine for thousands of years. Even sound within and around the canyon would change. The whole frequency of the place would be different as the elements adapted.

This is what happens when toxic heavy metals enter a child's midline cerebral canal. We see the child behaving in ways we don't expect because her or his brain is adapting to the extra materials blocking internal communication. It's learning to access different parts of itself.

Specially Evolved Brain Neurons

Children with ADHD and autism also grow specially evolved brain neurons, especially in the frontal lobe. These facilitate communication with others and intuitive abilities for "reading" people (e.g., being able to sense what someone is thinking and feeling). That might seem surprising, since children with ADHD and autism can exhibit antisocial qualities that make them appear to be shut off to others. Their laser-focus on themselves and their personal interests is actually a way to avoid being overwhelmed by the flood of information they're picking up from the people around them. The focus hides these children's powerful intuitive development.

Not only do new, evolved neurons grow in the frontal lobe, but they also develop in other parts of the brain. The new, evolved neurons are excitable—and cause most of what we witness as the issues around ADHD. This is even more true for many autistic children, who grow a greater abundance of these evolved and adaptable neurons. Either way, they require more electrolytes, trace mineral salts, and glucose, so as these new neurons develop, if a

child isn't getting what's needed to feed, reinforce, and develop these new neurons, it can lead to a more difficult struggle.

Age and Brain Development

This sequence of events—the toxic heavy metals accumulating in the midline canal between the left and right cerebral hemispheres (along with toxic heavy metal exposure in other parts of the brain), followed by the push to access unused portions of the brain (because communication energy and information cannot pass across the canal), followed by the development of numerous evolved neurons—typically happens no later than age four.

However, the toxic heavy metals, such as mercury and aluminum, can be removed from the child's brain through the tools and cleansing techniques in this book at any point up to, roughly, early adulthood. If this is done, the child's intuitive nature will remain, while the removal of the heavy metals will most likely end the child's ADHD or autism. This is a win-win, allowing the child to be extraordinary and yet be spared the difficulties associated with having these conditions. Some behaviors that might have been considered symptoms will likely reveal themselves to have been simply patterns and habits developed for survival with ADHD or autism. You may see improvements in many areas of your child's well-being while some of these patterns linger (for example, in the areas of communication and sensitivities). It will take new experiences and time without the toxic heavy metals for these to shift.

In early adulthood, the midline between the cerebral hemispheres closes up. The left and right cerebral hemispheres start to squeeze together, limiting the free and easy flow of energy and childlike, free-spirited information between the left and right sides of the brain. This is the normal process of growing up. It's the body's way of turning one's focus to the responsibilities of adulthood. But it also traps any toxic heavy metals such as mercury that are residing in the canal between the two hemispheres.

If you're an adult with ADHD or autism, this means you'll probably continue having some form of the condition unless you diligently try to keep removing the toxic heavy metals from your system and avoiding new exposure. For most people, ADHD and autism can be viewed not as a negative, but just as living differently from the mainstream. That said, if you have severe ADHD or autism that interferes with your life and relationships, you can follow the advice in the next section to lessen its effects.

Similarly, if you're a parent, the next section will tell you what can be done to address your child's ADHD and/or autism.

ADDRESSING ADHD AND AUTISM

Doctors typically prescribe amphetamines to treat ADHD. That's counterintuitive, because amphetamines are stimulants, which are the last things you'd think would calm down an overactive child or help one who struggles with focus.

Prescribing amphetamines reminds me of the practice in the late 19th and early 20th centuries of giving children Mrs. Winslow's Soothing Syrup to calm them when they were misbehaving. The concoction did quiet the children rather quickly—because it contained morphine. Eventually, when it was determined that giving children this narcotic was dangerous, the product was taken off the market.

When doctors prescribe amphetamines to help children focus for short periods, it does work most of the time—though medical communities don't know why.

The key to this mystery is the exceptional development that's taken place in your child's brain. Accessing normally unused portions of the brain and the growth of numerous evolved, adaptable neurons requires two to three times the usual amount of glucose and trace mineral salts, which are the brain's primary foods. (Glucose is most important to the brain, and trace mineral salts second most important.) The chances are your child isn't getting enough glucose or trace mineral salts to the brain, and that's partly responsible for much of her or his ADHD-related behaviors. Amphetamines stimulate the adrenal glands to produce adrenaline, which the brain accepts in place of glucose and trace mineral salts to fuel its activities. To override the toxic heavy metals such as mercury and aluminum in the brain, the adrenaline forces electrical nerve impulses to fire at an alarming rate. This helps stabilize your child's ADHD and helps your child focus, though only temporarily. The medication can also be hit-or-miss—that is, highly unpredictable in how your child responds.

Also note that if a child is struggling from a pathogen such as the Epstein-Barr virus or shingles virus, it can create a mild elevation of inflammation throughout the body, even if other viral symptoms have not developed yet. That mild inflammation can be enough to create brain fog and/or focus and concentration issues that are misconstrued as ADHD. In these cases, the adrenaline that an amphetamine triggers will reduce that inflammation temporarily, making it seem that the prescription is "working."

Amphetamines create a huge burden on the adrenal glands (not to mention all the organs regularly flooded with adrenaline). If this drug use goes on for years, eventually the adrenal glands are likely to "burn out" and become unstable, leading to a host of problems. I often hear from young adults who have adrenal malfunction, severe fatigue, and high anxiety as a result of prescribed amphetamine burnout. This is especially common in women.

A better long-term solution for both ADHD and autism is to make sure you provide ample fresh fruit—preferably organic—for your child to consume. This will give your child the highest quality glucose possible in a form that's easily accessible to the brain. (See Chapter 20, "Fruit Fear.") Get creative with making fruit a habit, for example, by blending frozen bananas to make a snack the consistency of ice cream.

Providing your child with the highest quality trace minerals is another important step. The most beneficial option is fresh celery juice, even if you start out with small dosages. (For celery juice amounts for children, see the table in Chapter 21.) Celery juice is a complete electrolyte. If celery juice is not an option, try coconut water (that's not pink or red), which has trace mineral salts and is high in electrolytes. A simple third option—while not the same, still beneficial and easy—is to make a homemade lemonade by squeezing lemon in water and adding raw honey.

Right now, a diet trend for ADHD and autism management is to cut out grains and sugar. This is a wise decision—*only* if fruit is taking the place of the other sugars being eliminated. Another trend is the high-fat ketogenic diet. Once again, doctors who fear sugar recommend this one. It's not an advisable path. Any improvement your child displays will be temporary, and only because the high levels of fat force the adrenal glands to release more adrenaline than they would with other diet techniques, allowing your child to focus better at times. In the end, it will likely result in adrenal fatigue and even neurotransmitter deficiency. It's not enough to offer diet and food recommendations that are guessing games. When you understand *why* a child is struggling with ADHD or autism and how the brain works, only then can you understand what's needed and choose the proper tools. If your child doesn't get fruit sugar (in its natural form), she or he will continue to struggle with symptoms of ADHD and autism or, years later, develop new, additional symptoms.

This might give you some perspective if your child is drawn to high-sugar foods or extremely high-calorie starches such as french fries and battered, fried foods; it's the brain telling her or him it wants glucose. The problem is that in addition to having the worst kind of nourishment-deprived sugar, junk food typically contains lard or rancid GMO oils, which stop the sugar from reaching the brain. So unhealthier versions of such "treats" do nothing for ADHD or autism.

In fact, beyond steering your child clear of traditional sweets, you ideally want to cut *all* wheat products and gluten from her or his diet. Medical communities don't know why it's important for children who are struggling with the symptoms of ADHD and autism to eliminate gluten. They believe there could be an allergy, or that gluten creates inflammation, or that there could be a genetic issue with a child that does not allow for the digestion and assimilation of gluten. There are a lot of theories. The truth is that those with ADHD or autism are often struggling with viral and bacterial infections. *Streptococcus* is the leading bacteria in children with ADHD or autism, and it's unknown to medical research and science that bacteria feed on gluten. So strep thrives on gluten, and that's what can raise inflammation levels and create other digestive issues and symptoms. Gluten itself does not create or raise inflammation.

If possible, you also want your child to avoid any foods and additives that have toxic qualities, such as corn, canola oil, MSG, aspartame, citric acid, nutritional yeast, and natural flavors. (See Chapter 19, "What Not to Eat.")

You'll also want to keep your child away from any other types of toxins and poisons—especially toxic heavy metals. (See Chapter 18, "Freeing Your Brain and Body of Toxins.") Always question everything your child is exposed to, including medical treatments.

Finally, see if you can put your child on a daily diet of the herbs, supplements, and foods that follow. In all honesty, in about 85 percent of cases, children with ADHD or autism won't want to cooperate. So if you feel your child would benefit from the items below, see if you can tap into inventive ways to make them seem appealing (or camouflage them). Engage your child in the process, too, by gearing your approach to her or his unique desires and personality. A mother or other primary caregiver has the most insight into how to speak to her or his child's best interest. Every child is wonderfully unique and amazing in every way, so just play things by ear and do your best.

Healing Foods

Diet is key to recovery from ADHD and autism. Some fruits, leafy greens, herbs, wild foods, and vegetables in particular are especially beneficial for, variously, flushing out toxic heavy metals and other toxins, healing brain tissue, restoring neurotransmitters, supporting healthy neuron signal transmission, providing glucose to the brain, calming the mind, and strengthening the central nervous system, as well as lowering and killing off pathogens such as viruses and bacteria. These healing foods include wild blueberries, cilantro, potatoes, apples, celery, bananas, spinach, melons, winter squash, sweet potatoes, tomatoes, broccoli, pears, mangoes, blackberries, avocados (in small amounts), strawberries, Atlantic dulse, and hemp seeds (in small amounts). Incorporate as many of these foods into the diet as you can.

Also look for the Heavy Metal Detox Smoothie recipe in Chapter 23. Try to incorporate this smoothie whenever possible.

Note that a child usually doesn't have the appetite for the full amount that the Heavy Metal Detox Smoothie recipe yields. To figure out the right portion for your child, think about a glass of apple juice—how much will your child usually drink? Eight ounces? Ten or twelve ounces? Wherever you land, that's an appropriate amount of Heavy Metal Detox Smoothie to give your child. You can either reduce the recipe accordingly—for example, cutting it by half or two-thirds (making sure to keep the five key ingredients in there, if possible, in proportionate amounts)—or make the full recipe and drink the leftover that your child doesn't want. Or you can give your child the ingredients separately within a 24-hour window.

Healing Herbs and Supplements

A very helpful place to start for anyone dealing with the symptoms of ADHD or autism is with fresh celery juice on an empty stomach and, later in the morning or day, the Heavy Metal Detox Smoothie—which incorporates two of the supplements below, barley grass juice powder and spirulina. (Remember, don't drink the celery juice and smoothie together. Always space out your celery juice at least 15 to 30 minutes from other beverages and food.) Again, for guidance on celery juice amounts for children, see the table in Chapter 21.

If you're looking for additional support, this list provides options. Please note that these supplements are all listed in **adult** dosages. You are welcome to take this list to your pediatrician to see what dosages are right for your child. **Before applying these, be sure to read Chapter 21, "Critical Guide to Supplement Protocols."**

Supplements for ADHD and Autism (Adult dosages)

Remember that you can take these adult dosages to your pediatrician to see what dosages are right for your child.

- **Fresh celery juice:** work up to 16 ounces daily
- **Celeryforce:** 2 capsules daily

- **Barley grass juice powder:** 1 teaspoon or 3 capsules daily
- **B-complex:** 1 capsule daily
- **Elderberry syrup:** 1 teaspoon daily
- **EPA and DHA (fish-free):** 1 capsule daily (taken with dinner)
- **GABA:** 1 capsule daily
- **Goldenseal:** 1 dropperful daily (one week per month)
- **Lemon balm:** 3 dropperfuls daily
- **Licorice root:** 1 dropperful daily (two weeks on, two weeks off)
- **Magnesium glycinate:** 2 capsules daily
- **Melatonin:** 1 to 5 milligrams daily (preferably at night)
- **Mullein leaf:** 1 dropperful daily (one week per month)
- **Spirulina:** 1 teaspoon or 3 capsules daily
- **Vitamin B$_{12}$ (as adenosylcobalamin with methylcobalamin):** 1 dropperful daily
- **Vitamin C (as Micro-C):** 2 capsules daily
- **Zinc (as liquid zinc sulfate):** 1 dropperful daily

CASE HISTORY:
Fruits of a Mother's Labors
2005

As a child, Jonathan had a hard time communicating with friends, family, and teachers. He didn't get along with his little sister. He could never seem to sit still, and focusing was a near-impossible feat. At age five, he was diagnosed with ADHD.

Jonathan's mother, Alberta, was his major support in life. For the next 13 years, she devoted herself to getting to the root of his issues, and to promoting his health and well-being. She kept a journal of every symptom Jonathan exhibited, every health-care professional they visited, every diet, and every medicine he received, such as popularly prescribed amphetamines.

Alberta's husband liked to joke that no matter how good a day Jonathan was having concentration- and hyperactivity-wise, he was just like Rudolph—he never joined in any reindeer games. Part of it had to do with Jonathan's peers leaving him out. Another factor was that Jonathan had more advanced and intense interests than the other children his age.

While Jonathan's behavior wavered between ADHD and mild autism, Alberta knew he was a brilliant, golden, intuitive being. After coming across the phrase "indigo child" in a book, she started referring to him as one.

She always held on to the memory of Jonathan as a seven-year-old, sitting in the back seat of the car wearing jeans, his blue sweatshirt, and his favorite sneakers that he said fit just right. As Alberta sat in the front seat recording the details of the meeting she'd just had with the school counselor, Jonathan started talking to himself. "Nobody understands me," he said. "I just need a little more time to adjust here in the world."

In Jonathan's early adolescence, Alberta found a functional medicine doctor who gave them some results. Dr. Duval said that Jonathan's ADHD and borderline autistic behavior had to do with intestinal flora issues—that is, lots of unproductive bacteria and not enough good bacteria. He believed grains were part of the problem, so he recommended removing all wheat, rye, oats, barley, and so forth from Jonathan's diet. He also felt Jonathan would do best without any processed sugars or dairy products, such as milk, cheese, and butter. He advised lots of leafy greens such as kale, along with other vegetables, some nuts and seeds, and liberal servings of meat, chicken, and fish. For supplementation, Dr. Duval prescribed advanced probiotics to address what he called an unhealthy intestinal environment, as well as immune-supporting supplements.

Jonathan was the rare kid who was eager to please when it came to food. Though Alberta heard from other moms that it was near impossible to influence their children's eating habits, Jonathan didn't mind cutting out wheat and eating lots of leafy greens like kale in its place, along with nuts and seeds and other foods Dr. Duval said were brain-enhancing.

Over the years, Jonathan's focus and communication issues improved enough to get through elementary school, junior high, and eventually high school. For various periods, Alberta homeschooled Jonathan and later hired tutors. Both moves were crucial to Jonathan's scholastic success.

At the age of 18, though, Jonathan still struggled with his symptoms. He and Alberta were trying to get him into college, and both were worried (though Jonathan wouldn't admit it) about how he'd perform away from home, without Alberta's constant support. It would take a miracle for him not to have to rely on prescribed amphetamines and other stimulants.

The past 18 years had been hard on Alberta. Yet she wouldn't have traded a minute of it for anything. Whenever she got frustrated, she remembered that seven-year-old in the back seat, hoping for the world to understand him. At parent-teacher night at Jonathan's school, Alberta got talking with a mother whose child was in a similar situation. That mother gave Alberta my number, and she booked an appointment.

Alberta got on the phone for our first call, and though Jonathan wasn't on the line, I was able to perform the scan on him. I told her heavy metals, predominantly mercury, were the culprits. The functional medicine doctor and other practitioners had been able to improve Jonathan by 40 percent of his healing capacity. They'd been able to take him only so far because they were missing the most important link: the toxic heavy metals.

Substantial amounts of mercury were caught in the midline canal between Jonathan's cerebral hemispheres. (Medical research won't explore this for another two or three decades.) Since Jonathan was 18 years of age, the cerebral hemispheres were starting to squeeze together and close off the canal—but there was still space enough to get radical results.

Alberta sounded relieved that she'd called me in time, but panicked about how things would have turned out for Jonathan if she'd called me just a year later. I assured her that even if Jonathan were older, we'd still be able to get results from detox methods.

Because fats in the bloodstream get in the way of preciously needed glucose reaching the brain, we reduced Jonathan's fat consumption, which had come in the form of animal protein. All these years, the heavy metal contamination in Jonathan's brain had meant that he needed twice as much glucose as he was getting. Alberta said that Jonathan had always been drawn to sweets and frequently seemed to focus better when eating them, though it tended to last only a moment before the processed sugars brought him crashing down hard.

I agreed with her observation and confirmed that processed sugars were not the way to go. Dr. Duval had been right about something—grains and dairy were not helpful, either. What Jonathan needed most were the true brain foods: wild blueberries and other berries, apples, dates, grapes, and any other fruit that Jonathan enjoyed. Vegetables and leafy greens such as kale were also important.

For supplementation, we focused on a high dose of spirulina (mixed with coconut water for glucose and palatability) coupled with two servings of cilantro daily.

"This will be a tectonic shift," Alberta said. "All these years, Jonathan hasn't been allowed to eat fruit."

"Kale and protein as the solution to all life's problems is a well-intentioned trend," I told her. "Kale's amazing, yet it provides a fraction of the brain benefit that fruit does. And we have to be wary of the fat hiding in animal protein. This new diet, with its combination of antioxidant-rich fruit sugar, lowered fats, plus spirulina and cilantro to remove heavy metals, will change Jonathan's life."

And it did. Three weeks into the protocol, Alberta left a message with my assistant. For the first time ever, she'd had an actual, in-depth conversation with her son. Not a monologue, a dialogue. He didn't talk at her, or cut her off, or abruptly leave the room. Instead he listened and responded, and they went back and forth like two functioning adults. Day by day, she said, she could sense the heavy metals leaving Jonathan's system.

"My jaw is on the floor," she told my assistant, tearing up. "You know, I'm getting near the end of the latest notebook I've been using to track Jonathan's symptoms and treatments. Maybe I don't need to buy a new one."

Jonathan noticed the difference, too. Within the first month, he was able to finish his college applications without gallons of coffee. He got into a top university, enrolled, and bonded with his roommate immediately over what a mom-like thing it had been for Alberta to send him off with a 15-pound box of dates.

Alberta also started sending him weekly deliveries from an organic fruit company. Jonathan was all too happy to roll his eyes over it—but he and his roommate snacked on the fruit every day. The glucose helped Jonathan power through his classes and even a few clubs he'd gotten involved in. By the time midterms rolled around, he was at the top of his game.

"When you understand why a child is struggling with ADHD or autism and how the brain works, only then can you understand what's needed and choose the proper tools."

— Anthony William, Medical Medium

CHAPTER 13

Posttraumatic Stress Disorder

Every single soul on this planet is dealing with some form of *posttraumatic stress disorder* (PTSD). This isn't just the fight-or-flight response to tragedy or the war trauma that veterans suffer from—that is, the well-known and documented extreme form of PTSD.

There's also an epidemic of hidden PTSD. Since this book was first published, that's become more true than ever.

This unknown form of PTSD, which is the focus of this chapter, is so rampant that almost everyone has it. It results from the unpleasant situations that we all have to deal with, ones that we may forget about consciously but not subconsciously. PTSD stems from millennia of hurt, too; its essence is in us from human history.

It's normal, and even healthy, to be terrified when your life or someone else's is in danger. Your fear triggers a fight-or-flight response that floods your body with adrenaline, temporarily giving you enhanced strength and heightened reflexes for dealing with the threat. Once the threat has passed, you may experience emotional aftershocks. This is the classic form of PTSD that therapists and psychiatrists recognize.

A client, Jerry, once told me of his son-in-law Mike's near-death experience when they were working together in construction. On the job one day, Jerry heard Mike screaming for help from across the site. Jerry raced to see what was the matter and found Mike trapped beneath a half-ton trailer. Mike had been fixing an axle when the blocks the trailer had been resting on gave out and the trailer pinned him to the ground, nearly crushing his chest.

If he stopped to call for help, Jerry knew it would come too late. So rather than dialing 911 and later having to tell his daughter that she'd lost her husband, Jerry went into survival mode. A burst of adrenaline filled his body. He proceeded to lift the thousand-pound weight off his son-in-law's chest enough that Mike could slide out. Mike survived.

Even though a miracle had occurred and everything was okay, Mike consistently had nightmares about being trapped under something heavy and screaming for help. And Jerry couldn't look at any type of trailer without feeling nauseated. After years of this, Jerry came to me for insights into how to heal. Both men had experienced what could obviously be deemed PTSD.

Then there are the day-to-day emotional wounds that add up. Insecurities, trust issues, fears, guilt, shame, and more: These all actually stem from past challenging emotional experiences. They are all a result of hidden PTSD. So, for example, when a person has a fear of committing to a relationship, it's showcasing that something happened earlier in life to create a certain level of posttraumatic stress disorder. You never know what happened in someone's past that's contributing to her or his present-day reaction.

PTSD can happen on so many different levels. I remember a hike I took once where I decided to go off the beaten path. As I veered from the trail, Spirit warned me not to do it. And yet, knowing that I was meant to go in the safe direction, I instead used my free will to follow my curiosity to a cliff. I crept to the cliff's edge and saw a terrace below that I could reach if I was careful. With no safety rails, I started to climb. Just as I was navigating the most treacherous ledge, with the ocean 100 feet below me, a fog thicker than clotted cream rolled in, and fast.

I could barely see my hands in front of me. Below, waves crashed into rock. I knew that if I slid forward or to the side just six inches, I would meet my maker. I was stuck.

For hours and hours, the fog remained. By nightfall, it was still just as dense. The temperature had dropped, and the light clothes I was wearing were soaked through from the mist. Falling asleep on the side of a cliff was not an option, so I stayed up, freezing, until dawn, when the haze lifted enough for me to see the footholds that would guide me to safety. I finally got back to the car, drove home, and tried to sleep.

As soon as I closed my eyes, all I could see was the cliff—with me on it.

Over and over, I saw the same image and felt panic at how close I'd come to the end. For someone with a daredevil streak, someone who liked to experience nature with a dose of adrenaline, the experience probably wouldn't have fazed her or him one bit. I know people who wouldn't flinch from being fogged in on a precipice—rock climbers, for instance, who regularly risk their lives free-climbing with no safety equipment. That's not me, though. I was shaken.

Luckily, I knew the secrets to recovery. With time and patience and the application of Spirit of Compassion's healing program, I moved on from the trauma before long.

UNRECOGNIZED PTSD

In recent times, we've become a society that's in favor of talking openly about subjects that used to be hush-hush. In the past, we pretty much had to shut up and be quiet about how we felt or we'd be sent to the asylum. If we acted out a little too much, we might even be eligible for a lobotomy.

It took centuries for war veterans to finally receive attention and treatment for the lasting stress of the traumas they had endured in battle. As a culture, we have a history of burying emotions with alcohol, drugs, food, and adrenaline-fueled activities. Expressing ourselves wasn't really an option until fairly recently, within the last 40 years. We live in a stressful age, but therapists, counselors, and life coaches abound now—and we're allowed to expand the definition and scope of PTSD.

As far as we've come, we're still lacking in our societal (and scientific) understanding of trauma and how the vicious cycle of PTSD truly unfolds. And although the stigma is not as bad as it once was, it hasn't gone away altogether. We still have more progress to make in how we relate to and support anyone who's been through any kind of trauma.

Posttraumatic stress disorder is something that occurs from any difficult experience. There are the more severe cases of PTSD we know about, the ones that result from experiences such as abuse or tragedy or kidnapping or witnessing a violent crime.

Then there are the under-recognized triggers. A child's parents divorcing could make her avoid marriage as an adult. A teenager who doesn't get a date for prom could start disliking all school dances. Turbulence on a plane ride could lead a person never to want to fly again. And I've heard many stories about food poisoning contracted at a restaurant franchise that lead people to squirm in their seats every time they drive by one of the chain's locations.

Other triggers include getting fired from a job, breaking up with a girlfriend or boyfriend, the experience of being betrayed by someone you trusted, small fender benders that don't even result in injuries, or a moment in life when you feel like you failed at something. There are no limitations to what can cause PTSD.

A client once told me that she hadn't been able to eat green beans and meatloaf since adolescence because it had been forced on her when she was a teenager at boarding school. Just the sight or smell of either food gave her flashbacks to her coercive headmaster. I've also known many women afraid to conceive after enduring difficult pregnancies in the past. These are forms of PTSD too.

Yet even in today's modern times of self-help, therapy, and emotional understanding, society isn't ready to refer to any of these under-recognized triggers as PTSD-inducing. Health professionals mostly reserve the term *posttraumatic stress disorder* for life-or-death experiences. This ignores the hundreds, if not thousands, of other incidents that alter (for the worse) the way someone experiences life.

That's what PTSD does, no matter the scale: it negatively influences the choices we make and changes the fabric of who we are.

One trigger that is all too rarely spoken about is illness. Many people develop PTSD just from having the flu for two weeks, never mind chronic fatigue for three months or neurological problems for years. The experience of these symptoms is one part of the story. A whole other cause for emotional damage is the doctor-shopping journey—the battery of tests, the constant MRIs and CT scans that don't reveal anything, the imaging scans that *do* reveal issues (whether or not they're the true cause of your symptoms), the despair of not finding relief or validation.

PTSD tends to pile up on top of itself. Once you've been sick for any period of time, and you start believing your body is letting you down, and you're lost in a non-diagnosis or a misdiagnosis or a diagnosis that leads to no healing, and the financial strain starts to build, and maybe you feel your hold slipping on your career or relationships—it makes you a likely candidate for a unique composition of posttraumatic stress disorders.

PTSD is a very real response to the illness of a loved one, too. Watching someone lose her or his vitality and cease to be able to perform the same role she or he once did in your life can make you feel vulnerable and powerless. Overextending yourself to care for someone can be taxing, too. Even if your loved one recovers, the moment they later sound groggy or develop a benign sniffle, it can dredge up those old fears and make you feel you're reliving that dark time.

Now we have PTSD from COVID. There are several varieties of it. This PTSD can develop from fear of getting COVID. It can come from losing touch with our community, friends, and family as interactions change, become more distanced, and life alters in so many ways. PTSD can result from contracting and becoming ill from COVID, whether it was a milder case or you had to fight for your survival until you recovered. There's also post-COVID PTSD—because not everyone who contracts COVID feels great on the other side of it. As you read about in Chapter 3, "Epstein-Barr Virus, Chronic Fatigue Syndrome, and Fibromyalgia," it's common to experience the onset or worsening of chronic symptoms after COVID, even though most of these symptoms are not COVID-caused; they're COVID-*triggered*. (That is, existing pathogens in the body can take advantage of the immune system crash from COVID. That's the true cause behind the majority of post-COVID symptoms.) Whether someone is struggling with a flare-up of chronic symptoms or experiencing brand-new symptoms after COVID, it can lead to this type of PTSD. Then there's the PTSD of running or working in businesses, such as restaurants and retail shops, open to the public. Cashiers and other grocery store employees, as well as flight attendants, transit workers, health-care providers, and those in many other public-facing professions, are struggling with

PTSD from encountering more impatient and stressed-out crowds. The list goes on—you can likely name other forms of COVID-related PTSD from your individual experiences. There's PTSD from managing childcare and eldercare in this new landscape, and from dealing with blurred boundaries between home, work, and school. There's PTSD from loss of a job and/or financial security due to COVID. There's PTSD from losing a loved one to COVID or a COVID-related circumstance.

It's possible to have PTSD and not realize it. If it originates from a subconscious memory, you may experience unexplained feelings of avoidance, or you may shut down in certain circumstances and not know why. Perhaps you find yourself driven to overeat sweets or seek out adrenaline-rush activities. Or maybe people have given you the upsetting labels "touchy," "prickly," "fragile," "wounded," "anal," or "oversensitive." These are all signs that something once happened—or happened over an extended period—to bring about a reaction now.

The medical establishment doesn't truly know yet what PTSD is. It doesn't know PTSD's range, and it doesn't know how it occurs.

In this chapter, you'll get answers.

You are not beholden to the unpleasant parts of your personal history. You are not destined to relive the same patterns of trauma over and over again. The people who've hurt you do not hold the power to haunt you for the rest of your life. The mishaps and chronic stresses do not have to define you. There's a way forward.

With the right nutritional, emotional, and soul-healing support, you can reclaim your vitality and go back to fully living your life.

WHAT REALLY HAPPENS

What happens on a physical and emotional level to cause PTSD?

Put plainly, it's a lack of glucose in the brain that occurs when someone experiences trauma. When there isn't enough glucose stored in the brain tissue to feed the central nervous system, emotional upheaval can create lasting effects. Contrary to popular science belief, though electrolytes do play a critical role in brain health, PTSD does not occur from a loss of electrolytes. Again, lack of glucose is the real cause.

Have you ever heard the expression "He has a thick skin" or "It's like water off a duck's back with her" to describe someone who goes through life untroubled by life's shocks and upsets? What's really behind these people's temperaments are ample glucose reserves in the brain. As a result, they can handle a heck of a lot of trauma without being affected.

Glucose is a protective biochemical critical to the brain because it places a veil of protection over sensitive brain and neurological tissue. Medical research has not yet tapped into an understanding of just how much glucose the brain requires to function in times of stress—and just how critical it is that there's ample glucose reserved in the storage bank of the brain. If glucose were converted into dollars, then one substantial traumatic event, like an accident, could be the equivalent of buying a new car. And a long-term trauma, such as an abusive relationship, could have the same effect on your glucose reserves that buying a new house would have on your bank account.

Glucose's protective veil is necessary for three reasons: First, glucose is needed to prevent brain cells, brain tissue, and neurons from becoming saturated by the acidic and corrosive nature of the adrenaline and cortisol released from anger, frustration, hopelessness, and fear. Second, glucose is there to stop the electrical storms in the brain that arise when trauma occurs, with electrical impulses firing off at an alarming rate, affecting brain tissue, neurons, and glial cells. Third, glucose prevents brain atrophy—which is critical, because otherwise, trauma can rush that process of brain shrinkage.

Think of the brain like a car's engine. Sweet like sugar, antifreeze runs through the engine. Without this coolant, the engine can overheat and become damaged. In the same way, when the brain doesn't have the coolant it needs—glucose—then the electrical impulses that run through the thousands of neurons in the brain can cause overheating and burnout.

Have you ever heard of eating sugar to calm the spice of a chili pepper? Sugar acts as an antidote to the pepper's heat units, preventing the gums, tongue, and roof of your mouth from becoming burned. In the same way, glucose (sugar) protects the brain. If someone's glucose storage is low, she or he could get PTSD just from a flat tire. On the other hand, someone with a high level of glucose storage could witness an armed robbery and tell the story to a friend over dinner that same day, unruffled. Whether glucose storage is low or high in part has to do with how much trauma a person has experienced in life. Someone could come into this world with more glucose and be able to sustain it because they haven't experienced too many hardships, so their reserves haven't been tapped.

Animals have a built-in understanding of glucose's importance. Here's something else you won't find in an Internet search: when two chipmunks are running across the road and a car runs over one of them, the surviving chipmunk will dart back into the road and drink the other's blood for a quick hit of glucose. It's an innate, natural response that the chipmunk was born with to prevent brain damage from its fight-or-flight adrenaline response.

Humans also intuitively understand sugar as a calming device. It's why many people turn to foods high in sugar as their first choice when going through an emotional hardship such as a relationship breakup. Plenty of people turn to sweets to soothe their wounds. They may just think they have an overeating problem and are particularly vulnerable to the temptations of sugary treats—whereas, really, they're subconsciously trying to address a physical debt.

And as another antidote to PTSD, people have started to replace sugar with adrenaline. There's an increasing number of adrenaline junkies who jump out of planes, engage in high-intensity sports, go zip-lining or bungee jumping, or dive off cliffs as a way of coping with suffering they may not even realize is there. Then there are rebound relationships—that new girlfriend or boyfriend someone may turn to for a boost of adrenaline following a breakup. These are all examples of using adrenaline as a quick drug to stand in for glucose.

The problem with these approaches is that what goes up must come down. A sugar high from packaged cupcakes (even vegan ones) is going to mean a crash later. And adrenaline highs lead to adrenaline lows. While an adrenaline high may feel healing and empowering in the moment, the surge won't last forever. You can end up with a bout of depression as the aftereffect of that adrenaline leaving your brain, cells, and tissue. These aren't the real solutions to our wounds.

We don't have to take risks in order to heal from PTSD. We don't have to gamble.

HEALING PTSD

Posttraumatic stress disorder, in its true definition, is the experience of lingering uncomfortable feelings (from mild to extreme) that result from any adverse encounter, and that limit a person in any way. These feelings include fear, doubt, insecurity, worry, concern, panic, avoidance, anger, hostility, hypervigilance, irritability, distractedness, self-loathing, abandonment, defensiveness, agitation, sadness, frustration, resentment, cynicism, shame, invisibility, voicelessness, powerlessness, vulnerability, loss of confidence, lack of self-worth, and distrust.

One of the most powerful ways to heal posttraumatic stress disorder across the spectrum is to create new experiences to serve as positive reference points in your life. The more of these you create, the greater your chances of putting PTSD behind you. Every new positive experience plants a life-giving seed in a garden of nutrient-thieving weeds.

These experiences don't have to be big. They don't have to be dangerous or risk-taking (nor should they be). And they don't have to look like much to anyone else. Just taking a walk in peaceful surroundings or trying one of the soul-healing meditations from Chapter 24 can help you restore your brain.

It's all about how you *perceive* each new experience, however tame. Keep a list of every new experience and journal each one, taking notes on how you felt. For example, when you took a walk, did you see any birds? What was the weather like? Was there a certain angle of light? What effect did it all have on your state of mind? It all matters. It's all part of being in the moment.

Or try putting together a puzzle. As you turn the pile of random pieces into a coherent whole, you'll be teaching yourself that order can emerge from chaos. Try painting, sketching, or drawing, too. These are powerful exercises that help orient us in the present moment and make us pay attention to beautiful details in the world around us that otherwise go unnoticed. The cathartic effects of art-making are potent.

Or perhaps call up a dear friend you haven't seen in years and ask her or him out to lunch. It will help reconnect you to essential parts of yourself. Or adopt a pet—every day will be new and filled with love. Alternatively, pick up a hobby. Surprise yourself; choose a skill area you never would have expected yourself to venture into, or one you always wanted to explore. Learn a new language. Take a vacation. One of the best things you can do is start your own garden.

No matter what you choose, journal about it all. Keep adding to your log of favorable experiences. It will help you become aware of the goodness life brings your way when you're not even looking for it, and it will help clear out the hurtful and harmful experiences from your consciousness. Spirit of Compassion always tells me this is an exercise that will pluck one unwanted weed at a time to free up space in your garden mind. This isn't hollow advice. When you've endured emotional turmoil at one time or another, whether it's ongoing in the present or has passed, it has probably shaken you and altered your perception of the world. You may find yourself re-experiencing those old memories as though they

were happening all over again—or re-experiencing the emotions they triggered without knowing why.

When you create new, constructive touch points for yourself—and pay attention to their positive effects on your state of mind—you train your brain, as though it's a radio, to access a healing frequency that is always available to you. And then when life becomes overwhelming, you can turn that internal dial to the restorative station to activate the impressions those positive experiences left on you, as though they're recordings of the original broadcasts.

When you're healing from PTSD, picture yourself as a tree that's been transplanted. Digging up the tree puts it in shock—just as whatever stressors you've experienced may have felt like they uprooted you. When you replant the tree in fresh, new soil, it's still traumatized, affected on all levels by losing its foothold. It will take months for the tree to recover from the change and reestablish itself.

In the same way, it can take a good three to four months on a Medical Medium PTSD-healing program to feel like yourself again. And just as nurseries offer nutrient-dense soil amendments to feed that tree in its new spot in the ground, you can nourish your central nervous system and cognitive function, as well as restore your heart and soul, with the nutrient solutions (i.e., healing foods and supplements) in this chapter.

Healing from PTSD requires support from loved ones, time, patience, and key nutritional elements. Part IV, "How to Finally Heal," will fill in more information.

Prayer, in whatever form brings you comfort, is another healing tool. You can also pray to specific angels by name to help you. The angel who best understands how the spirit and soul can be beaten down, and how they can be recovered, is the *Angel of Restitution,* and that's who you should call upon for the most direct aid with PTSD. (See Chapter 25, "Essential Angels.")

And to help mend the soul fractures that trauma can create, try the soul-healing meditations and techniques in Chapter 24. They can have a remarkable effect on the psyche by putting you back in touch with yourself, and restoring faith and trust.

You don't have to live in a tortured state of mind anymore. There's a way forward.

Healing Foods

In order to restore glucose to the brain—and build a glucose storage bin to prevent life disruptions from turning into PTSD—focus on incorporating the following foods into your diet: wild blueberries, melons, beets, bananas, persimmons, papayas, potatoes, tomatoes, sweet potatoes, figs, oranges, mangoes, tangerines, apples, raw honey, and dates. Incorporating leafy greens along the way would also be beneficial; spinach, cilantro, parsley, mâche, and butter leaf lettuce are very helpful. Incorporate as many of these foods into your diet as you can.

Note that the natural sugars in fruit, raw honey, winter squash, potatoes, and sweet potatoes are among the only sugars the body accepts for glucose storage in the brain.

Try to avoid eggs, milk, cheese, butter, and other dairy products as you seek relief from PTSD. Also consider keeping radical fats (such as nut butters, seeds, avocados, coconut oil, other oils, meat, chicken, and fish) to

a minimum—try this periodically, if you can, while recovering from PTSD.

Healing Herbs and Supplements

Before applying these, be sure to read Chapter 21, "Critical Guide to Supplement Protocols."

Supplements for Posttraumatic Stress Disorder (PTSD) (also known as Posttraumatic Stress Symptoms, or PTSS)

- **Fresh celery juice:** work up to 32 ounces daily

- **Celeryforce:** 3 capsules three times a day

- **5-MTHF:** 1 capsule daily

- **Aloe vera:** 2 or more inches of fresh gel (skin removed) daily

- **Ashwagandha:** 2 dropperfuls twice a day

- **Barley grass juice powder:** 1 tablespoon or 9 capsules daily

- **B-complex:** 1 capsule daily

- **California poppy:** 3 capsules or 3 dropperfuls daily at bedtime

- **Cat's claw:** 1 dropperful daily

- **CoQ10:** 1 capsule daily

- **Curcumin:** 2 capsules twice a day

- **D-mannose:** 1 tablespoon daily in water

- **Elderflower:** 1 cup of tea daily

- **EPA and DHA (fish-free):** 1 capsule daily (taken with dinner)

- **GABA:** 1 250-milligram capsule daily

- **Lemon balm:** 5 dropperfuls three times a day

- **Licorice root:** 1 dropperful daily (two weeks on, two weeks off)

- **Magnesium glycinate:** 2 capsules twice a day

- **Melatonin:** 5 milligrams at bedtime daily

- **NAC (N-acetyl cysteine):** 1 capsule daily

- **Nascent iodine:** 4 small drops (not dropperfuls) daily

- **Nettle leaf:** 3 dropperfuls twice a day

- **Peppermint:** 1 cup of tea twice a day

- **Spirulina:** 1 tablespoon or 9 capsules daily

- **Vitamin B$_{12}$ (as adenosylcobalamin with methylcobalamin):** 3 dropperfuls twice a day

- **Vitamin C (as Micro-C):** 2 capsules twice a day

- **Wild blueberry powder:** 1 tablespoon daily

CASE HISTORY:
Soothing the Soul from Hidden Trauma
1997

Jacquelyn had worked in the corporate world for over a decade. During that time, she'd proven herself as an extremely loyal and disciplined employee who was easy to get along with and who cared about her coworkers. After years of commitment, she'd been promoted to her dream job, project coordinator.

Though she wasn't technically a manager, Jacquelyn had been one of the first employees hired in her department 10 years earlier. Everyone knew that her experience made her the de facto boss in their division, and they respected her quiet leadership style. Whenever they finished a task, her coworkers would come to her desk to ask, "What can I do next to help you?" Every time she presented a finished assignment to the head of their corporate branch, they rooted for her to hit a home run. And she always did.

Jacquelyn's boss knew that she was one of the company's best workers, that she was eager to take on every project with a deadline of yesterday thrown on her desk, no matter how much after-hours work it required. The new position was demanding—and that was before all the drama.

Soon a new employee, Bridget, was hired in Jacquelyn's department. Bridget had worked for the company previously in human resources. Jacquelyn had been asking for more hands on deck for the busy season, and she figured the new addition would work to support her like the other people on the floor did.

At first, Bridget didn't seem to do much of anything, besides chat on the phone in a low voice and spend long stretches away from her desk. Then on the Friday of Bridget's third week, Jacquelyn arrived back at the office from a lunch break to find Bridget going from cubicle to cubicle, telling each of their coworkers, "You report to me now." If anyone asked why, she said, "I have the most experience."

Rather than confront her with everyone watching, Jacquelyn went to her desk and continued on as though nothing had changed. Her employees weren't eager to start turning in their work to this imposter Bridget, so they kept going as usual, too. Bridget approached Jacquelyn a couple of times during the afternoon to fuss about this or that detail she wasn't happy with in the checklist for their current project, but Jacquelyn just nodded each time and returned to the task at hand.

After the others had gone home, Jacquelyn approached Bridget, ready to put her in her place. Before Jacquelyn could open her mouth, Bridget told her she'd looked into Jacquelyn's past projects and they were all seriously lacking. The department needed an overhaul. Jacquelyn felt the room spin.

On Monday morning, after spending Saturday and Sunday catching up on work projects, Jacquelyn came into the office and noticed the room had been rearranged. A note was on her desk saying she was expected at her boss's office at 9 A.M. When she got there, her corporate branch manager and Bridget were deep in conversation, laughing. As soon as they saw Jacquelyn, their happy expressions faded. "Bridget, why don't you kick things off?" said Jacquelyn's boss.

Bridget proceeded to voice outlandish complaints about Jacquelyn, then produced a list of Jacquelyn's unmet responsibilities. Bridget claimed that the current deadline they were working toward was destined to be a disaster and told the branch manager there was no leadership in the department. At the end of the meeting, the boss told Jacquelyn they'd been working on creating a new manager position for Bridget, and effective today, it was official.

Staving off tears, Jacquelyn rushed back to her department and inquired among her staff about issues with the project Bridget had mentioned. Several told her that, yes, it was looking like they'd blow the deadline—because Bridget had insisted they stop their tasks and start over. One staff member became incensed on Jacquelyn's behalf and led her back to the boss's office. The staff member explained to the manager about Bridget's tactics to undermine Jacquelyn, yet the boss told him he must be fabricating the story. A few days later, Jacquelyn's advocate was fired.

For the next few months, the mental abuse Jacquelyn suffered at the office was worse than that in a high school cafeteria. Bridget made up more lies about Jacquelyn, spread gossip, and acted as a taskmaster. She'd frequently assign Jacquelyn something to do, then take it away. Though Jacquelyn didn't realize it, her brain was suffering physical damage from the repeated trauma.

Jacquelyn decided she'd take her complaint to her boss one more time—but she was turned away by his receptionist and told she needed to register a complaint with human resources instead.

As Jacquelyn's weekly complaints filled a file in the HR department, nothing was done to address Bridget's abusive behavior.

One day, Jacquelyn poked her head into the HR office to make sure she'd been following the proper procedure to get Bridget disciplined. The woman she spoke with told her that the complaints hadn't, in fact, been sent on to the branch manager. "Those descriptions didn't sound like Bridget." Suddenly it dawned on Jacquelyn that this was the department where Bridget used to work, and this HR person was her friend.

Jacquelyn spent her lunch hour on a walk, working up the courage to approach her boss about the HR conspiracy. But then she walked by the window of a restaurant and spotted Bridget and their boss dining together inside, all smiles.

For about the umpteenth time, Jacquelyn went home in tears and poured her heart out to her husband, Alan. He had been her witness through the chronic nightmares, anxiety, and insomnia. She was exhausted and burned out. Whenever she tried to have a moment's peace, she heard Bridget's voice in her head, berating her. She now felt worthless, and every hour of work was torture. After 10 years of effort and devotion, she might have to resign.

Jacquelyn contacted me, and before she spoke a word, both Spirit and I knew she was afflicted with posttraumatic stress disorder. When she did speak, anger, sadness, abandonment, and hurt came through in her voice.

Her identity had previously been as the hardest worker at her corporation. It was what made her feel she had a place in the world. Before her mother had died, she'd told Jacquelyn how proud she was that she'd gotten through college with flying colors and landed the job she had.

So Jacquelyn's PTSD was layered. It wasn't just about Bridget making the office an unpleasant environment; it was about Jacquelyn losing her sense of self. Jacquelyn's will and spirit were dwindling fast, and she was headed into a grave depression.

Alan got on the phone with us and said that he hadn't been able to say anything to comfort Jacquelyn. "It's like she has an allergic reaction every time I tell her she's capable."

"Do you have any vacation time?" I asked Jacquelyn. She said she had two weeks stored up, so I told her to request time off immediately.

Over the next 14 days, we implemented powerful restructuring of her spirit and soul.

To begin with, we searched for and revived things she'd once loved to do, long before her corporate identity had taken hold. We made a list of everything she'd ever enjoyed in life. Alan took out the old Scrabble set they'd played when they were courting each other.

The memory-imbued game alone was a powerful first step in reigniting Jacquelyn's spirit.

Jacquelyn also started a journal of the positive experiences she was enjoying during her time off. For example, walking the dog at night had once been her task, before she'd gotten too busy and Alan had taken over. Now she made note of how calming and quiet the neighborhood was at night, of how her dog stopping to sniff every tree reminded her to breathe, and of how so many people she passed greeted her warmly.

For more positive touchstones, Jacquelyn ordered DVDs of television shows she'd once loved. Alan suggested they start learning the waltz at a local dance school. They went to favorite restaurants they hadn't had a chance to visit in years. Then they decided on a weekend getaway to a bed-and-breakfast that held positive memories.

As the list grew and the pages in Jacquelyn's journal filled, she started to feel capable again. She felt an inner strength return, the essence of who she was—her soul. On a physical level, to replenish Jacquelyn's glucose stores, Alan had been cutting up melon for her in the morning and making her all-fruit smoothies in the afternoon.

At this stage, we talked about how miserable life must be for Bridget. She must be a very injured person to be so hateful, deceitful, and angry; it must be very hard to be her. We developed a way to feel sad for Bridget. Jacquelyn realized that despite her facade, Bridget wasn't empowered at all. Just the opposite. She had no power—which was why she felt the need to trample on Jacquelyn. This allowed Jacquelyn to see Bridget in a whole new light.

We discussed how Jacquelyn's place in the office had always been hers, and it still was. Her title hadn't changed. She had been there the longest and had the most respect in the department. Instead of absorbing Bridget's negative energy each day, Jacquelyn needed to find a way to shower her with caring, love, and positive energy.

At the end of the two weeks, Jacquelyn arrived at work and noticed Bridget sitting in her car with talk radio blasting—no doubt trying to drown out the negative messages she was hearing in her head. A sorrow came over Jacquelyn as she watched Bridget sipping her coffee and frowning, and she saw how pathetic Bridget's attempts at domination truly were.

Jacquelyn knocked on Bridget's window. "Do you want to go in to work with me?"

Bridget cocked her head. "Um, sure?"

As they walked into the building, Jacquelyn put her arm around Bridget. "You're a wonderful person, you know that? I see you're struggling, and I want you to know, I'm here for you."

Bridget appeared so shocked she couldn't come up with anything to say. Over the course of the day, Jacquelyn noticed Bridget didn't utter one snide remark.

After a few months, when the corporation went through restructuring, Bridget advocated for Jacquelyn to become head of the new creative department. Bridget probably got a bigger paycheck in her new, vague managerial role. Still, assured in the knowledge that she was probably much more fulfilled than Bridget, Jacquelyn learned to accept the gift she had been given and move forward.

CHAPTER 14

Depression

When I lost my childhood best friend to a car accident when he was 21, I was inconsolable. This guy had been my soul brother. He'd understood my gift of hearing Spirit and what kind of pressure that put on me growing up, and he'd taken me seriously. He was one of the only people on earth who got me. When I heard the news that he was gone, I felt like a car had slammed into me, too.

No matter what words of comfort Spirit offered, my wounds couldn't be soothed. I was hurt, grief-stricken, angry, afraid. And I felt for my friend's family as well. Watching them suffer this unimaginable loss while I dealt with the aftermath of my own shock, I went into a temporary depression. It was unlike any trial I had faced yet in life, even with my struggles growing up. Nothing made sense anymore.

In the past, I'd been able to help depression sufferers because Spirit of Compassion understood their plight, but I couldn't identify with them on a personal level. Now I'd been where they had been. The experience gave me a window into what others might feel when they faced their own trials.

Over time, I healed. I still look back on the loss of my friend with great sadness, but I don't reenter that headspace of despair. I learned we have to have patience with depression. Even if you've suffered with it for 5 years, 10 years, or more, you have to keep the hope alive that it won't always be like this. Faith is essential to recovery from depression. You *must* hold on.

If you haven't experienced depression personally, then you've surely known someone who has. We've all had loved ones or friends or workmates who have uttered the phrase "I'm depressed." Many who've never suffered through clinical depression confuse it with the everyday experience of being sad now and then, and don't understand why those struck by depression can't just "cheer up." The truth is, there's a world of difference between occasionally feeling down and having clinical depression. For some people, it's a feeling that can't quite be described, a general dampening of life. Others experience depression in its much graver form. It occurs on all different levels of severity for all different periods of time.

In medical research and science, and in medical communities, depression is still a condition with great mystery behind it. Depression has been perplexing people since humankind began. It's probably the most profound of all the mystery illnesses on the planet, never mind the universe, because its origin is in both our soul and physical body.

In this chapter, I'll reveal key causes and triggers of depression. I'll help you uncover the reason behind your imprisonment, and I'll help you learn how to break free.

Over 20 years ago, a client compared the onset of her depression to being let off a train in the middle of nowhere. The train pulled away, and she was stranded all alone, with no way home. No more trains were traveling through the station. She told me the depression felt like a loneliness that wouldn't leave her. That description has stayed with me ever since.

If you suffer from depression, I want you to know: the train is coming back for you. You don't have to wander alone anymore. Let this chapter be the train's headlights, signaling that it's getting close. If you follow the recommendations here, you can find your way home to a healthy state of mind.

DEPRESSION SYMPTOMS

If you have a depressive disorder, you're probably experiencing symptoms such as sadness; loss of interest in activities that used to provide pleasure; an unexplainable feeling in your heart, chest, or stomach that confuses and saddens you; feeling disconnected from yourself, in a crisis of understanding who you are; feeling out of body and lost; slow thinking, speaking, and/or movement; and even thoughts of self-harm.

As these symptoms indicate, clinical depression is a very serious condition.

When you experience depression, as hard as it may be, it's important to share what you're going through with those who care about you, and to let in their love and support. You can let go of any shame you feel about your depression. There are important aspects of it that medical communities haven't yet uncovered. As you read the sections that follow, you'll gain new insights into what's behind your symptoms—and what you can do about them.

IDENTIFYING AND ADDRESSING MAJOR CAUSES OF DEPRESSION

Most people assume clinical depression comes from emotional pain, such as severe sadness and/or suppressed anger. That accurately describes one type of depression, but this is a complex condition, and it can stem from a number of different root causes. While some are based in emotion (e.g., traumatic loss, betrayal), others are entirely physical (e.g., toxic heavy metals, Epstein-Barr virus).

What follows are the most common reasons behind a depressive disorder. Any of these issues by itself is powerful enough to cause or trigger depression. However, it's also possible to suffer from two or more issues simultaneously. Do your best to identify those causes or triggers that apply to you.

Traumatic Loss

The most obvious reason for depression is a severe emotional blow or series of blows. This typically involves loss.

Examples are a family member dying (loss of a loved one); a spouse cheating on you (loss of trust, and of a close relationship); getting fired from a job that defined you (loss of security and identity); experiencing an event that demolishes long-held plans (loss of direction and purpose); suffering an injustice that makes you decide the universe is cruel (loss of faith); and having reason to believe you're soon going to die (loss of your future).

Of course, different people react to situations in different ways. A loss that sends someone else into a depressive spiral might not affect you on the same scale, or vice versa. Such dissimilar responses are due in part to variations in sensitivities, personal history, and physical compromises. What matters most is the effect a loss has on *you*. If it fills you with feelings of intense emotional pain, helplessness, and/or hopelessness, that can be enough to initiate severe depression.

Medical research and science don't yet know that such traumatic emotions can create *micro-strokes* in your brain—that is, damage to brain tissue on a much smaller scale than that caused by conventional ischemic strokes, or even transient ischemic attack (TIA). These micro-strokes are so small that they don't show up on MRIs, CT scans, or any other imaging technology that we have today. They can result in numerous problems, including any of the symptoms of clinical depression. Fortunately, they can heal over time.

A major emotional shock can generate an actual electrical jolt in your brain. There's a reason why someone delivering bad news often warns, "You may want to sit down for this": we know intuitively that shock has a physical effect. The electrical impulse from a shock fires at a much more intense and rapid rate than normal. First, as we receive the shocking data, a charge builds quickly. Then It "explodes" out of the running gate, rushing through neurons throughout the emotional center of the brain and leaving behind a wake of leftover heat. The combination of this "explosion" and the leftover heat in the neurons can be so intense that it effectively "blows a fuse" in your brain, causing parts of it to switch off.

This shutdown is a safety mechanism designed to protect your soul (which resides inside your brain) from being too badly injured. Whether it's a betrayal, learning you've been fired from a job, or returning to your car to find the window smashed, an alarming experience can trigger an electrical pulse in the emotional center of the brain that's almost like a tidal wave crashing onto shore. Depression can result when a series of upsetting events over time prompts the safety mechanism to break down and go awry. For some people, a delayed depression response can occur even months later, when the problems themselves have already subsided.

Often, the safety measures cease proper function when upheavals add up. Picture a sand castle on the beach. The first line of defense against the rising tide is the wall you built around the castle—it stays standing against the first strong wave and holds the tide at bay for the first 20 minutes. Then a big wave hits and takes out the wall. That's okay, because you've dug a moat; the castle is still intact. For the next few minutes, all is well. And then a third swell rises—and takes out the castle.

When our mental safety measures have ceased normal operation, certain parts of the brain, the *I-can't-believe-it* emotional areas, may no longer perk back up. This can result in the feelings of numbness, burnout, or pessimism that so often accompany depression.

There's good news, though: we can rebuild our mental resources. With the right nurturing, our safety mechanisms can restore themselves so that we're able to experience life in an awakened state again, and to bounce back from unexpected events. Over time, we can heal our depression.

Traumatic Stress

Another major cause of depression is severe and *sustained* stress. While we all feel such pressure now and then—it's part of being alive—when you're suffering from intense stress for a prolonged period of time, it can create a burnout effect.

Some examples are being unemployed for months and continually worrying about how you're going to pay your bills, getting hit with a lawsuit that threatens to ruin you financially, going through a combative divorce, and enduring a major illness that makes you feel afraid and helpless.

While these are serious issues that cause sustained, traumatic stress for many people, little stressors can also feel traumatic when they pile up. We have to respect that everyone has a unique sensitivity level. While something like a letter getting lost in the mail may seem like no big deal to one person, to another, it may trigger a memory of the time a critical payment went missing en route to a creditor—or maybe it's one more thing he doesn't have time to deal with in the day.

Did you ever have an elder tell you that you just needed perspective? Maybe, as a teenager, you picked up your prom dress from the tailor on the night of the dance, found it was three inches too short, and got no sympathy from your grandfather: "There are children starving in Africa, and here you are crying about a *dress*?" Or perhaps you've had a broken wrist and complained to a colleague about the difficulty of taking a shower with a cast, only for her to reply, "Well at least you still *have* your arm." Chances are, these statements (more like chastisements) didn't help.

Sure, it can be beneficial to gain perspective on our suffering, to get outside of our heads from time to time and try to see our lives in the grand scheme of things. Rational thought doesn't always help with our emotional experience of a situation, though. We go through severe stresses in our earthly lives, and we go through less severe stresses. They're hard all the same. We have to honor the different reaction levels in ourselves and in one another.

On a physical level, these events trigger a fight-or-flight response that sets your adrenal glands to flood your system with adrenaline. That would be a good thing if you were about to fight for your life against a tiger or flee down an alley as a car chased you. But when you aren't able to physically flush out or burn off the adrenaline saturating the tissues of your vital organs—and especially your brain—it eventually creates damage that can lead to major depression. The adrenaline becomes a trigger that breaks down dozens of the most important neurotransmitters and even lowers melatonin production, setting you up for feeling lost at sea in a depressive fog and eventually causing sleep disorders, whether sleeping too much or not being able to sleep at all.

Adrenal Dysfunction

Depression can also stem from a purely physical cause. In such cases it may hit you out of the blue, leaving you dumbfounded about why you're feeling awful.

For example, as just explained, intense and/or prolonged emotions can flood your brain with corrosive adrenaline. Compare it to filling up your car at the gas station: your car needs the fuel to run, but if you overflow the gas tank, the petroleum will eat away at your paint job.

Even if you've never been rocked by such emotions, your brain can still suffer this harmful flooding if your adrenal glands are malfunctioning, and this can just as readily create depressive burnout.

To get a sense of whether this is an issue for you—and, if it is, how to heal your weakened glands—read Chapter 8, "Adrenal Fatigue."

Viral Infection

Medical communities don't know that millions of people suffer from depression as a result of a virus such as Epstein-Barr (detailed in Chapter 3) or Lyme disease (detailed in Chapter 16). Some varieties of viruses latch on to your nerves and continually inflame them. Viruses such as EBV and shingles also emit a poison, or *neurotoxin,* that further inflames your nerves and brain cells. This puts a strain on the central nervous system, sometimes disrupting the most fine-tuned signals throughout the brain . . . which can lead to depression. Even a mild viral load in the body that's causing undetectable inflammation and no other symptoms can create an underlying depression.

Heavy Metals and Other Toxins

Another type of depression is the *Everything-is-perfect* variety. Someone can have a loving family, the perfect job, a beautiful house, and feel gratitude for all of it. Yet a dark, unexplainable cloud can arrive and loom over all of it. It can cause a person to feel different, sad, not like herself or himself anymore—as though something is missing. It can make a person not want to get out of bed in the morning.

Those around such people often don't understand. "You've got everything," they say. "What's wrong with you?"

This type of depression is the result of toxins—not a bad attitude.

As a result of normal modern living, over time the body will accumulate toxic heavy metals, especially mercury, aluminum, and copper. For example, tuna and other seafood often contain mercury. Most soda cans are made of aluminum. And your tap water is probably carried into your home by copper pipes, and also filled with fluoride, a toxic aluminum byproduct.

These metals may eventually settle into the area of the brain near the thalamus and the pineal, pituitary, and hypothalamus glands. If an acidic environment inside the body increases throughout the years (because of foods someone is consuming such as vinegars, certain grains, processed foods, dairy products, eggs, and alcohol) and is coupled with a high-protein, high-fat diet, the metals will start oxidizing quickly, which causes a release of oxidative metal byproduct, which then creates a poisonous chemical pool that contaminates other brain cells and neurons and lowers electrical impulse activity. This disruption, in this particular area of the brain, can create a depressive disorder, which can sneak up on a person when least expected.

The oxidation isn't necessarily continuous. If the oxidative runoff from the toxic heavy metals happens on an occasional basis, you will experience depression only sporadically, with no apparent rhyme or reason for each episode.

Other toxins can also create neuron and neurotransmitter damage that disrupts your brain's ability to function. The toxins most responsible for depressive disorders include:

Pesticides and herbicides: you can encounter these chemicals when living near a sprayed yard (for example, from a neighbor's lawn treatment), garden, farm, or golf course; walking in a recently sprayed park; eating non-organic food; and so on.

Formaldehyde: this chemical is used in thousands of household products, and also used as a preservative in processed foods.

Solvents: the chemicals used in carpet cleaning, household cleaning, and office cleaning create gases that you breathe in every day. Breathing in gasoline fumes also creates exposure.

Food additives: MSG, aspartame, sulfites (used as preservatives in many foods), and other unnatural additives to foods can build up in your brain. Once they've begun triggering depressive episodes, even drinking a can of diet soda can set off a new attack.

Electrolyte Deficiency

To remain healthy, your body must maintain a certain level of electrolytes. These electrolytes help maintain and allow electrical impulses to travel throughout your body—especially your brain, which is the center of your body's electrical activity. People who have higher levels of mercury and other heavy metals in the brain need higher than normal electrolytes to balance them out. Toxic heavy metals tend to reduce electrolyte activity in the brain, because someone with toxic heavy metals in the brain needs more electrolytes and uses them up more quickly than someone without toxic heavy metals in the brain.

Imagine your brain as a car battery. When the chemical electrolyte solution in the battery is too low, it interrupts the flow of electricity within and keeps the car from starting. In the same way, when you run low on the electrolytes meant to be in the blood that's pumping through your brain (the battery), it can severely disrupt electrical activity and act as a trigger for depression. And like a car battery, you can recharge your brain from burnout—if you get enough electrolytes.

HEALING FROM DEPRESSION

As you've just seen, there are numerous triggers and explanations for depression. The most helpful thing you can do is address any particular cause(s) for your depression that you have identified. Just knowing what's behind your state of mind can have an enormously validating and healing effect.

It's also recommended that you take the herbs, supplements, and foods described in this section. Using these powerful Medical Medium tools, you can bolster your brain tissue, nerve cells, and endocrine system; detoxify yourself; and improve your mood. For more information on nutrition—which can have a profound effect on mental health—turn to Part IV, "How to Finally Heal."

There, you'll also find Chapter 24, "Soul-Healing Meditations and Techniques," and Chapter 25, "Essential Angels." Those pages contain exercises that can help you find peace and validation as you recover from depression and reclaim your life.

Healing Foods

Specific fruits, leafy greens, herbs, wild foods, and vegetables can help rejuvenate the brain, remove toxic heavy metals, replenish electrolytes, heal brain tissue, kill off and starve viruses, and/or address the nutritional deficiencies that exist along with depression. The ideal items to incorporate into your diet for the alleviation of your symptoms are wild blueberries, spinach, hemp seeds (in small amounts), cilantro, potatoes, bananas, papayas, ginger, parsley, sprouts, kale, brussels sprouts, artichokes, green beans, lettuces, melons, apples, celery, tomatoes, apricots, avocados (in small amounts), and walnuts (in small amounts). Incorporate as many of these foods into your diet as you can.

The Heavy Metal Detox Smoothie from Chapter 23 incorporates some of these healing foods and can be a very helpful tool when seeking relief from depression.

Try to avoid eggs, milk, cheese, butter, other dairy products, and gluten. These are foods that will feed viruses. By starting to remove them in favor of the healing foods listed above, you're taking away the viral fuel so that you can experience the peace you deserve.

Healing Herbs and Supplements

Before applying these, be sure to read Chapter 21, "Critical Guide to Supplement Protocols."

Supplements for Depression

- **Fresh celery juice:** work up to 32 ounces daily
- **Celeryforce:** 2 capsules three times a day
- **5-MTHF:** 1 capsule daily
- **Ashwagandha:** 1 dropperful daily
- **Barley grass juice powder:** 2 teaspoons or 6 capsules daily
- **B-complex:** 1 capsule daily
- **Curcumin:** 2 capsules daily
- **EPA and DHA (fish-free):** 1 capsule daily (taken with dinner)
- **GABA:** 1 250-milligram capsule daily
- **Hibiscus:** 1 cup of tea twice a day
- **Lemon balm:** 4 dropperfuls twice a day
- **Licorice root:** 1 dropperful daily (two weeks on, two weeks off)
- **L-lysine:** 2 500-milligram capsules daily
- **Magnesium glycinate:** 2 capsules daily
- **Melatonin:** 5 milligrams at bedtime daily
- **Nascent iodine:** 3 small drops (not dropperfuls) daily

- **Spirulina:** 2 teaspoons or 6 capsules daily

- **Vitamin B$_{12}$ (as adenosylcobalamin with methylcobalamin):** 2 dropperfuls twice a day

- **Vitamin C (as Micro-C):** 4 capsules twice a day

- **Vitamin D$_3$:** 1,000 IU daily

- **Wild blueberry powder:** 2 teaspoons daily

- **Zinc (as liquid zinc sulfate):** 1 dropperful daily

CASE HISTORY:
An Unexpected Answer to Happiness
2004

Ellen had been a happy person all her life. Friends and family called her the life of the party. She knew how to comfort anyone who was down or sad, and she was the rock of her marriage. She looked forward to the sun rising and loved to plan weekends, future vacations, and her three daughters' birthday parties. Ellen treasured life and was thankful for every day. She felt her life was perfect.

Then, at the age of 44, Ellen returned home from vacation with her family and immediately began to feel strange. She couldn't quite explain it, but it felt like part of her was missing. On top of feeling extra tired, she felt like she'd lost her spunk and passion for life. A sadness started to develop.

At first Ellen passed it off as the post-vacation blues, figuring it would pass. Over the next few months, there were times when it felt like it was getting better, then it would gradually worsen again. Ellen felt like she was losing herself. Her husband, Tom, was gravely worried. "I miss your cheerleader smile," he'd tell her. She'd always given off a bright light, and now it was dim.

Searching for answers, Ellen visited her doctor, who examined her and ran a complete hormone profile test. When Ellen's hormone levels came back normal, the doctor concluded that she must be suffering from depression and handed her a prescription for antidepressants. "See if this gives you any relief."

Ellen walked out of the office more depressed than she'd been when she arrived. The diagnosis and medication felt so foreign to her. When she shared the news with her family, they were as shocked as she was. She began to take the antidepressants, but without any explanation of why these new feelings were happening to her or how long they would last, she felt as if she were a prisoner to the medication.

She decided to seek professional counseling. The therapist was positive that stored emotions were holding Ellen back. Ellen worked on digging into her past with this wonderful, supportive counselor. The process felt productive, and helped give Ellen a support system she felt was critical to keeping her afloat during her depression—but the depression was still there.

A year after its onset, Tom decided to take Ellen away from it all with another vacation. He thought maybe it would create forward movement. Off the family went for 10 days—and Ellen felt a little better. She was chattering with her daughters again, planning costumes for school plays with them, and rising with the sun. She wasn't her old self, but she felt a 50 percent improvement. Sitting at the airport afterward, waiting for their flight home, Ellen told Tom the trip had been just the jump start she needed.

As soon as she began to unpack, though, after just a few hours at home, Ellen crashed. She curled up in bed and felt the depression wash over her stronger than ever before. The feeling stayed as the days passed, and she felt as if it would never go away. She began to cry often—when she was brushing her teeth, tying her shoes, or even waking up in the morning. She no longer had the energy to sit in the living room with Tom and her daughters to watch their favorite show on Sunday nights.

Unable to get Ellen over this hump, her therapist recommended she make an appointment with me. As soon as I started the reading on Ellen, Spirit alerted me to a high level of insecticides in her organs, along with traces of herbicides. I explained the findings, and Ellen suddenly got quiet.

"Are you okay?" I asked.

Ellen started to explain that her husband had the interior and exterior of their house treated by the pest company periodically. I asked Ellen for the treatment schedule, and she had Tom pick up from another phone. He explained that every time they went away, whether for a weekend trip to his mother-in-law's or for one of their longer vacations, he'd have the neighbor let in an exterminator to spray for insects. Monthly, he had a landscaping company treat their lawn and gardens with herbicides.

I insisted that Ellen, Tom, and their children move out of the house immediately to see if Ellen improved. While they stayed at Ellen's mother's house, Ellen started a healing food, supplement, and detox regimen — as described in this section, and in Part IV of this book—to rid herself of the chemicals and heavy metals in her system that were causing her depression. (Tom joined in, too, plus we did a modified version of this program to help their daughters cleanse from the toxins.)

Ellen came back to life. With the mystery illness solved, the healing protocol in place, her renewed confidence, distance from the pesticide exposure, and the added benefit of the emotions she had processed in therapy, Ellen felt better than ever. She and Tom decided to put their house on the market and start anew.

CHAPTER 15

Premenstrual Syndrome and Menopause

Through nearly all of history, women viewed *menopause* in a positive light. Although it was a reminder of getting older, menopause gently and painlessly ended the difficulties and inconveniences of *premenstrual syndrome* (PMS) and *menstruation,* often resulted in a heightened libido, and allowed for sex without the worry of accidental pregnancy.

Women in the past didn't turn to doctors for help with menopause, because they didn't experience notable physical problems or symptoms with it. Women almost always felt *better* in perimenopause, menopause, and postmenopause than they had before. It was a normal part of life that didn't require anything beyond acceptance.

Medical literature produced up through the 1800s very seldom even mentioned menopause. When it did, it almost never referred to menopause as symptomatic or as a hardship that required a doctor's care. Hot flashes and heart palpitations were practically nonexistent.

That all changed in the modern era, around 1950. Women born from 1900 on were the first ones to experience night sweats, hot flashes, fatigue, panic attacks, anxiety, hair thinning, and joint pain when they reached a certain age. In the middle of the 20th century, a tidal wave of women ages 40 to 55 were visiting their doctors with these symptoms—and doctors didn't know what to think.

Behold, mystery illness and the autoimmune confusion were born. Medical professionals had never been so bewildered.

Physicians reported the epidemic to pharmaceutical companies, and at first, the consensus was that it was all in women's heads—it was just crazy women syndrome. They had to be making up their symptoms, because otherwise it made no sense. It was all a cry for attention, a sign they were bored. World War II had recently ended. The thought was that the war had kept women so busy with worry, hard work, and taking care of their families while many men were away that now, women were reacting to having less to do. Women were told to join the PTA.

Yet through the 1950s, the wave of women experiencing memory issues, trouble concentrating, moodiness, weight gain, dizziness, and more grew larger. The pharmaceutical companies and doctors consulted again and decided that the one thing these women had in common was their age. The medical establishment decided the cause must be hormones—even though men were experiencing the same symptoms at the same time. Plenty of men were having hot flashes; they were just labeled "work sweat" (even if a man wasn't working when an episode hit) or "nervous sweat." Men dealt with other "menopause" symptoms as well—depression, growing waistlines, and forgetfulness, to name just a few. It didn't make news, though, because this was an era when men were taught to be stoic. The responsibility of being the breadwinners weighed heavily, so out of fear of losing their careers, they concealed their private physical issues.

Right away, a pharmaceutical company pursuit to exploit women and capitalize on the false discovery of female hormonal issues was born. By the late 1950s, the news was widespread that women must be suffering from hormone deficiencies. As the notion of this "women's issue" gained popularity, men felt even more pressure to keep quiet about their parallel symptoms.

Women had faced plenty of difficulties leading up to this point. They'd been oppressed and told to suppress emotions, and only in recent history had they gained the right to vote—to count as human beings. In the middle of the century, they still felt like they were fighting to have a voice. It was easy to take advantage of women by making them feel heard.

Doctors were baffled by women's mystery symptoms, but at least, finally, the doctors believed them. So even though medicine had gone in the wrong direction looking for answers, the theories were celebrated because they gave a name to women's health struggles. It was a well-intentioned effort by doctors.

To this day, doctors operate off this hormonal misinformation. Countless women hear that hormonal imbalance or menopause is behind their suffering.

It's not. Menopause is actually on your side. Believe it or not, the aging process slows down after menopause. That's not the message that's out there. Women think of menopause as the onset of aging and age-related health problems—when in fact it's just the opposite.

A woman's most rapid aging happens between puberty and menopause. That's because reproductive hormones can be steroid compounds that speed up the aging process. This time between puberty and menopause is also when the menstrual cycle is occurring, and as you read more about in Chapter 3, at both menstruation and ovulation, the immune system shifts from other areas of the body to focus more on the reproductive system. This happens at pregnancy and childbirth, too. That regular lowering of the overall immune system, while it serves a greater purpose, can create opportunities for the pathogens behind chronic illness to take hold. By reducing a woman's levels of estrogen and progesterone (which signal these immune system shifts related to the menstrual cycle), menopause helps safeguard her from cancers, viruses, and bacteria.

And here's the truth about osteoporosis: it's not that reaching postmenopause makes a woman more vulnerable to bone porousness. It's that osteoporosis takes decades to develop, so it just happens to show itself when a woman reaches a certain age. Medical communities mistake this coincidence for causation, saying that the reduced levels of estrogen in a woman's body contribute to her loss of bone mass. The reality is that osteoporosis starts to develop long before menopause. *Reproductive hormones* actually contribute to osteoporosis—because they're steroids, and steroids have a bone-dissolving effect. That said, estrogen and progesterone are a minimal reason for bone density issues. These hormones are one contributing factor among many, including infections of pathogens such as the Epstein-Barr virus, nutritional deficiencies, caffeine reliance, a diet that's not supportive, and toxic heavy metals (which have a strong effect in this area). Decades before menopause, a combination of these factors sets the stage for loss of bone mass—whether those bone density issues make themselves known when a woman is still young, or whether it's not until postmenopause that she's diagnosed with osteoporosis.

Let's look more closely at the history of the caffeine and diet factors. After the 1940s, caffeine truly got a foothold in women's lives. That's because women were starting to experience symptoms from the viral explosion—the very symptoms that led to the hormone blame of the era. For the first time in history, they had to rely on caffeine in a very real way in order to power through their symptoms of fatigue, brain fog, listlessness, malaise, depression, energy loss, and loss of motivation. The caffeine industry was truly born at this time and took advantage of this opening. For many women, this prompted years of caffeine use. Caffeine's stimulant effect kicked in fight-or-flight—more than women were already having in their lives—which led to the routine release of highly corrosive adrenaline, in turn contributing to the development of osteoporosis and other symptoms.

When the mysterious symptoms labeled as menopause started to take hold in the 1950s, women were also not being taught to improve their diets to counter any triggers they were experiencing, such as heightened stress or caffeine addiction or use. Doctors of the time were faced with patients experiencing brand-new symptoms, and their training couldn't explain it. Women weren't really given tools to counter anything; they were up against pathogens and weren't being taught how to level the playing field. And when women weren't feeling well—and on top of that weren't being heard or were misunderstood by doctors who didn't know why they were sick—this usually prompted a yearning for more comfort foods. These foods often weren't the best choices for people dealing with low-grade viral infections, although little did anybody know what was really going on. Answers were what women really needed, and still need—answers about why they're feeling a certain way and what to do in order to change that through tools such as healing foods and other protocols in the Medical Medium series. Women deserve to know the truth that menopause is on their side.

Reproductive hormones and the immune system shifts related to the menstrual cycle and reproduction are not bad. They're the reason women are able to bear children. Without these hormones, human life couldn't continue.

Yet the body knows its limits. It's willing to pay the price for the ability to create life, so long as it restricts childbearing to the years between puberty and menopause—because it wants to keep you safe.

Women are told reproductive hormones are the fountain of youth. The irony is that your youth wasn't in your 20s, 30s, or 40s. Your true youth happened before puberty. Reaching menopause is a way of reconnecting with that time. Menopause ends the reproductive system's cycle (and its drain on your body) and brings down reproductive hormone levels. It's the body's natural way of slowing down aging so that you can live a long, healthy life.

Menopause and life after menopause aren't anything to dread. Menopause itself isn't meant to be a difficult physical process, and the wave of younger women who've begun to experience symptoms categorized as hormonal aren't going through early menopause. Other factors entirely are in play—and there are powerful ways to address them. You *can* go back to living a healthy life and embracing life at every stage.

WHAT WAS *REALLY* BEHIND THE FIRST WAVE OF MENOPAUSE SYMPTOMS

Here's the real story: when women started to present symptoms in the 1950s that doctors and pharmaceutical companies attributed to the change of life, they were missing three other commonalities.

The first was viral. These women had all been born in the early 1900s, just as the Epstein-Barr virus (EBV) and other viruses were beginning to take root in the population.

EBV typically enters a woman when she is young and then spends decades building itself up to the point when it's ready to make itself known in the form of inflammatory illness. It just so happened that women affected by the first nonaggressive strains of EBV were in their 40s or 50s when the viral incubation

period ended and the symptoms began. (At the same time, thyroid inflammation started affecting a large number of women. For more on this, see Chapter 6, "Hypothyroidism and Hashimoto's Thyroiditis.")

So if you were born in 1905 and you'd contracted this new virus Epstein-Barr as a small child, by 1950 you'd be 45 years old and part of the first generation just beginning to experience symptoms of this epidemic viral infection. It was only a coincidence that this was the same age as perimenopause or menopause. Yet you'd probably hear that the reason for your hot flashes, night sweats, and fatigue was hormonal. If the viral inflammation presented earlier or later, you'd get the label perimenopause or postmenopause.

You didn't have to contract EBV at the beginning of life to exhibit symptoms by the 1950s. For example, you could have been born in 1900, contracted the Epstein-Barr virus in 1920, and still ended up with symptoms by 1950 or 1955. That's because newer strains of EBV had developed by the 1920s that were stronger and faster moving.

The second commonality among women who got the menopause tag in the 1950s was radiation exposure. Due to a colossal historical blunder called the shoe-fitting fluoroscope—a mistake that's been swept under the rug— women of this time were exposed to the most radiation ever seen in history. They might have been safer if they'd lived on the border of the Chernobyl evacuation zone in 1986!

Following the fluoroscope's invention, it was all the rage from the 1920s to 1950s for a visit to the shoe store to include sticking your legs and feet into this X-ray box. The idea was that the X-ray would help salesmen understand the bone structure of customers' feet to help get them the best fit for their cork-heeled shoes. Yet the dosage of radiation was unexamined and unregulated, and there were no doctors present at the store. It was just a shoe clerk pressing a deadly button at will and whim.

It happened at every visit to the shoe store, over and over again. Plenty of women tried on shoes as therapy, making a visit to the shoe store every other week. That could mean they had something like 800 radiation treatments in a lifetime. It resulted in severe radiation poisoning for millions of women.

By the time 1950 rolled around, the fluoroscope was quietly being removed from shoe stores, as if it had never been there in the first place. Modern medicine was beginning to realize at this time that radiation was dangerous, and I'm sure someone behind the scenes made the connection between women's unprecedented health struggles and their decades-long, repeated exposure to radiation—because it was obvious that tens of thousands of women were getting foot and leg amputations due to cancer. Radiation also lowered the immune system, allowing viruses to cause more harm and quickening additional symptoms.

Rather than point to radiation, though, think tanks selected menopause as the culprit—even though for these women's mothers and grandmothers and great-grandmothers, menopause had been a smooth transition.

At the same time, a third trigger for ill health was occurring: the explosion of DDT exposure. In the 1940s, DDT was used everywhere. It was sprayed on crops, in parks, and kids would even soap themselves up with the pesticide's suds for fun as the DDT truck drove by spraying throughout the suburbs. DDT salesmen would knock on the front door of every home and sell women cans of DDT to spray on their flowers and gardens. To prove its safety, the salesmen would even spray an apple with DDT, adding that it was a nutritious supplement. By 1950, DDT use was at its height, and the central nervous systems and livers of countless women had become overloaded with the toxin.

It's amazing to think that the risk was overlooked for so long. If it hadn't been for Rachel Carson's 1962 book, *Silent Spring*, which brought attention to the dangers of chemical pesticides and eventually led to a U.S. ban on DDT, the world might have continued to overlook the harm these pesticides were causing. As it was, critics attacked Carson and called her hysterical—the very term used for women's mystery symptoms at the time. Ultimately, though, she was vindicated. Everything she went through to bring the truth to light was worth it for the lives she saved.

(By the way, it's not a coincidence that when the massive chemical industry behind DDT took a hit from public awareness about its downsides, a new industry started to emerge and dominate: hormone treatment.)

Meanwhile, menopause became the scapegoat for dozens of symptoms that really had to do with completely different causes. Symptoms misattributed to menopause included night sweats, hot flashes, fatigue, dizziness, weight gain, digestive issues, bloating, incontinence, headaches, moodiness, irritability, depression, anxiety, panic attacks, heart palpitations, trouble concentrating, memory issues, insomnia and other sleep disorders, vaginal dryness, breast sensitivity, joint pain, tingling, hair loss or thinning, dry or cracked skin, and dry or brittle nails.

It should not have made sense to anyone that a healthy and natural life process would cause these problems—especially since it never had before. But hey, why bother considering 30 years of unregulated, intense exposure to radiation, DDT, and viral pathogens?

When women started to experience what were really viral conditions (ones often now called autoimmune), illnesses such as chronic fatigue syndrome, fibromyalgia, adrenal fatigue, hypothyroidism, other manifestations of the Epstein-Barr virus, lupus, heavy metal toxicity, liver dysfunction, and nutritional deficiency—all triggered by the modern era of viral, radiation, and DDT toxin exposure—medical research and science couldn't understand the real answers. (Even today, medical research and science don't consider these to be factors in menopause symptoms.)

It was the birth of the *It-must-be-in-your-head* argument, and when women pushed back against this non-diagnosis, because women's rights were growing stronger at this point, hormones were the perfect way to quiet women down and for doctors to comfort themselves. It was easier for doctors to say, "It's your hormones" than to admit, "I have no idea what's going on with you." Before 1950, a doctor's opinion was not considered the be-all and end-all. From 1950 on, though, modern medicine had its grip on society. For the first time in history, the doctor was heralded as God.

THE TRUTH ABOUT HORMONE REPLACEMENT THERAPY

Pharmaceutical companies actively encouraged the hormone trend when they realized billions could be made by demonizing menopause and creating drugs to "cure" it. In the early 1960s a major promotional campaign was launched claiming that "estrogen deficiencies" were the cause of most of the ills being felt by women before, during, and after menopause. Sales of products promising to replace the supposedly missing estrogen—called hormone replacement therapy (HRT)—skyrocketed.

HRT had actually been in the works for some time. When doctors started to diagnose women with hormone issues, pharmaceutical companies suddenly had a use for their steroid-based lab experiment. They sent patients the message, "We see your pain, so we developed this revolutionary treatment for you." In reality, they were just picking this as the perfect moment to release the products that had already been in development and hadn't had an application until now.

HRT products hardly ever produced any positive results, though. In rare cases, HRT did minimize some symptoms. However, HRT managed this not by genuinely addressing an imbalance in the body, but by acting as a steroid—that is, suppressing the immune system's response to viral inflammation, nutritional deficiencies, and exposure to toxins such as DDT.

In other words, HRT didn't make anyone healthier. On the contrary, in some cases it hid diseases by temporarily preventing the immune system from fully reacting to and combating them. So while it sometimes provided symptom relief, HRT allowed cancers, viruses, bacteria, and more to continue attacking women's bodies and aging them rapidly without their knowledge—at least, until the damage became so severe it couldn't be covered up any longer.

Suddenly, doctors were noticing cancer and strokes on the rise among the women taking HRT. It was just a glimpse of the true problems hormone replacement had been causing, yet it was enough to get attention. When the news was reported, sales dropped—for a while. Soon, another promotional campaign claimed that an adjustment to the products had addressed the problem, and HRT became popular again.

Then in 2002 an enormous clinical study called the Women's Health Initiative, which ran for over a decade and involved more than 160,000 postmenopausal women, caught on to more of the havoc that HRT had been wreaking and concluded that HRT substantially increased the risk of breast cancer, heart attacks, and strokes.[*] That is, hormone replacement therapy rapidly sped up the aging process. Once again, HRT sales plummeted.

When the findings came to light about HRT's dangers, it should have been banned. It should have prompted researchers to look into what was really behind women's mystery symptoms—and started them down the path to the discovery that hormones were never the problem.

Instead, another strategy came into the mix: bioidentical hormone replacement therapy (BHRT).

BHRT is much safer than the previous drugs used in HRT. Every doctor is smart enough to know that, at this point, BHRT remains experimental. It's at the beginning of a 30-year journey of trial and error, just as HRT once was. At least it's not starting from scratch. We have the history of HRT already behind us, which will allow doctors to watch newer hormone treatments more carefully, seeing their positives or any possible negatives.

Conventional trends in health care are so powerful, sometimes nothing can stop them. For doctors, these conventional trends can feel like following the Pied Piper—that is, following their best chance of keeping the peace with colleagues, protecting their livelihoods, and giving hope to patients seeking answers. It's a difficult balance. For women in a society that favors youth over wisdom, the pull is strong toward any trendy pill or cream that claims it's the fountain of youth. Not even bringing the truth to light will stop the hormone train.

If you're presented with both HRT and BHRT as options and still want to try one, I suggest you choose BHRT from a compounding pharmacy. Make sure you get your prescription from a highly skilled physician who's well versed in holistic health and can regulate and balance dosages with knowledge and precision—and who also views BHRT as a temporary, periodic Band-Aid rather than as an indefinite, lifelong treatment without dosage adjustments. There are some really great doctors who are highly skilled with alternative hormone treatments. They recognize subtleties in blood work, and they recognize

---

* Writing Group for the Women's Health Initiative Investigators, "Risks and Benefits of Estrogen Plus Progestin in Healthy Postmenopausal Women: Principal Results from the Women's Health Initiative Randomized Controlled Trial," *Journal of the American Medical Association* 288, no. 3 (2002): 321–333. doi:10.1001/jama.288.3.321.

the best times to draw blood. They're more understanding about symptoms that patients are suffering from, and they're open to other causes besides merely hormones. This does change the game for the better and offers women an opportunity to improve their health while adopting hormone treatments.

There are women who use HRT and get no relief, and there are women who use BHRT and get no relief. For over 25 years, I've seen women use both and get no results (except for accelerated aging, despite all claims that it will bring back their youth), and I've witnessed hundreds of frustrated doctors unable to get their patients better with hormone therapy. That's because neither form addresses the underlying health issues misattributed to menopause. When people feel like they're experiencing improvement with hormone therapy, it's because it's never prescribed by itself anymore; it's prescribed alongside loads of supplementation and an overhauled diet (meaning minimal processed foods and the removal of fried, greasy foods). It's the supplements and new diet that make women feel better. And there are reasons for that: through this guessing game process, some benefits occur as real causes happen to be addressed.

Hormone therapies, because they're steroids, act as immunosuppressant drugs. A patient's viral symptoms such as heart palpitations and hot flashes (which the doctor doesn't identify as viral) may calm down on BHRT, leading everyone to believe it's working. And consider the symptom vaginal dryness, which sometimes improves on BHRT. Vaginal dryness is a symptom of adrenal fatigue, not perimenopause or menopause—that's why this discomfort can trouble even women in their 20s and 30s. The BHRT steroids can potentially

prompt the adrenal glands to churn out adrenaline; this is what temporarily brings some women relief.

Yes, it's possible to have hormonal imbalances. Yet the symptoms doctors call menopause are really caused by all these other factors we've explored in this chapter, not an imbalance of reproductive hormones.

Saliva, blood, and urine tests are not always accurate in determining if a woman's hormones are balanced. These testing methods are fallible and often inaccurate. (Once again, a really good doctor who's seasoned with hormone therapies, knowing all the subtleties and nuances of when to test for hormones, when not to, and how to read them, matters greatly. If that same doctor is well versed in thyroid hormones, it's another win.) If the thyroid is underproducing hormones (that is, it's a hypothyroid), then the adrenal glands overproduce hormones to compensate. The interrupting nature of the overproduction of adrenaline confuses the viability and accuracy of blood tests that look at progesterone, estrogen, and testosterone levels. One way to get a more accurate reading when embarking on alternative hormone therapies, or any hormone therapies, is to make sure foods such as eggs, milk, cheese, butter, other dairy products, gluten, and even chicken and caffeine (coffee drinks, matcha tea, chocolate) are not in the diet. This will allow for a cleaner blood reading. Even if you only hold off on these foods temporarily, starting a few weeks before you get your blood tested, you're going to have a better chance of your doctors reading the signals with greater accuracy.

Body temperature fluctuations, bloating, dizziness, night sweats, heart palpitations, fatigue, and other issues listed in the previous section—these symptoms, viewed collectively, are brand-new to womankind as of the last 70 years. Reproductive hormones aren't to blame. There's a bigger picture being overlooked. I'm not trying to rain on anyone's parade here, poke the bear, or accuse well-meaning doctors of having anything but the best intentions for their patients. We are all working toward the same goal: women's health. We all want women to truly heal. That's all the information here is about.

It would be easier for me to repeat the conjecture and advice that's already out there. I can't do that in good conscience, though. The only way I sleep at night is knowing that I've listened to Spirit of Compassion, that I've offered people real answers and additional choices. Revealing the information in this chapter is worth it to me if it means it could protect you. I want to support you and your doctor in your health, to help you avoid chronic illness, cancer, and stroke, like I've successfully done for women all these years. I want you to live to 90 or 100. I want you to be happy and free.

Your life is precious. Your soul is precious. It's critical for every woman to know the truth about menopause. It's about having options, making informed decisions. Because if you don't understand the real story, how can you make the judgment call that's right for you?

Our choices get taken away from us when we are not given the proper options, information, and truth. There's a saying, "You always have a choice." Not when all the options aren't available to you! If the truth is hidden in a vault that you don't have access to, or lost in the past and forgotten, how can you make the right choice?

The details I provide in this chapter are meant to unlock that vault.

UNDERSTANDING MENOPAUSE TODAY

The disconnect between menopause and the symptoms I've described in this chapter has become clearer recently as the current-day illnesses affecting women have grown more aggressive. Rather than waiting several decades to strike until a woman is in her 40s or 50s, some viral strains and toxic loads are now affecting women in their 30s, 20s, and even in their teens. If this had been the case in the 1940s and early 1950s, if women of all ages had been presenting with mystery symptoms, maybe health professionals would have thought twice about blaming their troubles on menopause. Or maybe pharmaceutical companies and researchers would have concocted another game.

Why are doctors still not making the connection? They have no explanation for why an 18-year-old girl has "perimenopause symptoms"—or why a 25-year-old does, or a 30-year-old. Yet it's happening to these young women at an alarming rate; they're experiencing the same set of issues that used to only affect women in their 40s and 50s. These are the symptoms of Epstein-Barr virus, which causes thyroid disorders, liver problems, neurological symptoms, and more-—the same conditions that were behind the hormone, perimenopause, and menopause blame game that began in the 1950s. It was never menopause to begin with.

The prevalence of the same suffering in younger and younger women makes that clear. While shoe-fitting fluoroscopes and DDT have been phased out, women today are still surrounded by environmental toxins, pesticides, herbicides, heavy metals, and other technological-era pollutants—plus, old toxins passed down from previous generations still reside in us. At the same time, we've suffered epidemics of new forms of cancers, viruses, bacteria, and other illnesses born from the poisons of our modern age. Yet the truth gets buried deep beneath ego, greed, status, and stupidity.

Doctors didn't used to give 18-year-olds HRT or BHRT, by the way, although they're starting to now. They *still* prescribe birth control pills as the number one option when young women exhibit any symptoms—and birth control medication has a similar steroid-like effect of suppressing symptoms without addressing their cause. (Most likely, 18-year-olds will be prescribed HRT and BHRT more often in the future. Already, women in their late 20s and early 30s with virtually any symptoms are being offered BHRT, especially if birth control hasn't suppressed symptoms.)

Something else important to understand is that your doctor can't accurately test your hormone levels when you're suffering with the symptoms I described earlier, because they throw your system out of whack. Once again, it's imperative that the doctor you're using is highly experienced in looking at all aspects of a woman's health and is seasoned in knowing when to test, reading between the lines, and understanding blood results and their inconsistencies. When adrenals are underactive, it will knock the hormonal test off its tracks, too. The readings of estrogen and progesterone levels will not be accurate. Millions of women with underactive adrenals are getting back inaccurate hormone test results.

When a woman is prescribed BHRT and begins to improve, BHRT gets some of the credit. However, a doctor who recommends BHRT is often holistic-minded to begin with, and so she'll recommend a better diet (removing processed foods, eliminating gluten, and bringing in more salads and healthier fats) and plenty of nutritional supplements to clear up deficiencies at the same time. Again, the patient's switch to a healthy lifestyle is usually the real factor in her improvement. If you're experiencing symptoms like those described earlier in the chapter, you should aim to uncover the illness that's actually causing them. Reading the other chapters in this book is likely to help. So is the advice in the pages ahead. You deserve to be free from illness. You deserve to reclaim your life.

UNDERSTANDING PREMENSTRUAL SYNDROME

Symptoms such as depression, diarrhea, bloating, anxiety, insomnia, migraines, acne, body pain, anger, fatigue, and mood swings are often blamed on PMS.

That blame is inaccurate.

These symptoms, like the supposed symptoms of menopause, are actually from underlying health conditions such as a sensitive central nervous system; low-grade viral and bacterial infections such as EBV, shingles, and strep; intestinal tract disorders due to inflammation and food sensitivities caused by these chronic low-grade viral and bacterial infections; sluggish or stagnant liver; or heavy metal toxicity. They make themselves known at this particular time in a woman's cycle because the menstruation process takes up 80 percent of her body's reserves. The 20 percent left over cannot manage the health conditions that the immune system normally keeps at bay. (Again, for more on this, see Chapter 3, "Epstein-Barr Virus, Chronic Fatigue Syndrome, and Fibromyalgia.")

It's another prime example of how far medical communities still are from understanding women's health. Rather than pointing to the reproductive system as the reason for a woman's suffering at her time of the month, we should look at it as a messenger.

(Endometriosis, PCOS, PID, fibroids, and ovarian cysts are conditions that involve the reproductive system itself. Their causes are still unknown to research and science. For insights into what's really behind these conditions and what to do about them, see the Medical Medium book *Cleanse to Heal*.)

If you struggle with issues you've always thought of as PMS, use this book to explore what could really be causing your symptoms, and address that true cause. It's your key to a stress-free menstrual cycle.

ADDRESSING THE SYMPTOMS ASSOCIATED WITH PREMENSTRUAL SYNDROME, PERIMENOPAUSE, MENOPAUSE, AND POSTMENOPAUSE

The symptoms in this chapter that are usually, and falsely, ascribed to menopause are so broad that they can be caused by nearly any health condition. These include adrenal fatigue, food sensitivities, viral load, liver dysfunction, toxic heavy metals, low hydrochloric acid, weakened bile reserves inside the liver, a weakened immune system, an inflamed central nervous system, a range of toxins that have built up in the brain and liver, and chronic *Streptococcus* infections. And these underlying health conditions paint a much

bigger picture than just hormone problems. This section provides a set of herbs, supplements, and foods that address a wide range of viruses, bacteria, funguses, and other toxins that *probably* include whatever's creating your symptoms.

And keep in mind that diet can play a profound role in minimizing the symptoms discussed in this chapter. You'll find more information on how to support your body and overcome illness, including details on detoxification, in Part IV, "How to Finally Heal."

Healing Foods

When you're looking to boost the immune system and support the reproductive system, the best foods to concentrate on are wild blueberries, brussels sprouts, broccoli, cauliflower, butter leaf lettuce, red leaf lettuce, bananas, melons, papayas, blackberries, celery, mâche, artichokes, tomatoes, red bell peppers, asparagus, apples, spinach, black grapes, cucumbers, sesame tahini (in small amounts), avocados (in small amounts), hemp seeds (in small amounts), and lentils. They'll help by, variously, providing antiviral, antibacterial compounds and antioxidants, helping to cleanse the liver, preventing hot flashes, providing critical phytochemical compounds and nutrients to fortify vital organs, reducing inflammation by starving pathogens, and helping to keep the adrenals stable, which will help keep hormone levels balanced all through the body. Incorporate as many of these foods into your diet as you can.

The most important food to stay away from with any condition related to the reproductive system is eggs, which can worsen reproductive system conditions over time. Dairy products are second most important to avoid, and gluten is third. Learn more in Chapter 19, "What Not to Eat."

Healing Herbs and Supplements

These supplement lists offer general support for the symptoms often labeled as menopause and PMS. **Before applying these, be sure to read Chapter 21, "Critical Guide to Supplement Protocols."**

Now that you understand the bigger picture of what can cause these symptoms, also consider seeking out the information from other chapters to get additional help for your specific symptoms.

For supplements lists and dosages for endometriosis, PCOS (polycystic ovary syndrome), PID (pelvic inflammatory disease), fibroids, infertility, and reproductive cysts (including uterine cysts, ovarian cysts, vaginal cysts, and cervical cysts), refer to *Cleanse to Heal*.

Supplements for Everyday Liver and Health Maintenance

Your liver is responsible for producing some hormones and regulating hormone production. This supplement list will help you address general symptoms no matter your stage of life. If you're still menstruating, this list will also help you support yourself through the natural immune system shifts related to the menstrual cycle.

- **Fresh celery juice:** work up to at least 16 ounces daily
- **Celeryforce:** 1 capsule twice a day
- **5-MTHF:** 1 capsule daily
- **Aloe vera:** 2 or more inches of fresh gel (skin removed) daily

- **Barley grass juice powder:** 2 teaspoons or 6 capsules daily
- **Chaga mushroom:** 2 teaspoons or 6 capsules daily
- **Curcumin:** 2 capsules daily
- **Lemon balm:** 3 dropperfuls daily
- **L-lysine:** 3 500-milligram capsules daily
- **Magnesium glycinate:** 2 capsules daily
- **Nettle leaf:** 2 cups of tea or 3 dropperfuls daily
- **Spirulina:** 2 teaspoons or 6 capsules daily
- **Turmeric:** 2 capsules daily
- **Vitamin B$_{12}$ (as adenosylcobalamin with methylcobalamin):** 1 dropperful daily
- **Vitamin C (as Micro-C):** 4 capsules twice a day
- **Zinc (as liquid zinc sulfate):** up to 1 dropperful daily

Supplements for Hormonal Problems

- **Fresh celery juice:** work up to 32 ounces daily
- **Celeryforce:** 2 capsules twice a day
- **Ashwagandha:** 1 dropperful daily
- **Barley grass juice powder:** 2 teaspoons or 6 capsules daily
- **Hibiscus:** 1 cup of tea with 2 bags daily
- **Lemon balm:** 2 dropperfuls daily

- **Milk thistle:** 1 dropperful daily

- **Nascent iodine:** 6 small drops (not dropperfuls) daily

- **Nettle leaf:** 4 dropperfuls daily

- **Raspberry leaf:** 1 cup of tea with 3 bags twice a day

- **Schisandra berry:** 1 cup of tea daily

- **Spirulina:** 2 teaspoons or 6 capsules daily

- **Vitamin B$_{12}$ (as adenosylcobalamin with methylcobalamin):** 2 dropperfuls daily

- **Vitamin C (as Micro-C):** 2 capsules daily

- **Wild blueberry powder:** 2 tablespoons daily

Supplements for Menopause Symptoms

- **Fresh celery juice:** work up to 32 ounces daily

- **Celeryforce:** 2 capsules twice a day

- **5-MTHF:** 1 capsule daily

- **Ashwagandha:** 2 dropperfuls twice a day

- **Barley grass juice powder:** 1 tablespoon or 9 capsules daily

- **B-complex:** 1 capsule daily

- **Burdock root:** 1 cup of tea or 1 root freshly juiced daily

- **Cat's claw:** 2 dropperfuls twice a day

- **Chaga mushroom:** 1 tablespoon or 9 capsules daily

- **Curcumin:** 2 capsules twice a day

- **Dandelion root:** 1 cup of tea daily

- **EPA and DHA (fish-free):** 1 capsule daily (taken with dinner)

- **Ginger:** 2 cups of tea or freshly grated to taste daily

- **Glutathione:** 1 capsule daily

- **Goldenseal:** 1 dropperful daily (two weeks on, two weeks off)

- **Lemon balm:** 4 dropperfuls twice a day

- **L-lysine:** 4 500-milligram capsules twice a day

- **Magnesium glycinate:** 2 capsules twice a day

- **Melatonin:** 5 milligrams at bedtime daily

- **Milk thistle:** 1 dropperful twice a day

- **MSM:** 1 capsule daily

- **Nascent iodine:** 3 small drops (not dropperfuls) daily

- **Nettle leaf:** 4 dropperfuls twice a day

- **Raspberry leaf:** 1 cup of tea with 2 bags daily

- **Spirulina:** 2 teaspoons or 6 capsules daily

- **Vitamin B$_{12}$ (as adenosylcobalamin with methylcobalamin):** 2 dropperfuls twice a day

- **Vitamin C (as Micro-C):** 4 capsules twice a day

- **Wild blueberry powder:** 1 tablespoon daily

- **Zinc (as liquid zinc sulfate):** 1 dropperful twice a day

CASE HISTORY:
No More Sleepless Nights
1999

Valerie was 48 years old when she began to notice unusual symptoms. To begin with, she was having trouble sleeping through the night. At 3 A.M., she'd wake up and then lie in bed unable to sleep until 5:30 or 6:00, when she'd sometimes be able to nod off again. Valerie also started to experience occasional heart palpitations, daytime hot flashes, and night sweats, along with moodiness. She found herself being short with her assistant and coworkers at her interior design firm, and one day she overheard her 17-year-old daughter, Molly, on the phone with her older daughter, who was away at college. "Mom has gotten super insensitive. She seems angry all the time, and I swear it's not my fault."

Valerie decided to make an appointment with her general practitioner, Dr. Fitzgerald. He performed a complete exam and ran blood work. Everything, including Valerie's thyroid hormone levels, came back normal. Dr. Fitzgerald reported that he was pretty confident Valerie was experiencing the symptoms of perimenopause onset. He ordered a comprehensive hormone chemistry panel, the results of which indicated slight imbalances of her DHEA and testosterone levels, as well as declining progesterone and estrogen.

The prospect of trying hormone replacement didn't sit well with Valerie. She remembered her mother becoming sick from HRT in the 1980s. It had seemed to age her mother by 15 years in just a short time. Dr. Fitzgerald was aware of HRT's history, though, and assured Valerie that he only prescribed BHRT from a compounding pharmacy. Valerie agreed to give it a try, and for three months, she took the bioidentical hormones with no results. Dr. Fitzgerald made adjustments to the prescription and recommended another three months.

Though she agreed to continue with the BHRT, Valerie also decided to see another doctor for a second opinion. This physician advised Valerie to go on thyroid medication, even though her thyroid hormone levels were within normal range. Valerie opted to try it for six months, but soon after she started, she began to experience symptoms such as fatigue, depression, brain fog, more sleepless nights, and more frequent heart palpitations.

At this point, a friend recommended that Valerie give me a call. The first thing that came through in my reading was that, yes, Valerie had a thyroid condition. However, the thyroid medication wasn't addressing the issue—because the issue was viral.

The *virus* was causing her fatigue and brain fog. It was overburdening her liver, which was resulting in her sleep issues, hot flashes, and night sweats. It was creating a drain on her nervous system, which was affecting her emotions. And the viral byproduct in her bloodstream had created a sticky, jelly-like substance, which was getting caught in her mitral valve and causing Valerie's heart palpitations. It was a classic case of viral load being passed off as perimenopause.

Valerie immediately weaned herself off the BHRT and thyroid medications. She also started on a powerful antiviral food regimen—which included eliminating eggs and dairy—and used supplementation to correct deficiencies in the minerals such as zinc and iodine that truly mattered to her condition.

After one month with these changes, Valerie's health improved by 80 percent.

After three months, she was back to feeling normal.

Because we'd addressed the underlying issues causing her symptoms, Valerie's health restored itself.

Too often, doctors don't know about these root causes of people's illness, and so they get swept up in the hormone trend. Valerie had decided to ignore her hormone test panels and go by the results of how she felt. She and her family are happier for it.

"Menopause and life after menopause aren't anything to dread. Menopause itself isn't meant to be a difficult physical process, and the wave of younger women who've begun to experience symptoms categorized as hormonal aren't going through early menopause. Other factors entirely are in play—and there are powerful ways to address them. You can go back to living a healthy life and embracing life at every stage."

— Anthony William, Medical Medium

CHAPTER 16

Lyme Disease

For so long, I've wanted to bring the truth about Lyme disease to the public.

Yet even now, after decades of helping people, including doctors themselves, recover from Lyme, I'm almost reluctant to write this chapter. That's because Lyme comes with so much baggage—suitcases filled with mistaken theories, clinical misjudgments, and trendy misconceptions.

What I'm about to reveal is very different from what the belief about Lyme has been all along. I just want people to understand what Lyme disease really is, and how they can get better from it. I've been working and waiting patiently, teaching so many practitioners and other people about Lyme, all the while hoping that medical research would uncover the truth. But another year goes by, and another, and medical communities just follow more false leads.

No one has decades of their life to waste while they wait for answers about why they're ill.

If the real cause of Lyme doesn't keep reaching people, before Lyme disease gets to the next level, the truth will never have a chance to set them free. We are headed to the point in the next two decades where anyone who has a set of symptoms associated with rheumatoid arthritis, multiple sclerosis, fibromyalgia, myalgic encephalomyelitis/chronic fatigue syndrome, lupus, thyroid disorder, or any other condition truly caused by Epstein-Barr virus will be tested for Lyme disease with fallible tests—and told they have Lyme. The same will happen to anyone dealing with adrenal fatigue or chronic intestinal tract disorders.

To understand the Lyme confusion out there, imagine a snowball. Many years ago, it started rolling down a mountainside, getting bigger and bigger. Soon it started to engulf trees, wildlife, telephone poles, cabins—anything in its wake—picking up speed along the way. With enormous, almost unstoppable momentum gained from ignorance and confusion, it has swallowed up well-meaning practitioners and those who suffer from its symptoms—and it just keeps going. Now it's poised to set off an avalanche on the town of humanity.

The easiest thing for me to do would be to stand out of the way. But that's not how I work.

For the sake of the millions of people who could get swallowed up by the Lyme madness over the next 20 to 50 years—our daughters and sons, and the new generations of practitioners, doctors, and healers who will continue to operate with outdated hypotheses while also getting sick themselves with Lyme disease symptoms—I must do what I can to prevent the avalanche.

In this chapter, you will learn the truth about Lyme disease—and you'll learn how to protect yourself from the Lyme trap of the 21st century.

A LOOK BACK

Let's travel back in time for a moment to November 1975, when multiple children and young adults were developing symptoms, which alerted doctors to launch an investigation in the area around Lyme, Connecticut, that gave Lyme disease its name.

First let's remind ourselves of the technology back then: rotary phones on the kitchen wall, no such thing as voice mail, and Sony was just releasing its first VCR for sale in the United States. In the medical world, kids were getting their tonsils plucked out as if they were apples on trees, with no understanding of the underlying cause of tonsillitis. Even today, there's no clinical understanding of what's behind tonsillitis. While technology has made leaps and bounds, advancements in chronic and mystery illness have been at a near standstill. The symptoms that children and a few adults in the Lyme area started to experience—chronic fatigue, headaches, joint pain, and so on—were symptoms that had been seen for decades in every other town in Connecticut, not to mention every state throughout the entire country. Yet somehow in this area around Lyme,

the illness was treated as something new and unrecognizable. It's most likely because compassionate doctors were trying to go above and beyond their role, taking these symptoms more seriously on a personal level. Doctors, researchers, and townspeople began looking for a culprit—and landed on the deer tick, because one of the patients reported seeing a tick a few weeks before he fell ill. That's like a train derailing for reasons unknown, and a passenger mentioning a deer he saw grazing 50 miles back. The clues don't add up in either scenario. Even though no one could explain *why* a tick would give someone Lyme disease, a 17th-century-style witch hunt began. Based only on rumor, deer and the ticks that lived on them became the targets.

In 1981, an entomologist announced he'd discovered the missing link—a bacterium named *Borrelia burgdorferi* that the ticks passed along to humans through their bites. He was lauded for his discovery, which led to a series of bacteria-focused tests and treatments for Lyme disease.

It was the perfect "out" for medical authorities. No one liked ticks anyway, and the theory of a tick-borne illness fed into the fear of nature already present in society. Medical authorities felt they could give up on digging for the answer.

Unfortunately, all these "discoveries" were wrong.

This is what you won't hear anywhere else: Lyme disease is *not* caused by ticks.

And Lyme disease is *not* caused by *Borrelia burgdorferi* bacteria.

When the research was taking place in the 1970s and 1980s, you'd suppose researchers would have realized the problem was happening nationwide—and globally. And today, you'd think someone would wake up and realize that hundreds of thousands of people who have never been near a deer tick receive Lyme disease diagnoses.

As for *Borrelia burgdorferi,* it's a normal part of our environment that's carried by every human being and animal on this planet—including entirely healthy ones. Truth is, this bacteria poses no health risk . . . and has zero connection to Lyme disease. If someone with Lyme disease tests positive for *Borrelia burgdorferi,* it's meaningless.

Nonetheless, virtually all the efforts of medical communities for the past decades to devise methods of diagnosing and treating Lyme disease have been based upon the false premise that it's caused by ticks and bacteria.

When a mistaken theory starts to take on a life of its own, no one's going to want to admit the mistake and disprove it. It's the equivalent of building a house using a poorly drawn set of blueprints. A worker might recognize an issue with the plans, but second-guess himself because he doesn't want to cause a problem or jeopardize his job. In this situation, no matter how skilled the builders and no matter how intricate and beautiful the decorations, the first strong wind that comes along will blow the house down.

Similarly, medical communities' acceptance of false assumptions in the 1970s, 1980s, and 1990s has resulted in untold misery for patients who not only aren't helped, but in many cases are gravely harmed by well-meaning doctors acting on tragically inaccurate information.

Something else medical communities don't know is that there are multiple reasons that people experience symptoms associated with Lyme disease. The earliest version, which dates back to 1901, produced relatively mild symptoms. The disease mutated into more varieties and strains by the 1950s. It then began mutating into even more aggressive varieties, which leads us to the Lyme symptoms of the 1970s.

By that time, the disease had actually been disrupting the lives of people worldwide for nearly 60 years, with its symptoms always attributed to other illnesses, or simply considered "a mystery."

We still deal with these ailments today, and have names now for many of them, including myalgic encephalomyelitis/chronic fatigue syndrome, fibromyalgia, multiple sclerosis, ALS, thyroid disorder, lupus, Crohn's disease, Addison's disease, autoimmune disease, and many more. Yet they still cause widespread puzzlement and often account for Lyme diagnoses.

LYME DISEASE SYMPTOMS

The confusion about Lyme disease symptoms is vast. At this point, every autoimmune disease or mystery illness in this book and in existence has symptoms that have been linked to Lyme disease.

If you visit a Lyme specialist with *any* symptoms, or even a diagnosis, of MS, lupus, fibromyalgia, RA, CFS, or ME/CFS—we're talking mild to extreme and/or persistent fatigue; muscle pain, weakness, twitching, or spasms; restless leg syndrome; brain fog; burning skin; jaw pain; dizziness; migraines; anxiety; aches and pains; joint pain or swelling; or tingling or numbness in the hands and feet—you could be deemed to have Lyme whether tests come back positive or negative. Yet if you visit a doctor who doesn't focus on Lyme, you may get a totally different diagnosis. It all has to do with where the doctor's interest and attention lies.

I often tell people that visiting a Lyme specialist is like visiting a broom store—without realizing all they sell is brooms. You tell the clerk that you need supplies to scrub your shower tiles, clean up spills in the kitchen, and get rid of the streaks on the living room windows. It won't matter that all these tasks are beyond the scope of what the store sells; you'll walk out carrying a broom.

WHAT LYME DISEASE *REALLY* IS

As mentioned previously, medical communities originally believed that Lyme disease was caused by a bacterium named *Borrelia burgdorferi* transmitted by a bite from a deer tick.

Recently, doctors and researchers have started to realize they may have focused on the wrong bacteria for the last three and a half decades. New patients are now hearing about different decoy bugs such as *Bartonella* and the microscopic parasite *Babesia* (which is a hybrid, a cross between bacteria and parasite). And the new patients aren't being told about the long road others have been down with the *Borrelia* tag, about the traps along the way. They don't have the benefit of that perspective.

You should know, by the way, that *Bartonella* and *Babesia* are also harmless, and most of us carry them. They're once again bait-and-switch theories that promise an answer but deliver only conjecture. In case you're wondering, *Bartonella* and *Babesia* have never been clinically found in a tick in nature that wasn't attached to a human being.

Truth is, Lyme disease isn't the result of ticks, parasites, or bacteria. Lyme disease is actually *viral*—not bacterial or parasitical. When medical communities finally awaken to this truth, there will be hope for Lyme patients.

The true cause of what's being called Lyme disease varies in each individual. People who have different varieties of Epstein-Barr can have Lyme symptoms, as can people who have HHV-6 and its various strains. People who carry any of the different strains of shingles can exhibit Lyme symptoms, with the non-rashing varieties causing the most severe cases, including symptoms such as brain inflammation and other central nervous system weaknesses. It's the same for any number of herpetic family viruses. So many Lyme patients' blood work also tests positive for EBV, cytomegalovirus, or HSV-1 (the virus that causes fever blisters)— and so many patients have different mutations and strains of viruses in this herpetic family that don't even show up in tests. Many viruses don't show up in blood tests because they're in the organs, or they're low-grade infections. Any of the more aggressive varieties of these viruses can be behind a patient's Lyme symptoms. All the viruses I list above are, again, in the herpes family and can cause fever, headaches, joint pain, muscle pain, fatigue, neck pain, burning nerve pain, heart palpitations, almost any neurological symptom, and/or other symptoms that doctors think of as so-called Lyme disease. They can dramatically decrease a patient's quality of life and pose serious challenges if not properly treated.

Even if you're experiencing symptoms of any number of these viral infections, you might be able to avoid experiencing a full-blown mystery illness that gets the Lyme disease tag by keeping the virus in a low-grade or dormant state. And if you're already suffering from more severe symptoms tagged as Lyme, there's a great deal you can do to combat and overcome the illness.

HOW LYME DISEASE IS TRIGGERED

If you're experiencing an onset of viral infection and your immune system is unusually weak, you can come down with Lyme symptoms in a matter of days. Much more typically, however, you'll carry a virus without knowing it's in your system for years—possibly even decades—before it strikes.

Any number of the viruses we've talked about tend to hide in your liver, spleen, small intestinal tract, central nervous system ganglia, or other areas where they can't be detected by your immune system. The liver is where they mostly nestle in, many times never branching out and entering any other spots in the body. A virus can bide its time until some traumatic physical or emotional event, poor diet, or other trigger (which you'll read about shortly) weakens you and/or provides an environment that makes the virus stronger. It can then proliferate—increase in numbers—by having a feeding frenzy on stored toxins, such as mercury, that everyone has a certain level of within them. A virus can also release a neurotoxin during its feeding frenzy that starts to exacerbate symptoms, for example to inflame your central nervous system—which weakens your immune system's ability to fight it off. When we're triggered by an emotional experience such as a breakup of a relationship, our body floods with a variety of adrenaline associated with the emotional trauma. Excess amounts of this adrenaline can weaken the

immune system more and even feed some varieties of viruses such as EBV.

If you accumulate a toxic heavy metal such as mercury in your system, it will poison you and impair your immune system. At the same time, a virus that can cause the Lyme disease symptoms *loves* heavy metal toxins; they're favored foods that make it stronger. This double blow triggers the virus to leave its dormant state and begin growing its "army" of virus cells.

As another example, if you experience a death in the family, your stressful and painful emotions can lower the defenses of your immune system, because they prompt your adrenal glands to produce potent adrenaline blends that can be harsh on the system over a sustained period. At the same time, these excess amounts of harsh versions of hormones are another favored food for the virus. Severe stress is therefore a very common trigger for Lyme disease symptoms.

A tick bite is at the *bottom* of the list of common triggers—*not* causes—of Lyme, accounting for less than 0.5 percent of Lyme cases.

It's also worth noting that your overall health can play a major role. Even if two people have the exact same type of viral infection and are struck by the same trigger, the one who eats well, exercises regularly, and gets enough sleep might not become sufficiently weakened to activate the virus, while the one who doesn't have opportunities to take care of herself or himself might rapidly come down with Lyme symptoms.

Millions of people globally come down with symptoms of Lyme disease due to the following triggers (listed in order of prevalence). All of these triggers can send you doctor-shopping and eventually land you with a Lyme specialist, who, regardless of your test results, may give you the Lyme disease tag—without truly understanding what Lyme even is.

Most Common Lyme Triggers

The substances and circumstances below do not create Lyme disease. Rather, they can *trigger* existing viral conditions that have previously been dormant in the body—viral conditions that surface in the form of the symptoms medical communities collectively call Lyme disease. These triggers can push a viral infection that's been at the tipping point over the edge. Please be aware that delayed responses can occur. Symptoms can surface anywhere from shortly after trigger exposure to months later. The triggers are listed in order of prevalence, with the most common at the top and the very least common at the bottom.

1. **COVID:** can challenge the immune system, both by exhausting its reserves and by causing it to overreact. A weakened immune system can, in turn, provide an opportunity for dormant viral infections to gain strength and create new symptoms, or lead symptoms that someone had previously experienced to resurface. COVID is difficult on the central nervous system, and people who have suffered with neurological Lyme symptoms are often dealing with nervous system compromises already. Just like the flu, COVID can prompt a high fever, which can heat and strain nerves that are weakened, have recently healed, or are healing from the causes behind neurological Lyme.

2. **Mold:** if you have mold in a home or office, you're spending many hours each day inhaling the funguses. This can wear away at your immune system until a breakdown occurs. If someone else in a family, or a coworker, is exposed to the same mold and does not exhibit a symptom yet, it's important to know that they may not be as viral, or they may not have the same viruses or viral varieties as the person who does develop a symptom.

3. **Mercury-based dental amalgam fillings:** if you have old mercury fillings in your teeth (also called *silver fillings*), a well-meaning dentist may decide to remove them all at once for your safety. That's a mistake. It overstresses the immune system and should be handled one filling at a time, as the mercury tends to be stable where it is, while there's a strong chance the removal process will end up sending the toxic mercury into your bloodstream.

4. **Extensive blood draw:** when a larger number of blood vials are drawn, it can be stressful on the immune system—because the very immune defenses that are keeping the viruses behind Lyme symptoms at bay end up being drawn out of the body with the blood that's taken. Larger

blood draws tend to take away a substantial portion of a person's immune system that day, and it sometimes takes weeks to rebuild those portions of the immune system. Within those weeks that the full power of the immune system is not present to monitor the blood, viruses can get a window to strengthen and proliferate. Infections can travel from organ to organ with ease, because they're not being corralled, and that can lead to a flare-up of symptoms, whether a week, a few weeks, or a month later. I recommend doing smaller blood draws over more visits. If you're struggling with Lyme symptoms or any other condition labeled autoimmune, I recommend no more than four vials of blood at a time, and even consider fewer if you're very sensitive. A mistake made by well-meaning doctors is to draw a large number of blood vials with sensitive people.

5. **Mercury in other forms:** mercury from *any* source is poisonous. For example, frequently eating seafood, especially large fish such as tuna and swordfish that tend to contain significant amounts of mercury, can eventually push your immune system past the breaking point and lead to a viral infection. Always be mindful about mercury exposure. Even in today's modern times, we're always vulnerable to coming into contact with it, especially in the medical field. Do your research, and question what's being offered to you, your children, and the rest of your family.

6. **Pesticides, herbicides, and fungicides:** if you have poisons on your lawn or in your garden, or you live near a sprayed farm, park, or golf course, you're spending time every day inadvertently inhaling their fumes. This both damages you and feeds the viral infection with toxins that strengthen it.

7. **Insecticides in the home:** flying bug spray, ant spray, roach spray, and other poisons meant to kill insects end up poisoning you, too, and also fueling viral infection.

8. **Flu:** challenges the immune system by exhausting its reserves or causing an overreaction of the immune system, which depletes it more quickly than on a normal day. When the immune system is lowered, it can allow other viruses—the ones responsible for Lyme disease symptoms—to surface. Also, when you have a history of nerve inflammation and other neurological Lyme symptoms, the high fever of a flu can put stress on the central nervous system, leading nerves that are recently healed, sensitive, or inflamed to overheat—in turn leading symptoms to return. (Note that milder strains of COVID can present themselves like a normal flu.)

9. **Death in the family:** the emotional trauma of losing a loved one can both weaken your immune system and strengthen viral infections—which

feed on the resulting more corrosive "challenging emotion" hormone blends produced by your adrenal glands.

10. **Broken heart:** betrayal by a loved one, an unexpected breakup, a messy divorce, or anything that causes similar emotional trauma is a common trigger for viruses for the same reasons.

11. **Taking care of a sick loved one:** again, the emotional trauma can both weaken the immune system and strengthen viruses.

12. **Spider bite:** spider bites are actually much more common triggers for Lyme disease symptoms than tick bites, accounting for about 5 percent of cases from this list. If the bite leaves some of the spider's venom in your skin, an infection can result that weakens your immune system. Roughly 1 out of 5 times, it'll also produce a bull's-eye-like red rash.

13. **Bee sting:** like spider bites, bee stings are much more common triggers for Lyme disease symptoms than tick bites, accounting for about 5 percent of cases from this list. If the sting leaves some of the bee in your skin, an infection can result that weakens your immune system. Roughly 1 out of 5 times, it will also produce a bull's-eye-like red rash.

14. **"Virus-friendly" prescription medications:** viruses thrive on antibiotics, which at the same time weaken the immune system.

Medications such as benzodiazepines have a similar effect. If you suspect you have a viral infection, see your doctor and reassess the medications you're on.

15. **Overprescribed medications:** even if a medication is necessary for you in moderation, a prescription for too much can throw your immune system off-kilter, opening the door for a viral attack. Or if you have multiple doctors prescribing different medications, they can combine into an overwhelming cocktail for the immune system.

16. **Recreational drug abuse:** illegal and legal drugs that contain toxins can simultaneously throw off your immune system and provide fuel for a viral infection.

17. **Financial stress:** worrying about losing your job, not being able to pay bills, and even possibly becoming homeless can lead to a number of strong challenging emotions—including fear of failure, fear of dying, loss of self-image, stress, and shame—that can weaken your immune system's ability to fend off a viral infection.

18. **Physical injuries:** if you twist your ankle, are in a car accident, or experience some other physical injury, it can wear down your body to a point where the virus feels emboldened to strike. That's doubly true if you require an operation to fix the damage—because surgery is usually accompanied by antibiotics.

19. **Summer swimming:** when the weather is warm, red algae can accumulate in lakes or along the ocean shore. The loss of oxygen they create encourages the growth of bacteria, which can weaken your immune system and trigger a virus to come out of dormancy.

20. **Runoff:** toxic heavy metals and other toxins can run off from old land dumps into nearby lakes, especially during hot summer weather. Swimming in these lakes exposes you to the toxins, and lowers your immune system's ability to fight off viral infection.

21. **Professional carpet cleaning:** traditional carpet cleaners use chemicals that are highly toxic for you. Plus many carpets contain toxins already, so the "cleaning" is adding poisons on top of poisons. If you spend a lot of time indoors, you'll breathe these toxic fumes for most of each day, which can both weaken your immune system and feed viruses. Avoid this by buying "green" carpets and organic cleaners, and/ or by using a modern "green" carpet cleaning service. Even these are questionable. If you're very sensitive, consider removing your carpets.

22. **Fresh paint:** most fresh paint fills the air with toxic fumes. If you're in a home or office without a lot of circulation, you can end up weakening your immune system and triggering a viral infection.

23. **Insomnia:** any sleep disorder disrupts your body, which over time can trigger a viral infection.

24. **Tick bite:** while medical communities are wrong in believing ticks *cause* Lyme disease, tick bites can be *triggers* for Lyme symptoms. As with spider bites and bee stings, an attack that leaves some of the creature in your skin can result in an infection, which in turn weakens your immune system. And if you have an underlying virus and the timing is perfect, a bite can be all you need to instigate a breakout of viral infection. This infection has nothing to do with *Borrelia burgdorferi*; *Borrelia* is *not* the bacterium that's in this infection. Again, contrary to popular belief, the tick is the *least* common trigger on this list, accountable for less than 0.5 percent of Lyme disease cases.

Even if one of these triggers awakens a dormant virus, it may take a while before the virus completes its war preparations—such as growing an army of "soldier" cells—and launches its initial assault. Not one of these triggers can actually infect you with the viruses that cause Lyme symptoms, nor can they infect you with the various bacteria that are falsely associated with Lyme disease.

If you're suffering with what doctors call Lyme disease, then chances are you were harboring a virus in your body for years before you got sick. There's a roughly 75 percent chance that one or more of the above triggers occurred within three months to a year of the onset of your symptoms.

ANTIBIOTICS

Medical communities' mistaken belief that Lyme disease is caused by bacteria (and recently parasites) is one of the greatest mistakes in modern medical history. It has kept so many generations dealing with viral infections from getting the true help they need. I call this the Lyme trap.

The way doctors usually deal with Lyme disease is to prescribe antibiotics, because they're aiming to destroy *Borrelia burgdorferi* and other bacteria such as *Bartonella*, as well as parasites such as *Babesia*—which actually have nothing to do with Lyme disease and aren't a health threat. *Borrelia*, *Bartonella*, and *Babesia* do not attack the central nervous system, and symptoms of an inflamed central nervous system are the number one issue among all Lyme patients. This is now labeled *neurological Lyme*. Until medical communities learn the truth, they will continue to prescribe antibiotics for Lyme and neurological Lyme that yield no positive results and leave a wake of damage. That's not merely ineffective. It's dangerous.

Powerful varieties of antibiotics hammer a Lyme patient with a double blow. And because Lyme patients usually have inflamed neurological systems from viral infections in the herpes family, these harsh antibiotics bruise already sensitive nerves. Some doctors are under the mistaken impression that the pain and other symptoms a patient experiences in this circumstance are a sign of progress—an indication of a beneficial *Herxheimer reaction*, that is, bacterial die-off as the body detoxifies. *Borrelia*, *Bartonella*, and *Babesia* are easy kills. In reality, the symptoms indicate something is very wrong.

Antibiotics tend to be harsh on the gut and liver. They can also kill good bacteria in your gut that are part of keeping a balance within your intestinal environment. If a doctor places you on an aggressive antibiotic for two or more weeks, then even if you take probiotics daily, your gut might need a year or more to recover from the damage. Some guts will never be the same, even if the antibiotic is administered intravenously. (For more on gut health, see Chapter 17.) The liver tends to absorb and store the antibiotics, resulting in short-term liver shock and stress. That storage of the antibiotics within the liver can also feed the viral infection responsible for Lyme.

The viruses that cause Lyme disease symptoms *love* antibiotics. And aggressive antibiotics do for viruses what mother's milk does for a baby: make them grow bigger and stronger.

Because the only significant natural enemy of the viral infections that cause Lyme symptoms is the immune system, taking an antibiotic that both compromises the immune system and supercharges the virus is like trying to put out a fire by pouring a barrel of gasoline on it. Yet it's the standard way doctors have always treated Lyme disease. Taking large doses of aggressive antibiotics can transform a relatively mild case of Lyme disease into a severe health crisis, even if that health crisis is delayed, occurring months after the administration of the antibiotics. Tragically, this still happens every day.

With integrated Lyme specialists now comprehending some of the damage that aggressive antibiotic treatment has caused for more than 40 years, they're starting to lower dosages of antibiotics and couple them with natural nutritional support, including natural intravenous vitamins. Before we give them a medal for the realization, though, we need to recognize that medicine is still decades away from understanding that *no antibiotics are needed*—because Lyme is viral. Popular alternative treatments such as ultraviolet blood irradiation therapy (UBI) don't help either, because they work on the misguided theory that the problem is bacterial and in the bloodstream. In truth, the viruses that cause Lyme disease symptoms are mostly neurological, and they never cause Lyme symptoms when they're in the blood. It's when the viruses are in the organs and central nervous system that they cause their trouble.

As long as doctors believe the problem behind Lyme symptoms is bacterial, they'll be lost at sea in a fog, chasing a ghost ship—at the expense of potentially millions of people. It's worth noting that viruses that create Lyme disease symptoms do have many cofactors. These include: the over 50 groups of *Streptococcus* and their hundreds of strains, *E. coli, Mycoplasma pneumoniae, H. pylori, Chlamydophila pneumoniae*, and/or *Staphylococcus*; plus toxic molds and unproductive fungus. *Bartonella* and *Babesia*, the bugs that have become popular recently in the Lyme field and which are no more harmful than *Candida*, are also cofactors.

Note that these cofactors do not *create* the symptoms known as Lyme. To understand how medical communities misunderstand these cofactors as causes, imagine two armies in battle, one army (the medical communities) chasing down a retreating army (bacteria). When the first group of foot soldiers finally reaches the troops they've been pursuing and has them surrounded on all sides, they'll discover that those weren't bayonets they saw in the distance—they were flagpoles, trumpets,

and drumsticks. The army went after the wrong guys. All this time that the foot soldiers thought they were chasing down their enemy, they were really following an infantry band. In this same way, medical research has been pursuing the messengers (bacteria), while the real adversary (viruses) sneaks by unnoticed.

Most of the real damage is caused by the viral infections that are not discovered in the patient—or, if they are discovered, pushed aside as a nonissue. The cofactors aren't the threat.

Further, the particular bacteria (mainly *Streptococcus*) that are cofactors for the viruses behind Lyme disease symptoms are usually resistant to antibiotics, and become even more highly resistant over time, leading to bladder infections, other UTIs, chronic sinus infections, ear infections, strep throat, sties, and acne. If you have Lyme symptoms, this is all the more reason to strenuously avoid antibiotics.

There's an exception to this rule: it's okay to use mild antibiotics to fight an infection. For example, when a normal skin infection occurs from a spider bite, bee sting, or a tick bite that leaves part of the creature lodged in your skin, your body fights against infection by creating a ringed rash, or red "bull's-eye," around the area. (This bull's-eye is the ultimate misconception about Lyme disease.)

In this situation, taking a less aggressive antibiotic is okay; the long-term risks of antibiotics are trumped by the short-term risk of the infection. Let's be clear, though: The infection itself is not Lyme disease. And it is *not Borrelia burgdorferi* within the infection. These bull's-eye infections are just normal staph infections that result from foreign debris getting beneath the skin's surface through a puncture wound.

For the record, *Borrelia* has never been found and cultured from a bull's-eye, nor has *Babesia* or *Bartonella.*

TESTING FOR LYME TODAY

There are various ways medical communities diagnose Lyme disease. These are two of the common tests: *enzyme-linked immunosorbent assay* (ELISA), which detects antibodies to the *Borrelia burgdorferi* bacterium; and *Western blot,* which seeks to find antibodies to several proteins of *Borrelia burgdorferi.* Both are based on the false assumption that Lyme disease symptoms are caused by *Borrelia burgdorferi . . .* which they're not. It's therefore common for a patient to have Lyme symptoms but receive negative results from these tests.

Advanced laboratories have started to discover that these tests never worked to begin with. As they try to develop better tests, though, they are still operating under the same old theory that bacteria and/or parasites are the cause of Lyme. If we go back to that faulty blueprint analogy, it's like trying to build a whole new house with the same plans as before—without fixing the critical mistakes in the plans' conception.

If you've recently received a Lyme diagnosis from an integrative or functional medicine doctor, there's a good chance she or he mentioned they no longer rely on ELISA or the Western blot. Your doctor may have said, "We need to send your blood to more advanced Lyme labs." When the results came back, your doctor most likely said that the Lyme titers (measures) of your blood work indicated antibodies, or that partial positives appeared for bacteria such as *Bartonella* and parasites such

as *Babesia.* (If you have the flu, a staph infection, EBV, or even *Candida,* there's a good chance you'll trip a false positive test result for Lyme.) Nowadays Lyme disease tests are even moving backward in technology. Lyme labs scan blood for signs of inflammation in any form, and if there's an indication that there *is* inflammation, then it will be reported that the patient has Lyme disease. The lab report the patient receives will still associate that inflammation with particular bacteria, leading the patient and even doctor to think it's definitive—never realizing it was only an inflammation test. The bacteria wasn't physically found under a microscope.

This is the sly way of diverting from the fact that patients have been wronged for decades, as medical communities went after the incorrect culprit. What these compassionate doctors don't realize is that these new *Bartonella* and *Babesia* leads aren't really progress—because they work off the same mistaken premise as always. Rather than understanding the bacteria and parasites as harmless cofactors, they point to them as the disease itself.

And since it's exceedingly rare for a patient with Lyme symptoms to have actually been bitten by a tick, medical professionals now tell stories about how Lyme disease can come from a mosquito, deerfly, or horsefly that may have bitten a patient years ago. Many medical professionals who are diagnosing Lyme disease are not even uttering the words "insect" or "tick."

There's an off chance that a bite from a deerfly or horsefly could act as a trigger for viral symptoms to come to the surface, in the manner that the other insect bites mentioned earlier can. However, pointing to these insects as actual causes of Lyme disease is once again acting on the old, misguided theory—and adding to people's fear of being out in nature. It's no more advanced than saying ticks are to blame.

The only upside to these recent developments is that medical communities are broadening the scope of what they look for with Lyme. They're coming to see it's not just one thing, and that *Borrelia burgdorferi* was a faulty hypothesis. Yet researchers are still looking in the wrong neck of the woods—literally. I predict that as the years go by, still other bacteria will be blamed for Lyme, and the true viral culprits will be ignored.

And if you're sick with Lyme disease symptoms, do you have 20 years for research to figure out the real cause?

The truth is that medical communities haven't yet discovered most of the genuine cofactors of Lyme, such as the over 50 groups of *Streptococcus* bacteria. And in the case of *Babesia* and *Bartonella,* beyond the truth that doctors don't realize their part in Lyme disease symptoms is nonexistent, there are multiple problems with testing for them.

First, you can have a viral infection that causes Lyme disease symptoms but not have these cofactors, in which case you'll test negative. Second, you can harbor these cofactors but not have them picked up by the tests—which are far from infallible—and so again receive a negative result.

But the biggest issue is that more than half of the population carries around *Babesia* and *Bartonella* (which are not harmful by themselves), along with hundreds of other harmless bacteria. As a result, you can be entirely healthy and yet test positive. Since medical tests often give a patient who has Lyme symptoms negative results and a patient without Lyme symptoms positive results, they're not very useful.

If you tested 100 healthy people with the newest, most advanced Lyme tests from the best labs—and those tests are still just inflammation tests at this point—more than 50 of them would test positive for Lyme. The titers for those 50-plus study subjects would indicate antibodies present for the bacteria medical communities say are behind Lyme disease.

Because of this book series, together with the years I spent working with doctors before publishing books, medical communities are more aware of the Epstein-Barr virus than ever before. Patients are now bringing this and other Medical Medium books to their doctors' offices, asking if they have EBV and not Lyme. This has prompted many doctors to test for EBV on a regular basis—anyone they suspect has Lyme disease, they'll also test for EBV. And they are often finding EBV infections. Rather than realizing that the answer is in front of their eyes, though—and realizing that neurological symptoms attributed to Lyme cannot be caused by bacteria, only by viruses such as EBV—these doctors will often believe the patients have both Lyme *and* EBV, not able to accept that the EBV infection and Lyme symptoms are one and the same. It goes to show that the old belief system that Lyme disease is caused by bacteria still dominates.

And remember, you can still have EBV even if it doesn't show up in a test. If your doctor runs a blood test for EBV and it comes back negative, or if it only comes back showing EBV antibodies that your doctor says indicate *past* infection, the virus could still be hiding out in your liver or another organ, causing your symptoms.

The most effective way to determine if you have a viral infection causing Lyme symptoms is to focus on your history and symptoms. If you've experienced one of the common triggers by which viral infection is activated; *and* you are or have been experiencing viral symptoms such as twitching, spasm, fatigue, brain fog, memory loss, nerve and joint pain, and other neurological symptoms; *and* you've eliminated other likely causes for how you're feeling—then there's a strong chance you're suffering from a virus that creates Lyme disease symptoms. As I mentioned earlier, it's most likely one of the many strains in the herpes family such as shingles, HHV-6, Epstein-Barr, or cytomegalovirus.

These viruses can all trigger false positives in the new, progressive Lyme disease lab tests, because they create inflammation. The viruses create byproducts, debris, and the famous spirochetes (which are viral casings mistaken for bacteria), and all of this elevates inflammation, which can trip up the fallible testing systems of Lyme labs by making a patient's illness appear to be bacterial. Blood labs are like any other company—they're open for business. They want to stay afloat, protect their livelihoods, and so a certain amount of profit-minded perspective guides their motivation. We can't trust claims about amazing new lab tests as absolute fact. And there's a big disconnect between blood labs and the doctors who order tests from them; doctors often aren't told how the labs come up with their results. Keep this in mind, and be cautious about what "facts" you believe.

If you have taken antibiotics and experienced the viral backlash, or if you haven't undergone treatment but experience the symptoms I've described in this chapter,

the odds are immense that you can recover your health by patiently and scrupulously following the directions in the next section. Over time, you should be able to destroy 90 percent or more of the virus's cells, allowing your immune system to send the virus back into a comatose-like, dormant state . . . and free yourself of Lyme.

ADDRESSING LYME DISEASE

When chronic symptoms of Lyme disease interrupt people's lives, it can be devastating. Most patients have seen multiple doctors and have received either no answers or a diagnosis such as MS, fibromyalgia, RA, Sjögren's syndrome, migraines, lupus, CFS, or ME/CFS. When one of these patients finally visits a Lyme specialist, the Lyme disease diagnosis can feel like a relief; it can feel like they've finally uncovered the mystery.

Globally, millions of people with symptoms of what are really viral infections are instead being treated as if their illnesses are bacterial—and they're receiving the Lyme label. It's becoming the most grievously misunderstood affliction of our time. As it gains momentum, it will become the most popular diagnosis of the future. Patients and doctors alike will be overwhelmed by the validation that this designation seems to provide, even if it doesn't make sense.

The tag "Lyme disease" will remain a label for a mystery illness that no one realizes is due to viral infection. The tag is not an answer to what's ailing you. Any name could have been put in the place of Lyme. For all the insight that name gives, you might as well just call it *cheese disease*, or *I-don't-feel-well disease*.

As we've explored in this chapter, it's critical to understand what's truly behind Lyme symptoms so you can protect yourself and your loved ones from the Lyme trap.

If you're 40 years old today, it won't be until you're 65 or 70 that the medical establishment starts to realize the mistake in how it's been conceiving of and treating Lyme disease—and that's being optimistic. However, if you follow all the steps described in this section daily without fail, you can force your viral infection back into its dormant state and render it harmless.

How long this process takes will depend on a variety of factors, such as whether you have one virus or a variety of viruses, whether they're more aggressive or less aggressive, and whether you have recently taken antibiotics, are in a healthy environment or a toxic one that can be a trigger and feed the virus, and are in the early or later stages of the illness. Since this book's first edition was published, countless people have already used this chapter to find relief from their Lyme disease symptoms. By working with and customizing Medical Medium protocols, you can take yourself as far as you need to go.

And don't stop with the recommendations in this chapter. Also turn to Part IV, "How to Finally Heal," where you'll find details on heavy metal detox and other tools you need to help you rid yourself of Lyme symptoms. The information you need to free yourself from the Lyme trap—or sidestep it altogether—is in this book.

You have the ability to heal. Your body *wants* to truly heal, and to be well. If you give your body what it needs and take away the unproductive elements, you can tap into your core healing power and recover.

Healing Foods

Certain healing fruits, leafy greens, herbs, wild foods, and vegetables can help your body ward off or recover from the viruses behind Lyme disease symptoms. Asparagus, wild blueberries, radishes, celery, cinnamon, garlic, apricots, onions, potatoes, winter squash, broccoli, cauliflower, cilantro, parsley, apples, oranges, grapefruit, papayas, bananas, tomatoes, spinach, and lettuces are among the best to focus on, as they can variously aid in killing viral cells, detoxification, repairing brain cells, recovering the central nervous system, and other healing processes. Incorporate as many of these foods into your diet as you can.

Also take care to avoid the foods in Chapter 19, "What Not to Eat." When dealing with a virus-caused symptom or condition, it's critical to begin the process of removing at least one or two of the foods that feed the virus. If you need to take your healing even further, try to gravitate toward removing all the foods that feed the virus.

Healing Herbs and Supplements

Before applying these, be sure to read Chapter 21, "Critical Guide to Supplement Protocols."

Supplements for Lyme Symptoms (including Neurological Lyme)

- **Fresh celery juice:** work up to 32 ounces twice a day if possible; if not, work up to 32 ounces every morning

- **Celeryforce:** 4 capsules twice a day

- **5-MTHF:** 1 capsule twice a day

- **Barley grass juice powder:** 2 teaspoons or 6 capsules twice a day

- **Cat's claw:** 3 dropperfuls twice a day

- **Curcumin:** 3 capsules twice a day

- **Glutathione:** 1 capsule daily

- **Lemon balm:** 4 dropperfuls twice a day

- **Licorice root:** 1 dropperful twice a day (two weeks on, two weeks off)

- **L-lysine:** 5 500-milligram capsules twice a day

- **Mullein leaf:** 4 dropperfuls twice a day

- **Nascent iodine:** 3 small drops (not dropperfuls) twice a day

- **Nettle leaf:** 3 dropperfuls twice a day

- **Raw honey:** 1 to 3 teaspoons daily

- **Spirulina:** 2 teaspoons or 6 capsules daily

- **Vitamin B$_{12}$ (as adenosylcobalamin with methylcobalamin):** 3 dropperfuls twice a day

- **Vitamin C (as Micro-C):** 8 capsules twice a day

- **Zinc (as liquid zinc sulfate):** up to 2 dropperfuls twice a day

CASE HISTORY:
The Lyme Trap
1997

Stephanie was a happy stay-at-home mom who took care of her husband, Edward, and their two children. When Edward left her for a younger woman, Stephanie was forced to get a job selling cosmetics. Unfortunately, her boss enjoyed torturing staffers with the threat that they'd be fired if they didn't produce daily results.

The pain of betrayal by her husband, the physical and emotional toll of working a day job while also trying to raise her kids on her own, and the stress of worrying about losing that job and becoming homeless provided multiple triggers for the onset of infection by a virus that had been lurking in Stephanie for years. Within a month, it woke up from its dormant state.

The virus left its hiding place in Stephanie's liver and invaded her central nervous system. Stephanie started to feel exceptionally tired and sluggish, and her mind became foggy.

Concerned, Stephanie went to her family doctor for a checkup. Her doctor conducted a physical exam and ran blood tests, but found nothing unusual. "It's just stress," the doctor told her. "Simply stop worrying, and you'll be fine."

Stephanie's high level of fatigue and mental confusion persisted. And as the virus reproduced and worked its way into the nerves of her legs, arms, and shoulders, Stephanie began to feel neurological symptoms she'd never experienced before. She was especially troubled by pain in her left hip and knee, which was interfering with her daily routine of jogging. All of a sudden she was almost tripping on her left leg, as if it no longer worked properly.

Stephanie returned to her family doctor, who still couldn't find anything wrong. With her joint pain in mind, he sent her to a rheumatologist.

The rheumatologist gave Stephanie another careful physical exam and blood tests, with a focus on rheumatoid arthritis. He couldn't find anything wrong either. "You're perfectly healthy," the rheumatologist concluded. "Stay calm, get enough rest, and these issues will go away by themselves."

As much as Stephanie wanted to believe this, her symptoms not only persisted but expanded. Stephanie felt tired all the time, no matter how much she slept. The pain in her left shoulder became acute. Her left hip and leg grew weaker, giving her a slight limp. And she developed a mild case of anxiety.

While sharing her woes with her friends, one of them said, "What you're describing sounds a lot like what my cousin Shelly has. She was diagnosed with Lyme disease."

"Lyme disease?" Stephanie said. "I live in the city. I haven't been in a forest or within miles of a deer for years. How would I get bitten by a tick?"

"I don't know," said her friend. "But no one else is helping you, so you might as well see a Lyme doctor. What do you have to lose?"

This made sense to Stephanie, so she saw Dr. Nartel, a Lyme specialist.

Dr. Nartel took Stephanie's blood to run two types of tests: ELISA and Western blot. Both tests primarily look for antibodies reacting to the presence of *Borrelia burgdorferi* bacteria. Stephanie's problem wasn't *Borrelia burgdorferi*, though; it was a virus, so the results of both of her tests were negative.

Dr. Nartel was experienced enough to know these tests can't be counted on, even though he didn't understand why. So unlike Stephanie's previous doctors, he took her symptoms seriously. "What you're describing is consistent with Lyme disease," he told her. "I recommend you go on a thirty-day treatment of antibiotics, which you'll take daily in pill form. If you really do have Lyme disease, this will kill the bacteria causing your illness."

That made sense to Stephanie: finally, a diagnosis and validation. She readily agreed.

During the next month, Stephanie felt no difference. However, the antibiotics killed not only the bad bacteria, but the good bacteria in Stephanie's gut, which actually weakened her liver's immune system long term. The antibiotics also inflamed the walls of Stephanie's intestinal lining, causing painful gastritis and spasms.

Dr. Nartel had anticipated some of these issues by also prescribing probiotics. They weren't enough to counteract the side effects of the medication. Stephanie had trouble digesting food, lost her appetite, and periodically felt a burning sensation in her stomach.

After another month, Stephanie's fatigue and joint pain were worse than before her treatment. So was her memory fog . . . which now also included periodic memory loss.

Seriously concerned, Stephanie conducted extensive research via books and the Internet. If she didn't have Lyme, she concluded that she might have CFS, fibromyalgia, lupus, or even MS. Since Dr. Nartel couldn't help, she decided to try a different Lyme specialist, Dr. Maizon.

Dr. Maizon ran a broader range of blood tests than Stephanie's previous physicians and also used a lab that tested more extensively. One of the results turned up positive for *Babesia* and *Bartonella*—which wasn't surprising, considering the different types of bacteria and parasites a person can carry around even without Lyme disease symptoms. Still, Stephanie didn't know that *Babesia* and *Bartonella* are harmless and had nothing to do with her central nervous system issues, so she relaxed because she felt she was in more experienced hands.

When Dr. Maizon told her, "We need to do a one-to-three month course of intravenous antibiotics, and we'll use a substantially stronger medication this time," Stephanie readily agreed.

The stronger antibiotic, which was much more aggressive, took her to a whole new level of pain and suffering. It fed and strengthened the viral infection the way coal fuels a fire.

After two months on this more aggressive antibiotic, Stephanie's fatigue, joint pain, brain fog, and memory loss became so severe that she had to quit her job. She also developed nerve pain and spasms throughout her body. She couldn't fully care for her kids, as she needed to spend a large portion of each day in bed.

Dr. Maizon assured Stephanie that her getting worse wasn't cause for concern. "It just means the antibiotics are working," he said. "We call this situation a Herxheimer reaction. It happens when dying bacteria release their toxins faster than your system can flush them."

What Dr. Maizon didn't know was that if the problem had been bacterial, as he thought, the antibiotics would have made a substantial difference for the better. The explanation he offered is actually a trendy rationalization that medical communities have concocted to explain why patients get worse under a treatment that's supposed to make them better.

In reality, Stephanie was experiencing sensitive, inflamed nerves being further irritated by aggressive antibiotics, as well as an increased viral load. Still, Stephanie believed her doctor . . . and grew increasingly ill.

After a third month on antibiotics, Stephanie had a deep feeling that if she continued the treatment much longer, she'd die. She dropped Dr. Maizon. But with her immune system compromised and the viral infection greatly strengthened, she stayed chronically ill.

Stephanie turned to yet another Lyme specialist, who prescribed natural treatments: multivitamins, vitamin D, coenzyme Q10, and lots of fish oil. This doctor knew from past experience not to be so heavy-handed with antibiotics, so when Stephanie noticed no change with just the supplements, the specialist recommended adding only low dosages of the antibiotic medication. He argued that she'd been on too high a dosage before, but low dosages daily for three months would bring about her recovery.

Stephanie's Lyme had begun as a mild case, and might have stayed that way if she had steered clear of antibiotics. But the more she took, the more she paved the way for her Lyme symptoms to reach their full potential. Now, choosing to give antibiotics yet another try effectively handed her unidentified virus a loaded gun. After six weeks, Stephanie experienced brain inflammation and nerve pain so extreme that it brought her to what she felt was beyond crisis management. She had to struggle to even speak.

She let go of her current doctor, and in a panic visited a series of new alternative doctors.

Considering the gravity of her symptoms, one of them decided she didn't really have Lyme disease after all, but Lou Gehrig's disease (ALS).

Another declared she had multiple sclerosis.

And yet another told her she had Guillain-Barré. (In fact, Stephanie did have a form of Guillain-Barré—which medical communities think is a distinct disorder, but is actually just another name for viral nerve inflammation that affects the brain. This is a prime example of how much confusion revolves around Lyme.)

Finally, Stephanie went to an alternative doctor who happened to be a client of mine. He referred Stephanie to me as an emergency case.

After doing a reading and scan, the first thing I did was ease Stephanie's mind about her condition. "Yes," I said, "I'm very familiar with this illness. It wasn't caused by a tick, horsefly, or spider bite—or by bacteria. Spirit says it's a strain of a non-rashing shingles virus in the central nervous system causing brain inflammation, and the antibiotics you've been taking have been making it much stronger."

Just knowing what was really going on lifted a great weight from Stephanie and gave her the opportunity to start healing. At the same time, she was furious with the doctors who had transformed a relatively mild unidentified viral infection into a nearly fatal condition. Had she been treated with the appropriate natural methods, she would've been spared a full year of agony.

"You're entitled to be angry," I said. "You should also know that your doctors were genuinely trying to help. They were operating under the wrong assumptions that started 20 years ago about the nature of this illness. Thousands of others have gone through the same trials. What matters now is that you know the truth and can recover and heal."

Stephanie went on the foods, herbs, and supplements recommended in this chapter, and followed the instructions in this book for the 28-Day Healing Cleanse. There was a great deal of damage to undo. After six months, she resumed normal household chores, and required only a two-hour nap midday to maintain energy. After nine months, she was active outdoors again: walking without limping, driving her kids to soccer practice, gently romping around with her dog. After a year on her natural program to eliminate the viral symptoms behind her Lyme diagnosis, Stephanie felt better than she had before starting on the aggressive antibiotics.

Over time, she was stronger than she had been before the very first mild antibiotic. Stephanie finally recovered her full health, started jogging again, and resumed her normal life.

What Stephanie went through was a nightmare. Millions of people with Lyme disease globally undergo a similar ordeal. Tragically, many of them end up suffering greatly.

The good news is that virtually all of this pain and suffering can be avoided when the true nature of Lyme disease is understood . . . and the actual illness is addressed with the on-target methods covered in this chapter and the rest of this book.

"Thanks to readers who went into action with the information here, this book has prompted medical research and science to recategorize Lyme disease. While labeling Lyme as autoimmune still does not represent a full understanding of Lyme symptoms, this recategorization is a way for medical research and science to admit, 'We don't understand this as well as we thought we did'—and that's a major shift toward progress. It's testament to the people who read here in *Medical Medium* that Lyme disease is viral, not bacterial, who brought that information to their doctors, and who applied the healing protocols here and got results. It's also thanks to the doctors who have educated themselves with this material as they work to help patients. Many doctors have even applied the healing protocols in their own lives."

— Anthony William, Medical Medium

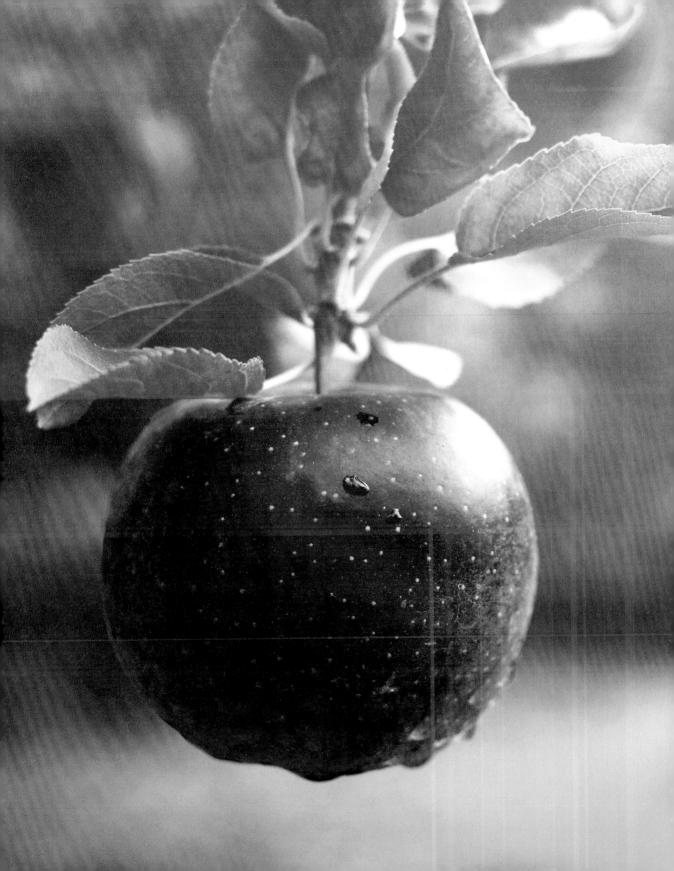

PART IV

HOW TO FINALLY HEAL

"Remember, Medical Medium is not just one protocol. That's why millions around the world have already gotten their lives back. There's a track record of this information changing lives. If you put the commitment, time, and effort into reading the books and understanding the various protocols, you have the ability to customize your own personal protocol within this information so you can go as far as you need to go."

— Anthony William, Medical Medium

CHAPTER 17

Gut Health

No one knows what really happens when food enters the stomach. The digestive system is a miracle and phenomenon beyond anything that anyone can perceive. Even with a medical understanding of the way some of it functions, the digestive system remains a great mystery.

Everyone knows we bite into a piece of food, chew it, swallow it, then it enters the gastrointestinal tract, some sort of breakdown occurs, and we expel it. We know that this is how we get nutrients. And we know that sometimes the process doesn't go so well, and stomachaches develop, or intestinal discomfort, or worse.

Just because medical science has discovered digestive enzymes, though, doesn't mean it has developed a comprehensive understanding of digestion. It doesn't mean medical science knows the difference between Jack the Ripper and Santa Claus when it comes to what we eat and how our bodies process it.

Digestion is the least founded part of the study of human physiology. While we walk around pretending that it's straightforward and science has it all figured out, it remains the most enigmatic element of how our bodies operate.

Unlike certain illnesses, where I can tell you that in a few decades, research will most likely make the discoveries it needs to make—discoveries of some of the information that's in this book—gut health is another story. Its secret workings may never be uncovered by medical communities on this earth—no matter what theory or terminology they use to make it seem understood at an advanced level—which is why this chapter is essential.

Your gut is one of the key foundations of your health, because you can consume important healing foods as tools. That makes caring for your digestive system the perfect place to start your journey of healing from the inside out.

Your gut includes the stomach, small intestine, large intestine (which includes the colon), liver, and gallbladder. The gut is responsible for ensuring that you absorb the nutrients of the food you eat, properly expel waste and toxins, and maintain a strong immune system through assimilating immune-building compounds from certain foods.

Yet not only is it critical for these everyday functions, your gut also holds a life force of its own. Food does not digest just from the physical process of food breakdown (a process scientific study hasn't fully pieced together); there are also critical spiritual and metaphysical factors involved in digestion. That's why enlightened beings on the planet employ eating techniques such as slow and thorough chewing; mindful, present eating; prayer before, during, or after meals; and becoming one with your food.

Imagine a river flowing inside your colon. Deep in the riverbed (the colon's lining), thousands of different strains of bacteria and microorganisms are there to maintain a homeostatic balance so that the river water doesn't become toxic (i.e., so the gut doesn't become septic and poisonous).

Just as a river has a spirit, the gut harbors much of the human spirit, too. That spirit is your essence of self, your will, and your intuition.

Have you ever heard the term *gut instinct*? Or *gut reaction* or *gut feeling*? Then there's "What does your gut tell you to do?" and "What are you, gutless?" and "I felt gutted." There's "I just about busted a gut," "I hate his guts," "I ran my guts out," and "You've really got guts." How many gut-related idioms are out there? It's because we understand on some level just what an integral role it plays in our lives, far beyond physicality. We understand that it's part of the core foundation of who we are emotionally and intuitively.

Your gut is where some of your strength is. It has emotional pores, and because of this, certain emotions can have an effect on whether your digestive system functions in peace or turmoil. This is why certain stressful situations can worsen acid reflux or trigger stomach spasms.

Poor gut health can keep someone busy with stomach and intestinal tract symptoms, not allowing them to be at peace enough to explore their intuitive abilities.

People are kind of like apples. You can have a shiny, perfect-looking apple that has a rotten core. That's like when someone's gut is spawning a lot of harmful bacteria, and maybe she or he has an immoral character, but you'd never guess from appearance. You can also have an apple with imperfections on the outside, yet on the inside it may have the most solid, healthy core you can find. Such a salt-of-the-earth, decent person may not have a happy resting face, or may not dress in vogue or seem like much fun on the surface, yet may possess a gut filled with good bacteria.

People can have anywhere from 75 to 125 trillion microorganisms residing in the gut. This can comprise bacteria (good, neutral, and bad), microbes, mold, yeast, fungus (both beneficial and nonbeneficial), mycotoxins from different varieties of fungus and mold, worms, and viruses. If not properly dealt with, pathogens in the gut can alter and block your natural instincts and create a breeding ground for an unlimited variety of illnesses—unless you know how to take control with the tools in this book.

This chapter covers what most commonly goes wrong with the gut, including leaky gut syndrome, poor digestion, acid reflux, bloating, intestinal infections, irritable bowel syndrome, gastric spasms, gastritis, and general pain in or near your stomach. It provides critical information about these conditions well beyond what's known by medical communities. It also debunks a number of unproductive gut health fads and trend "remedies" and offers simple steps you can take to genuinely heal your gut and restore your health.

UNDERSTANDING LEAKY GUT SYNDROME

One very confusing condition in medicine is *leaky gut syndrome,* also called *intestinal permeability*. The names themselves are perplexing; they're terms that different medical communities use to describe different conditions and theories.

When it comes down to it, there are three sides to the leaky gut syndrome story. Let's look at the first side: the conventional medical community's understanding. Most conventional doctors and surgeons use the term *leaky gut* for a critical intestinal disease that perforates the lining of the intestinal tract or stomach and causes severe blood infections, raging fevers, and/or sepsis. They have that right. True leaky gut is a very serious ailment that causes extreme pain and misery.

True leaky gut could stem from ulcers embedded deep in the stomach lining. Or it could result from bacterial strains of *E. coli* developing pockets in the intestinal tract lining; or superbugs like *C. difficile* causing *megacolon*; or from *hemorrhaging, abscesses,* or *diverticulosis*. The name *leaky gut* can be properly applied when one of these conditions breaks through the lining of the gastrointestinal tract and allows the pathogens and intestinal matter to leach into the bloodstream.

Another way that true leaky gut can occur is when a colonoscopy goes wrong and punctures the colon. (People have come to me who had very long hospital stays due to this.)

No matter the cause, true leaky gut results in dire symptoms.

The second side of the story is the alternative, integrative, functional, and naturopathic understanding of *leaky gut syndrome*. These medical communities use the term to describe a condition in which some believe mold, funguses like *Candida*, or unproductive bacteria thrive and burrow tiny holes in the linings of the intestine and cause micro levels of toxins to leak directly into the bloodstream, resulting in a multitude of symptoms. There are different variations of this belief, and they all mimic each other.

This theory behind leaky gut, no matter the variation, needs some adjustment.

While it's true that a toxic gut environment, including unproductive bacteria and nonbeneficial fungus, can contribute to various symptoms, referring to this as leaky gut is misleading. If these pathogens were truly breaking through the gastrointestinal lining in even the slightest way, then severe symptoms such as high fever, blood infection, extreme pain, and/or sepsis would result. *Leaky gut* should only be used to describe actual perforation of the digestive tract walls.

So why are tens of thousands of people who have fatigue, aches and pains, constipation, digestive discomfort, and acid reflux being told they have leaky gut or intestinal permeability by alternative practitioners?

Because there's something real going on, and this misunderstood catchphrase is the best theory the practitioners can offer. In the conventional medical world, millions of patients receive the tags IBS, celiac, Crohn's, colitis, gastroparesis, or gastritis to label these sorts of symptoms—yet the conditions remain mysterious. Or they experience gut symptoms and receive no diagnosis.

There *is* an explanation for these mystery gut problems that aren't actual leaky gut. I call it *ammonia permeability*, and it's the third side to the story.

Ammonia Permeability

Please do not confuse ammonia permeability with the recently trendy term *intestinal permeability*. Intestinal permeability is just a new name, meant to give the illusion of progress, for the old theory of leaky gut.

Ammonia permeability is a real occurrence. To comprehend what it is, you must first learn a few things about how your body processes food.

When you eat, the food quickly travels down to your stomach so it can be digested. (If you're chewing slowly enough for saliva to mix with the food, digestion will begin its initial stage in the mouth.) For dense protein-based foods—e.g., animal meat, nuts and seeds, and legumes—digestion in the stomach largely occurs through the action of your stomach's *hydrochloric acid* coupled with enzymes, which break the protein down into simpler forms that can then be further digested and assimilated by your intestines.

This is a relatively smooth process if your stomach contains normal levels of hydrochloric acid.

If your hydrochloric acid levels have become low, however, your food won't be sufficiently digested in your stomach. This is common when you're eating under stress or pressure. When the proteins reach your lower intestine, they won't be broken down enough for your cells to access their nutrients, and instead the food will just lie there and rot. This is called *gut rot*—putrefaction that creates *ammonia gas* and can result in symptoms of bloating, digestive discomfort, chronic dehydration, or oftentimes no symptoms at all. That's just the start.

In some people, good hydrochloric acid diminishes and bad acids take its place. A person could live with this condition for many years and not notice. Eventually, though, the bad acids can travel up the esophagus. (If you're experiencing acid reflux, these rogue acids are causing it, not your stomach's hydrochloric acid. This is a very common confusion; the medical world sees all stomach and intestinal acids as the same.)

A related issue is that the lining of your gut creates mucus in an effort to protect you from the bad acids. If a lot of mucus is coming up your throat for no apparent reason, it's probably your gut struggling to keep you safe because the rogue acids are trying to eat away at your stomach and esophagus lining . . . and it's a signal that you've got a problem that needs to be addressed. The mucus can also travel down the intestinal tract and stop proper absorption of nutrients. Mucus can also be formed in other ways, such as pathogens feeding on gluten, eggs, and dairy products.

Let's go back to that ammonia gas, though. This is the key piece of information: when food decomposes in your intestinal tract and produces ammonia, this toxic gas has the ability to float, ghost-like, out of your intestines and directly into your bloodstream. This is what I call ammonia permeability. This ammonia gas can also enter into the hepatic portal vein, which carries it up into the liver. Once this ammonia gas saturates the liver, it tends to be released out of the liver, either back into the bloodstream or into the gallbladder and back into the intestinal tract.

It's the ammonia gas that creates most of the havoc associated with leaky gut syndrome. It doesn't have to do with infections or punctures of the small intestines or colon. And it isn't *Candida* yeast or bacteria expelling toxins through the intestinal walls, either.

Millions of people walk around with digestive health problems, and the culprit is ammonia permeability. As I've said, what many alternative doctors diagnose as leaky gut syndrome has nothing to do with holes or other imperfections in your gut; it has nothing to do with acids or bacteria leaking out. It has nothing to do with the lining of the small intestinal tract or colon weakening or thinning out.

Rather, ammonia gas in your intestines is drifting into the bloodstream . . . which then carries the gas throughout your body. Besides the gut symptoms I mentioned earlier, ammonia permeability, if really severe, can result in malaise, mild fatigue, skin problems (such as dry skin), dental problems, restless sleep, anxiety, and so much more.

At this point you might reasonably ask, "If this all happens because of too little hydrochloric acid in the stomach, what causes *that*?" It's important to note that when someone has ammonia permeability, there's already liver dysfunction, usually in the realm of a stagnant, sluggish liver. Low hydrochloric acid levels in the stomach begin with a liver not functioning optimally—in part, not producing enough bile to break down fat, so that on top of proteins rotting in the digestive system, you also have fats from your food going rancid in the gut. That is, low bile production leads to extra demand on the stomach glands to produce hydrochloric acid to help break down food, which eventually depletes them, leading to low hydrochloric acid and ammonia permeability.

Beyond this underlying liver dysfunction, the number one reason for a deficiency of hydrochloric acid is *adrenaline*—which contributes to a stagnant, sluggish liver in the first place, too.

What is also not known is that there isn't just one form of adrenaline. Your adrenal glands produce 56 different blends in response to different emotions and situations. And the ones associated with difficult feelings such as fear, anxiety, anger, betrayal, hatred, guilt, shame, depression, and stress can be severely compromising to a variety of areas of your body—including your stomach's supply of hydrochloric acid. So if you've been chronically stressed or upset, that can be enough for adrenaline to slowly hinder and deplete the stomach glands that produce your hydrochloric acid—at the same time hindering and depleting your ability to properly digest food. Different levels of stress and emotions that we experience in our everyday lives can act as a trigger, weakening certain parts of the immune system. Plus, adrenaline saturating the intestinal tract hinders good bacteria and microorganisms. Most people going through an emotional challenge tend to choose foods, out of comfort, that do not support the immune system—and can even potentially feed pathogens both inside the gut and outside of it.

Also often wreaking havoc with your stomach's hydrochloric acid are *prescription drugs*. Antibiotics, immunosuppressants, antifungals, amphetamines, and a variety of other medications our bodies haven't adapted to can disrupt the stomach glands' ability to produce hydrochloric acid. Prescription drugs can weaken the liver over time, too, putting more stress upon the stomach glands.

Your hydrochloric acid is likely to be affected if you overeat any type of protein, such as animal meat, nuts, seeds, and/or legumes. (If the protein comes from greens, sprouts, or other vegetables, it doesn't have the same effect.) Eating a lot of foods that combine fat and sugar (such as cheese, whole milk, cakes, cookies, and ice cream) can have the same harmful effect on hydrochloric acid.

Both these categories of food require much more work to be digested than fruits, leafy greens, herbs, wild foods, or vegetables do, placing a huge strain on your liver and the rest of your gut. This can eventually "burn out" the liver, simultaneously burning out your stomach glands that produce hydrochloric acid and putting stress upon the pancreas, which weakens digestive enzymes. If you're eating high-protein meals (for example, chicken, fish, meat, nut butters, nuts, or seeds) and you're experiencing symptoms of low hydrochloric acid such as bloating, stomach discomfort, constipation, sluggishness, and/or energy loss, then eat the animal or plant protein sparingly and limit it to one serving per day. Keep in mind, these are foods that have higher fat content, which puts a further strain on digestion—in part because they force the liver to overproduce bile, exhausting its reserves.

There is good news in all of this. You can recover your hydrochloric acid, support bile production, and strengthen your enzymes with a miraculous herb that's sold everywhere.

Rebuilding Hydrochloric Acid

The way to fix ammonia permeability (which, as we've just discussed, is often mislabeled as leaky gut syndrome or intestinal permeability)—and the first step in addressing virtually any other gut health issue—is to rebuild your stomach's ability to produce hydrochloric acid, restore your liver, and strengthen your digestive system.

There's an amazingly simple and effective way to do this: daily, on an empty stomach, drink a 16-ounce glass of fresh *celery juice*.

This may not be the answer you were expecting. It may not seem like celery juice could be *that* beneficial. But take this very seriously. It is one of the most profound ways, if not *the* most profound way, to restore digestive health. It is that powerful. And keep in mind: while there are many juice blends out there nowadays that are fantastic for your health, you need to drink your celery juice straight (not mixing anything with it) if your goal is to restore proper digestive function. You'll join millions of people who have started drinking celery juice since this book was first published.

Do not be derailed by the simplicity of this. Think of it like being assigned a 10-page paper on one specific aspect of daily life in a certain historical time period. If you hand in a paper that's an overview of the era, with only two lines about that one part of daily life, the teacher won't be impressed by all the extra facts. She'll wonder why you didn't go in-depth on the one topic she assigned.

That's how your stomach feels when it's trying to restore hydrochloric acid. A juice blend of 20 different ingredients, only one of which is celery, will be a distraction. In this case, simplest is best. The stomach, stomach glands, intestinal tract, and liver want celery juice, and celery juice alone, so they can do their deep repair in this area. It's a secret method that can turn around the life of a person with a gut disorder.

Here's how to do it:

- Wash a fresh bunch of celery in the morning while you still have an empty stomach. (It's also an option to wash your celery the night before.) Anything else in your stomach will disrupt the effect of the celery juice.

- Juice the celery. Add *nothing* else, not even water or a squeeze of lemon, as any other ingredient will disrupt the effect of the celery, too. I recommend straining the celery juice to remove any grit or stray pieces of pulp.

- Drink the juice immediately—before it can oxidize, which reduces its power—for best results. After your celery juice, wait at least 15 to 30 minutes before consuming anything else.

- If it's not an option to drink your celery juice immediately after juicing, try to drink it within the morning you juice it. (If you keep celery juice refrigerated in a sealed container, it will still have powerful benefits for 24 hours. And if you have no choice but to keep it for longer, it's still worth juicing it ahead and consuming it when you can.) If you need to make or drink your celery juice later in the day, wait at least 60 minutes after your previous meal so your stomach is relatively empty again. For more specific guidance about timing, see "Celery Juice as a Medicinal" in Chapter 21, "Critical Guide to Supplement Protocols."

(You can also make your celery juice with a blender. In that case, wash your celery, chop it into roughly one-inch pieces, then place it in a high-speed blender and blend until smooth. Do not add water; use the blender's tamping tool if needed. Strain the liquefied celery well. A nut milk bag is handy for this.)

Celery juice works because celery contains unique sodium compositions, and these mineral salts that I call *sodium cluster salts* are bonded with many bioactive trace minerals and nutrients. Celery juice is also anti-pathogenic. Most people walking around with digestive symptoms that are impeding their quality of life are dealing with the presence of pathogens such as viruses and bacteria. When celery juice's sodium cluster salts enter into the body, they break down and destroy viruses, nonbeneficial bacteria, unproductive fungus, yeast, and mold upon contact. In the case of viruses and bacteria, sodium cluster salts weaken and break down the membrane wall that surrounds them. So not only does celery juice help to restore the liver and digestive system, it helps to rid the causes of many of someone's symptoms. If you drink the celery juice first thing in the morning, it will strengthen your digestion of the foods you eat for the rest of the day. And over time, the sodium cluster salts, minerals, and nutrients have the unique ability to completely restore your stomach's hydrochloric acid by rebuilding your stomach's gastric glands.

For a comprehensive understanding of the power of celery juice, see the Medical Medium book *Celery Juice.*

You should also know that it's common to have not just one gut issue, but several related gut issues at once. The rest of this chapter empowers you to deal with other gut problems.

REMOVING TOXIC HEAVY METALS FROM YOUR GUT

In our modern era, it's virtually impossible not to take in a certain amount of toxic heavy metals, such as mercury, aluminum, copper, cadmium, nickel, arsenic, barium, and lead. These heavy metals often accumulate in your liver, gallbladder, intestines, and/or brain. Since heavy metals tend to be heavier than the water that's inside your digestive system and blood, they sink down and settle into the intestinal tract—just like gold settles at the bottom of a riverbed.

Toxic heavy metals are poisonous, and if they begin to oxidize, their chemical runoff will mutate and damage whatever cells are nearby. However, the biggest issue with heavy metals is that they're prime food for bad bacteria, viruses, funguses, parasites, and worms. That means these metals are likely to attract and serve as a feeding ground for *Streptococcus*, *E. coli* and its many strains, *C. difficile*, *H. pylori*, and especially viruses. When these bacteria consume the toxic heavy metals, they release a toxic gas, while viruses release a neurotoxic gas upon consuming toxic heavy metals. Both these forms of gas attach themselves to the ammonia gas and travel through the intestinal lining. In other words, the ammonia permeability takes on a friend, and that friend is heavy metal contamination. The ammonia permeability makes it easier for the toxic gas to get through the intestinal lining.

Do not confuse mycotoxins (fungal toxins) with permeability, however. It's currently unknown to practitioners that some pathogens create neurotoxins when they consume heavy metals—and that these neurotoxins are very different from mycotoxins. Mycotoxins cannot create the neurological symptoms that neurotoxins do; mycotoxins tend to stay in the intestinal tract and get eliminated through defecation. Keep this in mind as you hear more and more about mycotoxins in the coming years. They are not the culprit in autoimmune disease. I don't want you to get swept up in a misguided trend—this is about you getting better and not distracted by the barrage of catchphrases out there.

Once the pathogens I mentioned above settle in, they'll start inflaming your gut—by saturating and, in some cases, nesting in the linings of your intestines, colon, or especially your liver. Bacteria and viruses will release poisons in your liver and intestinal tract directly via the bacterial toxins and viral neurotoxins they produce, and indirectly via their waste byproduct and toxic corpses. This is how most people develop illnesses and disorders such as IBS, Crohn's disease (mystery inflammation of the gastrointestinal tract), and colitis (mystery inflammation of the colon—which is typically a chronic infection of the shingles virus described in Chapter 11 coupled with *Streptococcus* bacteria).

Under a microscope, these byproducts of dead viral matter and cast-off viral casings often look like parasitical activity. This throws off many analyses of stool samples and results in numerous misdiagnoses, which means that it's often a mistake when someone is diagnosed with a parasite. This is a huge confusion in gut health today.

(Parasites are vastly different from viruses and bacteria. They can't live and breed inside someone long term; instead, they're usually acute—and sometimes highly toxic. This means that when you're exposed to a parasite, your immune system has to kill it off and your body has to flush it out within a short time period, just like food poisoning. In truth, many food poisoning cases are acute parasitical infections, either from a living parasite or a dead and cooked one. Some parasites, once they're dead from cooking, become foodborne toxins that can trigger the body into expelling them with diarrhea and/or vomiting. The agony someone experiences with a parasitical infection in the gut eventually subsides by either killing off or ridding the parasite. Your body doesn't get used to a parasite; that is, a parasite doesn't stay in you while you go back to life—which is the opposite of how most viruses and bacteria work. As for worms, it's a mistake to classify them as parasites. Some worms can stay inside the host, living inside the intestinal tract and even organs while the host is living life—maybe even a good-quality life, exhibiting no symptoms. When people suffer with neurological symptoms such as fatigue and many others, they'll often get diagnosed as having a parasite when really, neurotoxins produced by viruses are causing the symptoms. If you find this confusing because you've heard that some people get chronic symptom relief from parasitical treatments, know that those treatments are hit-or-miss guessing games. When your diet changes and you're randomly picking different herbs to try, you may by chance reduce your low-grade viral infection, getting some relief accidentally.)

While heavy metals can lead to problems if not addressed, they're relatively easy to rid from the gut. (You have to work a little harder long term to get them out of the brain and liver.) So if you have any kind of gut illness, or even chronic digestive distress, it's best to play it safe by assuming heavy metals are at least part of the problem and taking the steps to remove them.

Here are some powerful options to remove toxic heavy metals from your intestinal tract:

- **Cilantro:** eat one cup a day of this fresh herb as is, sprinkled on salads, or in a smoothie.

- **Parsley:** eat a half cup a day of this fresh herb as is, sprinkled on salads, or in a smoothie.

- **Spirulina:** if it's in powder form, mix 1 teaspoon daily into water or a smoothie, or take 3 capsules daily.

- **Barley grass juice powder:** mix 1 teaspoon of the powder into water or smoothie daily, or take 3 capsules daily.

- **Wild blueberries:** eat one cup of frozen wild blueberries a day, or add 2 teaspoons of powder to water or smoothie daily.

- **Garlic:** eat 1 to 2 fresh cloves a day.

- **Sage:** eat 2 to 3 medium-to-large fresh leaves (or 5 to 6 small fresh leaves) a day.

- **L-glutamine:** mix 1 teaspoon daily into water, or take 3 capsules a day.

- **Plantain leaf:** brew this herb to make tea and drink a cup a day.

- **Lemon balm:** brew this herb to make tea and drink two cups a day.

- **Apples:** eat 1 to 2 a day (blended is okay). Apples' pectin binds onto the heavy metal toxins that the herbs and other options in this list are uprooting.

THE GUT'S NATURAL PROTECTION

It's so far undiscovered in medical research that we're born with tiny, furry hairs that line the entire intestinal tract. This fur-like hair (not to be confused with villi, microvilli, or plicae circulares) is microscopic, just a little bigger than bacteria itself. These furry hairs have a grippy action, so when peristalsis occurs, they help by removing substances that are moving through the intestinal tract. At the same time, the hair helps protect your gut from invasion by viruses, bad bacteria, funguses, and worms. It's also there as a safe haven that harbors billions of good bacteria as well as antiviral, antibacterial compounds that are only found in fruits, leafy greens, herbs, wild foods, and vegetables.

Until the 19th century, this hair normally lasted for a person's entire lifetime.

Since the Industrial Revolution, though, we've been assaulted by environmental toxins, prescription medications, and other chemicals that can scorch the gut; the heavy metals described in the previous section; and the stress of modern living and its accompanying scalding adrenaline. As a result, your gut's hair lining may be largely burned off by the time you reach age 20. This contributes to some of the mild gut health problems that people struggle with today.

The reason medical science hasn't discovered this hair is because most intestinal surgeries are performed on people age 30 and above. By this point, it's long gone. And in intestinal biopsies for babies, this microscopic, furry lining just isn't on the radar.

If you do have any of this protective hair left, you can help save and bolster it by eating foods that are especially healthy for your gut. These include quality lettuce (e.g., romaine,

red leaf, and butter leaf); ancient herbs such as oregano, thyme, and peppermint; and fruit, with an emphasis on bananas, apples, papayas, melons, figs, and dates.

Also take care to steer clear of foods that can harm your health. For a detailed list, see Chapter 19, "What Not to Eat."

RESTORING GUT FLORA AND MAXIMIZING B$_{12}$ PRODUCTION

Beneficial microorganisms in your gut produce most of your body's supply of vitamin B$_{12}$. But this doesn't happen just anywhere in your gut. The *ileum,* the final section of your small intestine, is the main center of this B$_{12}$ absorption and production. It's also where *methylation* starts.

Whenever it's needed, vitamin B$_{12}$ is absorbed through the walls of your ileum via microvessels that are capable of absorbing B$_{12}$ and nothing else. The B$_{12}$ gets absorbed and sent up the hepatic portal vein highway into the liver, where the liver can store the B$_{12}$ and also put it to good use by sending it throughout the body. It's the B$_{12}$ produced in the ileum that's most recognized by the brain and rest of the body. Specific enzymes produced by your pancreas prohibit any other toxin or nutrient from being absorbed by these ileum blood vessels, and thus block them from entering your bloodstream.

Science has yet to discover this information.

Virtually everyone on the planet is dealing with a B$_{12}$ deficiency and/or a methylation issue. These issues show up in a few different forms. First, when methylation goes wrong, it can prevent true bio-absorption of critical micronutrients and trace minerals. Second, a methylation issue can interrupt the conversion process of non-active, bulky vitamins and other nutrients into smaller, bioactive versions that can be absorbed by the body. Third, a heightened level of the amino acid homocysteine, caused by a toxic liver or an elevated pathogen load in the body that creates a lot of toxic byproduct, can interfere with methylation, preventing proper conversion and absorption of nutrients.

You produce all the vitamin B_{12} you need when the ileum has abundant beneficial microorganisms of a specific kind. Sufficient beneficial microorganisms also make methylation strong, but everyone is short on these microorganisms—that is, micro-probiotics that live naturally on certain foods, enter the gut when we consume them, and fill the ileum. You can't buy these bioactive microorganisms in probiotic supplement form at the store, or get them from fermented foods and drinks.

When you're suffering from low hydrochloric acid, heavy metal toxicity, and/or ammonia permeability, plus you're missing this unique variety of microorganism, your gut's vitamin B_{12} production plummets or stops altogether.

You can't rely on B_{12} blood tests, because medical labs can't yet detect the levels of vitamin B_{12} in your gut, organs, and especially your central nervous system. While taking a B_{12} supplement can fill the bloodstream, so that your B_{12} levels will show up on blood tests as sufficient, that doesn't mean the B_{12} is entering the central nervous system, which critically needs B_{12}. So regardless of what blood tests exhibit, always take a high-quality B_{12} supplement. (Look for it as methylcobalamin—ideally, blended with adenosylcobalamin—rather than as cyanocobalamin. With methylcobalamin and adenosylcobalamin, your

liver doesn't have to do any work to convert the B_{12} into a usable form.) Keep in mind that if you get a blood test that shows your B_{12} is elevated above normal and you're not taking a B_{12} supplement, this means that the B_{12} in your body is not methylating, absorbing, or easily entering deep into organs or the central nervous system. Or you could start taking a high-quality B_{12} supplement, get a blood test, and then hear that your B_{12} level is high. That doesn't mean to stop taking B_{12}. You want it readily accessible so that your central nervous system has every opportunity to absorb it. Lack of B_{12} is a very real deficiency with very real health consequences. And as mentioned earlier, almost every person on the planet is B_{12} deficient in some way.

Also, take steps to restore your gut's normal levels of productive microorganisms. Cultured probiotics sitting on the shelves of the health food store or fermented foods that claim to have beneficial bacteria aren't the answers here. There is no study or research that can show these microorganisms entering into your gut and performing. It's a guessing game. The truth is that most, if not all, of these microorganisms will die in your stomach before they descend and reach the small intestine. And factory-produced probiotics never reach that last part of the small intestine, the ileum—which is the region that needs them most.

There *are* probiotics that stay alive in the gut and are responsible for restoring the intestinal flora, including in the ileum. These are still barely known after the three decades I've spent teaching about them, and we take them for granted. We don't even know they're there. Yet they are remarkably powerful and can change your health and life in ways unimaginable. When people have good gut health, it's most often because they've accidentally and occasionally consumed these naturally occurring, life-giving probiotics and beneficial microorganisms.

Where can you find them? On fresh, living foods.

The special probiotics that live on fruits, leafy greens, herbs, wild foods, and vegetables are what I call *elevated microorganisms,* or sometimes *elevated biotics,* because they harbor energy from God and the sun. Elevated microorganisms are not to be confused with soil-borne organisms and probiotics derived from soil. Elevated microorganisms are the most gut-renewing option there is. They are the very microorganisms that the ileum harbors, and they create the B_{12} that the body, particularly the brain, most recognizes.

A top source of elevated microorganisms is sprouts. Alfalfa, broccoli, clover, fenugreek, lentil, mustard, sunflower, kale, and other seeds like them, when sprouted, are living micro-gardens. In this tiny, nascent form of life, they're teeming with beneficial microorganisms that will help your gut thrive.

Again, these beneficial microorganisms are different from soil-borne organisms and "prebiotics." Elevated microorganisms are always found aboveground, on the leaves and skins of fruits, leafy greens, herbs, wild foods, and vegetables.

If you have access to your own garden (that you don't treat with chemicals), or you grow indoor food plants or sprouts, you can eat some of the fruits, leafy greens, herbs, wild foods, and/or vegetables you grow to get elevated microorganisms into your diet. The key here is to eat the food you're growing fresh, raw, and not scrubbed or cooked. (Although a

gentle rinse without soap can be safe.) Millions of revitalizing probiotics and microorganisms exist on the surfaces of these foods.

It's imperative to use your judgment about when it's safe to eat unwashed fruits, leafy greens, herbs, wild foods, and vegetables. Only do it when you know the growing source and are sure that there are no toxins or other contaminants that could make you sick. At the moment in history that this book edition goes to print, giving items that you haven't grown yourself a good wash is very important. If you can grow items in your own garden (that isn't treated with pesticides or other lawn chemicals), then as I mentioned, that's one option for getting access to elevated microorganisms. Container gardening (whether indoors or outdoors) is also an option. So is growing herbs in pots on your windowsill. Or you can grow sprouts from nearly anywhere—your setup can be as simple as the right seeds, a clean jar or bowl, and a strainer. Try to get a little bit of these elevated microorganisms wherever you can.

When you pluck a piece of kale from the ground, you can see a film in the pockets of the leaf. This isn't soil or dirt or soil-based organisms. This film is made up of elevated microorganisms—a naturally occurring probiotic that hasn't yet been washed off. (Not to be confused with a manure-caked piece of kale, which it's best if you thoroughly rinse off.) When you eat the leaf of kale, the pockets of good microorganisms get folded and trapped, so they often bypass the stomach. When they're released in the intestines, these millions of microorganisms have phenomenal effects on digestion and the immune system, as they find their way down to your ileum and replenish your B_{12} production and storage bank.

A raw, unwashed piece of kale straight from an organic garden—or a handful of sprouts from a countertop garden, or a fresh, pesticide-free apple plucked from the tree—outshines every single soil-based or lab-created probiotic and fermented food available. If you've eaten just one of these items that's coated with elevated microorganisms just one time in your life, it has protected you to some degree, without your awareness. And the more fresh, chemical-free, wax-free fruits, leafy greens, herbs, wild foods, and vegetables from safe sources that you eat without scrubbing or cooking, the more benefits you get.

Note that *prebiotics* have recently become popular. What the theory really translates to is eating certain fruits and vegetables that support productive microorganisms in the gut. This can never be measured or determined on any scientific scale. Truth is, every fruit, leafy green, herb, wild food, and vegetable that you can eat raw supports the entire gut's environment.

One common practice is to take quality store-bought probiotics or soil-borne probiotics, although keep in mind that even the most high-quality ones aren't all that helpful. Regardless of what you try out there, it's always best to try to ingest the elevated microorganisms from living fruits, leafy greens, herbs, wild foods, and/or vegetables at some point in your life—or as many times as you have an opportunity to do so. Nothing can compare to ingesting the elevated microorganisms on the skin or leaf of a fresh fruit, leafy green, herb, wild food, or vegetable.

If rejuvenating gut flora (or microflora) is what you're aiming for, this is one of the best ways to do it. Elevated microorganisms serve as one step to restoring your microorganism balance. It's also one step in healing so-called MTHFR gene mutations and other methylation issues. Note that the medical communities' label "MTHFR gene mutation" is inaccurate, though. People with this condition do not actually have a gene defect; rather, their bodies are experiencing toxic overload from toxins and low-grade viral infections inside the liver that are preventing the liver's job of converting nutrients to bioavailable micronutrients. These powerful elevated microorganisms, along with addressing the underlying viral infection and cleansing your liver, can lower homocysteine levels and virtually reverse an MTHFR gene mutation diagnosis.

Once you've reestablished your stomach's hydrochloric acid, removed toxic heavy metals from your gut and foods that feed pathogens from your diet, cleansed your liver to restore bile reserves, and supported your gut's ability to make vitamin B_{12} by restoring elevated microorganisms, any gut health problem you have has the foundation of what it needs to heal.

MAKING SENSE OF FADS, TRENDS, AND MYTHS ABOUT THE GUT

There are a number of gut health trends, both in and out of mainstream medicine, that are really unproductive—and sometimes reckless. When we're unwell, we often become desperate, willing to try anything, which makes it easy to be persuaded by the variety of trendy treatments out there. Take caution, though. What follows are descriptions of some of the most popular fads, along with why you should steer clear of them.

Hydrochloric Acid Supplements

There are supplements that claim to provide your stomach's missing hydrochloric acid in pill form. While these are well intentioned, there are two problems with them.

First, they aren't helping your stomach create hydrochloric acid on its own.

Second, and more important, the manufacturers of these supplements don't realize that your stomach's hydrochloric acid isn't composed of just one chemical. While science hasn't yet discovered this, your stomach houses a complex blend of *seven* different acids. (In the future, this book will prompt research into this, and the truth will start to surface in sources other than this book.)

The supplements offer only *one* of the seven acids that make up your stomach's digestive hydrochloric acid, so they're a very incomplete solution.

Even worse, they can *hinder* your stomach's rebuilding of its digestive fluids by creating a chemical imbalance that overwhelmingly favors just one of the seven acids in the blend. And the supplements still don't duplicate the specific nature of that particular acid created by your stomach glands. Until this is properly researched and understood, hydrochloric acid supplements are not a good option.

These supplements are unlikely to do you any great harm. However, you're tremendously better off drinking a glass of celery juice daily. It's only with celery that you'll fully restore your stomach's store of hydrochloric acid and reclaim your gut health.

Sodium Bicarbonate and *Candida*

A lot of people are championing *sodium bicarbonate*—aka baking soda—as a treatment. They believe the culprit behind gut problems is *Candida,* based on the longtime trend of *Candida* diagnoses. They figure that sodium bicarbonate, which is heavily alkaline, will somehow stop *Candida* . . . which they believe thrives in an acidic environment.

Nearly every link in this chain of reasoning is wrong. The one exception is that, yes, many bugs do like an acidic environment, because many bugs create the acidic environment. However, *Candida* is not the cause of gut health issues; it's the messenger. When your gut is dysfunctional as a result of toxic heavy metals and other toxic troublemakers, you can develop pathogenic infections from a number of sources. *Candida* is merely a side effect, and typically not a serious one. (For more on *Candida*, see Chapter 9.)

Sodium bicarbonate is ineffective against *Candida* anyway. More broadly, sodium bicarbonate does *nothing* to help your gut. On the contrary, it's abrasive and will only create an imbalance. If you take a large dosage of sodium bicarbonate, any combination of the following is likely to happen:

- **Gastric spasms,** i.e., a twisting and tightening of your intestinal tract and colon.

- **A homeostasis crisis for your body,** which must strain mightily to reestablish balance after so much alkaline is abruptly dumped into it.

- **A toxic crisis for your body,** because while sodium bicarbonate is perfectly safe in small amounts, past a certain level it becomes an irritant to your stomach and intestinal tract, especially if you already have inflammation from a condition. In some cases this causes diarrhea, vomiting, severe bloating, and/or other discomfort.

- A *worsening* of bacterial and fungal infections, because sodium bicarbonate puts such a strain on your intestinal tract, which can weaken your immune system.

- A *worsening* of your digestive issues, because sodium bicarbonate destroys your hydrochloric acid and thus contributes to a misdiagnosis of leaky gut syndrome. It also interferes with the absorption of food in your intestines.

There are many negatives to sodium bicarbonate as a "remedy." I've seen a lot of people struggle after using it.

Diatomaceous Earth

Another fad is trying to heal the gut by consuming *diatomaceous earth,* also called *diatomite.* This is a soft sedimentary rock that crumbles into a fine white powder. Some people believe diatomite has the ability to kill parasites and clear toxins from the gut.

However, it doesn't do a single useful thing for your gut. It can actually be quite dangerous for your health, if you're sensitive and have a health condition.

Diatomite clings tenaciously to the sides of your intestinal tract and colon, and severely interferes with their ability to absorb the nutrients from your food. On top of that, it

damages your hydrochloric acid and kills good bacteria. In some cases it causes initial vomiting and diarrhea, followed by long-lasting gastric spasms and pain.

In other words, it has all the bad effects of sodium bicarbonate, only to an even worse degree. Plus it can take some time to shake loose from your intestinal tract. So don't even think about taking diatomite or consuming food-based diatomaceous earth.

Gallbladder Flush

Yet another trend is trying to purge your gallbladder of gallstones and toxins by drinking various odd concoctions, such as a glass of pure olive oil, or olive oil mixed with herbs and/or lemon juice, cayenne, or maple syrup.

People believe these oil-based concoctions work because within a day after they drink one, they see what appear to be gallstones in their stool. What they don't realize is that they're seeing the *oil* they drank. When a large amount of oil is dumped into your body, your digestive system uses mucus to form it into little balls (sometimes in multiple colors, depending on what foods are in different parts of your intestinal tract) that can be easily expelled. This is to protect an overburdened liver. (Keep in mind, this information applies when people believe they have liver stones, as well.)

I've run across people who have done gallbladder flushes for years, multiple times each year, and still report hundreds and hundreds of large gallstones. If gallbladder flushes really worked, this would have to mean there were thousands of stones in the gallbladder—a tiny organ that could fit in the palm of your hand. It's not humanly possible for someone to produce or harbor that many gallstones. If you *were* to flush out a gallstone, it would probably become caught in your gallbladder's duct. You'd then be headed to the hospital for emergency surgery.

Gallstones are made up of protein, bile, and cholesterol. You don't have to choke down a pint of olive oil—and potentially create a crisis—to purge them. The best way to get rid of gallstones is to lower your consumption of dense proteins (which are rich in fat and include plant-based proteins such as nut butters) and eat a diet that emphasizes sodium-rich vegetables, leafy greens, herbs, fruits, and wild foods that contain healthy bio-acids. By incorporating more spinach, kale, radishes, mustard greens, celery, lemons, oranges, grapefruit, and limes into your meals—and by drinking a glass of lemon water every morning and every evening—you can start the stone-dissolving process.

One safe and amazingly effective option for dissolving gallbladder stones and restoring the liver is straight celery juice on an empty stomach. Or a small amount of asparagus juice is very effective: you can juice a handful of fresh, raw asparagus along with whatever other juice ingredients you like. (Remember to keep celery juice on its own—you're not adding asparagus juice to your celery juice.)

The best way to *prevent* new gallstones from forming is to follow the advice in this book for creating and maintaining a healthy gut.

Fermented Foods

Let's go back in time, before refrigeration was invented. For millennia in various parts of the globe, you would take your last crop of the season and, in order to survive another winter, throw the fruits and vegetables into pots. These harvests would then undergo a mysterious process that prevented total decomposition and instead preserved the foods. In Russia, for example, they threw cabbages into vats and let them dissolve until they were practically mush, creating what we know as sauerkraut.

This fermentation was critical—without it, people would have starved to death. No one had a supermarket to pop into on their way home from work, or a freezer or refrigerator to preserve their food supply.

In the present day, fermented foods have taken on a revered status—they're celebrated as a boon to health. That's not quite correct.

There's a misconception that because fermented foods helped humans along for thousands of years, they have health benefits. Truth is, fermented foods were about survival. A self-preserved food was the difference between life and death by starvation. It's better to view these edibles as an important historical stopgap, rather than as a health aid.

The so-called probiotics in fermented foods are not life-giving. The bacteria in them thrive off the decay process—in other words, they thrive off death, not life. When an animal dies in the woods, the bacteria that start to engulf its flesh are in the same category as the bacteria used to preserve fermented foods of all kinds.

They're in a different category of bacteria from the beneficial type we covered earlier in this chapter. The elevated microorganisms on living fruits, leafy greens, herbs, wild foods, and vegetables thrive on life, and are therefore restorative to your gut, because *we* are alive. They have a life force that the bacteria in fermented foods do not.

When we think of beneficial bacteria, we often think about yogurt. We've been conditioned to believe that the probiotics in yogurt support our gut health. If you're struggling with a health condition, though, yogurt is not a positive food to consume; dairy feeds all pathogens. Plus, if it's pasteurized yogurt, the pasteurization process has killed the probiotics anyway. The beneficial bacteria that do thrive in raw, living yogurt cannot withstand hydrochloric acid and therefore die in the stomach, never reaching the intestinal tract. Besides, beneficial bacteria from yogurt have no bearing on the pathogens that cause chronic illness. Good bacteria and bad bacteria don't go to war with each other. Neither do good bacteria and viruses. You can have all the good bacteria you want, and any viruses and/or unproductive bacteria in your system will still cause problems.

The vast majority of fermented foods—kimchi, sauerkraut, salami, pepperoni, soy sauce, kombucha tea, and so on—breed bacteria from foods that are no longer alive. Such bacteria are useless for your gut.

For most people, these bacteria do no harm; they're simply passed through the digestive tract and quickly expelled by the body as unnecessary. I'm not opposed to consuming them.

Some people's bodies respond more harshly, however, perceiving the bacteria as foreign invaders and overreacting in efforts to banish them. This can result in bloating, stomach pain, gas, nausea, and/or diarrhea. Even if this occurs, though, it's a temporary situation that ends once the bacteria's flushed out.

So if you like fermented foods, it's fine to keep eating them for their unique flavor. And if fermented foods upset your stomach (as they do for so many), or if you just don't like them,

don't eat them. They don't provide a lot of health benefits to your gut.

And if you think they have major benefits, you're being misled. The hydrochloric acid in our guts is extremely sensitive to the bacteria on fermented foods, so it kills the unproductive bacteria even if it's harmless; it sees it as the enemy. This is in stark contrast to the life-giving bacteria from freshly picked living foods. The beneficial bacteria on a piece of kale straight from the garden is virtually indestructible by hydrochloric acid—so that's one of the tools where you should turn your focus if you're looking for the true boon to gut health.

Apple Cider Vinegar

If you're concerned about a gut health condition of any kind and you're looking for cures, steer clear of the apple cider vinegar myth.

Don't get me wrong. Apple cider vinegar (ACV) is by far the most beneficial, healthiest, and safest of all vinegars. It's better for you than cleaning vinegar, white and red wine vinegars, balsamic vinegar, rice vinegar . . . And apple cider vinegar is ideal for external use, such as addressing skin rashes, scalp issues, and even wounds. But any vinegar taken internally can act as an irritant to any gut health issue and will ultimately be detrimental. Apple cider vinegar (like all other vinegars) puts stress upon the liver, causes chronic dehydration, wears down the enamel on the teeth, and weakens stomach glands, which produce hydrochloric acid. If you have any kind of digestive system symptom or disorder, ACV can worsen the condition and cause additional bloating.

If you can't resist vinegar, use high-quality apple cider vinegar, preferably with "mother" in it, which means it's unprocessed, living vinegar.

CASE HISTORY:
Able to Eat Again
2011

Since she was a teenager, Jennifer's stomach had been sensitive. She would often get stomachaches, as well as occasional constipation and diarrhea. Jennifer could never foresee how her stomach would react to what she ate. As she was growing up, her unpredictable loss of appetite had been a frequent source of friction at the family dinner table.

She spent years visiting doctors. One told Jennifer that she must just be seeking attention. In reality, attention was the last thing she wanted. Her true desire was to be free of pain and discomfort so she could focus on things she loved, like volunteering at the local animal rescue.

Finally, when she was 25, a gastroenterologist diagnosed her issue as irritable bowel syndrome. Though the specialist didn't say so, all this label meant was that Jennifer was dealing with a mystery illness.

She found it comforting to have a name for her symptoms, but she still wasn't finding relief.

Jennifer turned to alternative medicine. She found a great practitioner who noticed she was allergic to wheat gluten and dairy products such as milk and cheese. He recommended she eliminate these foods from her diet and take plenty of probiotics. However, he also concluded that she must have *Candida* and warned her off all processed and natural sugars, including fruit.

For six months, Jennifer tried the doctor's diet regimen: chicken twice a day, lots of fresh vegetables, and salads with tuna or hard-boiled eggs. Jennifer was strict about the food guidelines—though about once a month, the desire for something sweet would take over and she'd succumb to a piece of cake at her grandmother's house. She did notice some improvement—she no longer had diarrhea. Yet she still struggled with bouts of constipation, stomach cramping, bloating, and pain.

Frustrated, Jennifer decided to seek out a new alternative doctor. This one told her that not only did she have an allergy to wheat and dairy and an issue with *Candida*, but he was positive she had leaky gut syndrome. He put her on a diet of only meat, chicken, eggs, fish, and leafy green vegetables—that is, almost all protein. She was to eat no grains or beans of any kind and no starchy vegetables, though she was allowed the occasional Granny Smith apple. To treat the *Candida* overgrowth and leaky gut syndrome, the doctor also prescribed an herbal intestinal cleansing product.

For eight months, Jennifer stayed the course—with no positive results. Instead, she was now becoming fatigued, beset by brain fog and more constipation, and her bloating was at the point that it was making her look what she called "preggers." She felt unattractive, and it was always a challenge to find a place where both she and her vegetarian best friend could eat. After a decade of struggling with her digestive system, Jennifer decided isolation and suffering were her lot in life.

Then one day Jennifer's mom mentioned her troubles to a friend, who referred Jennifer to me. Immediately in my initial reading, Spirit informed me that Jennifer had virtually no hydrochloric acid left, and this was causing ammonia permeability. The proteins putrefying in her gut were creating the ammonia gas—resulting in inflammation, pain, and the bloating that she thought made her look pregnant.

Jennifer also had heavy metals in her intestinal tract, and the microorganisms that are crucial to the health of the lower small intestine, including the ileum, were nonexistent. It was true that Jennifer was allergic to wheat and all other grains and gluten, as well as beans, corn, canola oil, and eggs, so she needed to avoid them. She'd also started to develop an allergy to animal proteins because they were not breaking down and digesting in her gut. Further, her liver was sluggish and struggling from an overburden of animal fat.

Right away, I advised Jennifer to start drinking two 16-ounce glasses of fresh, plain celery juice a day.

"My last doctor had me on a green juice blend," she said. "How is this any different?"

I explained that juice blends don't restore hydrochloric acid levels. Only straight celery juice taken on an empty stomach can do that.

To stop stressing the liver with too much fat, we lowered Jennifer's animal proteins to one serving every other day. In its place, we brought in vegetables, fruits, leafy greens, herbs, and wild foods, most notably avocados (in small amounts), bananas, apples, all kinds of berries, papayas, mangoes, kiwis, lots of butter lettuce, and spinach, as well as a quarter cup of fresh cilantro in each of her salads to detox from heavy metals.

In contrast to the last diet Jennifer had been on, which was nearly all animal protein and virtually no fiber, the fruits in this new plan helped push food through her inflamed intestinal tract, which gave her some immediate relief from the constipation.

After one week, Jennifer's "preggers" bloating had decreased substantially.

After one month, she had no more constipation.

And after three months, the pain, cramping, brain fog, and fatigue were gone.

Her hydrochloric acid had restored itself, and the ammonia permeability had stopped. Jennifer's liver had also been freed up to process fats and store sugars properly, which had allowed her to lose the extra pounds she'd gained over the years.

She'd also spent the summer eating fresh, organic, unwashed kale and tomatoes from her grandmother's garden. The elevated microorganisms on the surfaces of these vegetables replenished the flora in Jennifer's gut, particularly the ileum, and allowed her body to start producing B_{12} again.

In the fall, Jennifer started working full-time at the animal shelter. She and her best friend renewed their bond and now spent Friday nights preparing Medical Medium meals for a growing group of pals from the shelter staff.

Jennifer's vitality is back. She can now eat the occasional "prohibited" food at a party or a friend's house, and her body won't pay the price. She never had leaky gut syndrome, nor an overgrowth of *Candida*—though they're two alternative diagnosis trends that lead countless people astray.

"Unlike certain illnesses, where I can tell you that in a few decades, research will most likely make the discoveries it needs to make—discoveries of some of the information that's in this book—gut health is another story. Its secret workings may never be uncovered by medical communities on this earth—no matter what theory or terminology they use to make it seem understood at an advanced level— which is why this chapter is essential.

Your body has been waiting patiently for you to discover this information. It's ready to work with you. It's ready to reignite its healing powers. It's ready to heal."

— Anthony William, Medical Medium

CHAPTER 18

Freeing Your Brain and Body of Toxins

Never before in our history have we been exposed to so many poisonous substances. These include the heavy metals mercury, aluminum, copper, lead, nickel, arsenic, and cadmium; air pollution such as chemtrails; pharmaceuticals; nanotechnology chemicals sprayed on almost everything manufactured; pesticides, herbicides, and fungicides; plastics; industrial cleaners; petroleum; dioxins and toxic algae blooms in our oceans; and thousands of new chemicals introduced into our environment every year. These poisons saturate our water reservoirs and fall down from the sky.

The majority of these substances are so new that it'll take decades before science recognizes how dangerous they are to our health. And those risks will only be discovered if funding and common sense go in the right direction, which is unlikely. Most industries' MO is to put chemicals into our environment—and deal with the consequences down the road.

Most of us are carrying around toxins that have been with us for almost our whole lives and have burrowed deep inside us. Many of us have had these toxins from the very beginning. It's these old poisons that can sometimes be the most dangerous. Toxic heavy metals, for example, can oxidize over time and kill the cells around them.

Toxins pose multiple threats. They directly poison your body, damaging your brain, your liver, your central nervous system, and other vital areas. They weaken your immune system, leaving you vulnerable to illness. And worst of all, they attract and feed cancers, viruses, bacteria, and other invaders that can instigate a serious health condition. In fact, these toxins, together with pathogens, are the cause of our current epidemic of cancer. These toxins are also behind many other illnesses, such as Alzheimer's disease.

This chapter identifies major toxins and how you can avoid them so you don't continually accumulate new ones. Living in this world, it's impossible to steer clear of everything harmful, so we'll focus on minimizing exposure to the extent possible. We'll also cover how to remove the toxins already in your body to protect you from potential illness and disease, making it easier for your immune system to recover and support you.

You always have the opportunity to turn things around. The pages that follow will empower you to take control over your well-being so that you can ensure many healthy years ahead.

MERCURY

For close to 2,500 years, man tried to claim that mercury was the fountain of youth. It was called the ultimate cure for all disease, the secret to living forever, and the source for eternal wisdom. In ancient Chinese medicine, mercury was so revered that countless emperors died from mercury elixirs that healers vowed would end all their problems—which I guess you could say they did, if you take a morbid view of things.

Mercury wasn't only a favored medicine in East Asia. All throughout England and the rest of Europe, mercury elixirs were celebrated. Mercury concoctions became all the rage in the Americas too. For a time in the 1800s, medical universities in the U.S. and England were turning out doctors fast, and the number one protocol they taught students was to give a glass of mercury water to any patient who was ill—regardless of age, gender, or symptoms. This "treatment" was an especially common method to force a miscarriage and to treat what was labeled

as "female hysteria," which translated to a woman speaking up for herself.

The 19th century wasn't exactly the Stone Age. It had been established that mercury was a dangerous toxin that destroyed the life of anyone who played with it, consumed it, or even touched it. For centuries already, people had borne witness to the millions who died from mercury exposure. So why was it still favored?

One factor was the great industrial demon that sat behind mercury. That alone was enough for it to be pushed as the top cure-all trend. There were interest groups pushing it forward.

The mercury movement finally hit a speed bump in the mid-1800s. Doctors had become more accessible than ever before in history to people from all walks of life—which seemed like a good thing. Yet as increasing numbers of people went to visit these new medical school grads, observers caught on that more and more of these patients were coming down with uncontrollable shaking, fevers, madness, rage, body tics, jerking, and gibberish talk. It became obvious that a visit to the doctor could result in poisoning.

For example, a wife and mother of five might have sent her husband to the doctor to help the husband with his gout. Upon arriving home, her husband would be delusional, yelling out children's rhymes as his eyes twitched. After just one experience like this, a family would have had enough.

Following this widespread realization, there was a 25-year ghost-town period for medical businesses. People preferred to risk the fate of whatever was ailing them; they knew that a visit to the doctor would give them a lower chance of survival. Medical universities hit an all-time funding low.

This was exactly the break natural practitioners and healers needed to gain some credibility. For this brief time, early forms of homeopathy, chiropractic treatment, and other varieties of alternative medicine exploded in popularity.

Finally traditional doctors' offices caught on and started advertising that they no longer offered quicksilver (liquid mercury) drinks, and traditional medicine gained back some credibility.

Yet the demon behind mercury still wanted the population to get plenty of exposure, so it worked on other hidden and inventive ways to get it into people's systems. Not only were industries dumping mercury into every river, lake, and waterway possible, but other forms of mercury-containing medicine were born by the turn of the 20th century. Plus, dentists were still using mercury amalgam fillings.

Hat production was one of the industries that relied on mercury—in the form of a solution used to speed the felting process. This is where the term *mad as a hatter* comes from; the average hatmaker survived only three to five years after starting work at a factory. And it wasn't just the workers who were exposed. Every man who wore a felt hat in the 1800s and the first half of the 1900s would get an infusion of mercury when his brow sweated. (Which reminds me: don't try on antique hats at the thrift store.)

Almost all mental illness of the time was from mercury poisoning. The asylums of the 19th and early 20th centuries were filled with people experiencing madness and convulsions. And what was the treatment protocol? Mercury concoctions to drink, or mercury pills

to swallow. Abraham Lincoln's depression severely worsened from the use of mercury pills—a depression that had likely started from a few glasses of "medicinal" mercury elixirs.

The Dirty Secret

What does this have to do with you? Why am I going on like this about mercury? Because it's the dirty secret we're not supposed to talk about, and we have mercury in our brains and bodies from generations of ancestors who were exposed to it. You're not supposed to know about what mercury has done to shape history, right up to this present moment. Mercury can be toxic even in tiny doses you can't see. And there's no hazard sign saying, "BEWARE—MERCURY."

If it were up to the mercury demon, we would think mercury was harmless, even good for us. Better yet, mercury would be entirely hidden, and we wouldn't even know it existed. Mercury never goes away—unless you take specific steps to detoxify it. It gets passed on from generation to generation, for centuries. It's practically guaranteed that your great-great-grandparents and other ancestors tasted mercury elixirs. Your parents have mercury in them, and they got it from their parents. That same mercury got passed along to you at conception. Some of us have mercury in us that's a thousand or more years old.

Mercury casts an evil and soulless shadow that has engulfed so many. This toxic heavy metal becomes a part of us, and that reflects itself in our health.

Greed, carelessness, darkness, and ignorance are the major factors that have allowed mercury to prey on the population. A mercury mine owner of the past likely didn't care if workers only lived six months to three years after starting at the mine—because there was money to be made.

What good has mercury ever done? None. It's done *nothing* for us. Absolutely nothing. It's an unnecessary, dangerous neurotoxin. It could have been replaced in its medical and industrial uses with something safer.

Is mercury gone yet? Is the nightmare finally over? Have we come to our senses and learned to avoid it at all costs for the sake of humankind? For the sake of our health and well-being? For the sake of our children?

Nope. It's just that it's out of sight and out of mind. There's still plenty of mercury to be had. It's constantly at our fingertips, in ways that are extremely controversial.

Just as a result of modern living, over time your body will accumulate toxic heavy metals such as mercury. We're continually exposed to this toxin, because it slips through the cracks. Figuratively, it slips through the cracks of our health-care and industrial systems. Literally, mercury absorbs into the cracks of the brain. All of us have some level of mercury inside our bodies. It's unavoidable.

Why should we care?

Because mercury is a top fuel for viruses, cancers, and bacteria. Mercury exposure is a factor behind inflammation and can take people hostage by causing or contributing to a vast number of symptoms and conditions, including depression, anxiety, ADHD, autism, bipolar disorder, neurological disorders, epilepsy, depersonalization, Parkinson's, ALS, MS, Lyme disease symptoms, tingles, numbness, tics, twitches, spasms, seizures, hot flashes, heart palpitations, hair loss, memory loss, confusion, insomnia, loss of libido, fatigue, migraines, and thyroid disorders.

How often are people told they've brought a condition like depression upon themselves? It's all part of mercury's blame-the-victim game. Those depressive symptoms are the mercury speaking for the patient without her or his consent.

Sometimes mercury moves past the hostage phase and takes someone out, resulting in death by Alzheimer's, Parkinson's, dementia, or stroke. It's that serious. Mercury has injured or killed well over a billion people.

No one likes Alzheimer's; it's a frightening, terrible disease. Yet it's rapidly becoming common—and it's 100 percent mercury-caused. You heard that here first: mercury is 100 percent responsible for Alzheimer's disease. You will never in your lifetime hear the truth about that anywhere else.

(Everyone has a different combination of toxic heavy metals inside their brains. In Alzheimer's, aluminum is commonly present along with mercury, and when that's the case, aluminum in the brain will play a role and contribute to the disease. That said, you can also have Alzheimer's without aluminum, whereas you can't have Alzheimer's with aluminum and no mercury. For the specific symptoms of this disease, mercury must be present.)

The medical industry will never blame mercury for that condition or any other—because then fingers would be pointed in the direction of the Mercury Man, whose true name is unknown. He's responsible for the original and very first good ol' boy industry, which wants the medical industry to continue to use mercury in their medical treatments involving children and adults.

And I've only covered the basics when it comes to the dirty secret of mercury.

If we can't stop the mercury demon from enticing people even today to expose us and our children to this toxic heavy metal, then we can take power into our own hands by becoming aware of situations that could bring us harm. To shield yourself and your family, you have to question *everything*, researching and asking if there is mercury involved in medical treatments.

We can also take full control over our health by ridding our bodies of the mercury we've accumulated from the generations before us and from present-day exposure. We can make simple Medical Medium detoxification protocols part of our daily routine.

Your life is precious, sacred, and important. You deserve to know how to protect it.

Seafood

One of the many ways we take in mercury is through seafood. It's in all fish, but typically at higher levels in tuna, swordfish, shark, and any other large and oily fish. That's because our oceans are polluted with mercury, and eventually the mercury runoff from factory manufacturing (left over from the past and still accumulating today) finds its way into someone's tuna salad, tuna casserole, or sushi.

You can mitigate the risk by eating small fish, such as sardines and mackerel. Wild salmon is also safe enough to eat in small amounts, if you're someone who keeps fish in your diet.

Dental Amalgams

Dental amalgam fillings are another common source of exposure to mercury. So many of us have these silver fillings in our mouths, or have had them at one point.

It's becoming popular to get all mercury-based fillings removed at a holistic dentist's office. This may seem sensible, like the right thing to do, but you have to be very careful about the process. Getting all of your amalgam fillings removed at the same time can lead to an extremely high level of mercury exposure, regardless of the best techniques and protection available at the dentist's office. The exposure can put a heavy load on the immune system and also feed viruses, making the exposure a trigger for many kinds of health conditions, whether existing ones that flare up or new ones that develop from a dormant virus becoming active.

I know people who've had 10 fillings dug out at once, and as a result, their blood platelets dropped so low that they almost died.

It's best to remove metal fillings only when an individual tooth requires it—such as if the filling becomes unstable, or the tooth is damaged. If your teeth and fillings are all in good order, and you're still anxious to have the amalgams removed, then get only one taken out at a time. Schedule at least a month between each removal.

If you've already had all your metal fillings removed, then it's time to do some cleanup to protect yourself.

And if you get new cavities, select the safest filling option available—and make sure it doesn't contain mercury. Know that anything is better than a filling that contains mercury.

Heavy Metal Detox

The best way to remove heavy metals is to consume the following five items every day:

- **Barley grass juice powder:** draws out heavy metals from your liver, spleen, intestinal tract, pancreas, and reproductive system. Barley grass juice powder prepares the toxic heavy metals for complete absorption by the spirulina.

- **Spirulina:** draws out heavy metals from your brain, central nervous system, and liver and absorbs heavy metals extracted by your barley grass juice powder.

- **Cilantro:** helps remove toxic heavy metals in the stomach, intestinal tract, liver, and gallbladder.

- **Wild blueberries:** draw heavy metals out from your brain. Also heal and repair any gaps that the toxic heavy metals create, which is especially important for your brain tissue. This is the most powerful food for reversing Alzheimer's. (If you can't get frozen or fresh wild blueberries, wild blueberry powder is an option.)

- **Atlantic dulse:** binds to toxic heavy metals. Unlike other seaweeds, Atlantic dulse is a powerful force for removing toxic heavy metals out of deep, hidden places in the small intestine and colon—it seeks out toxic heavy metals from pockets inside the intestinal tract linings and other places in the gut, binds to them, and never releases the heavy metals until they leave the body.

You should consume all five of these foods and supplements within 24 hours of one another for optimal effect. If you can't fit them all in, try to eat three daily. All five of these powerful heavy metal–removing foods leave behind critical nutrients for repairing heavy metal damage and restoring the body.

Your first choice for getting these five key components into yourself is to drink the Heavy Metal Detox Smoothie from Chapter 23 daily. Don't skip it altogether if you don't have all the ingredients; make it with the ones you do have. For example, if you run out of cilantro, dulse, and frozen wild blueberries, you can still incorporate spirulina, barley grass juice powder, and wild blueberry powder into your smoothie, and it will be highly beneficial.

If the Heavy Metal Detox Smoothie is not an option, here's an example of how you could fit the five ingredients into your day: eat a bowl of (thawed) wild blueberries, add cilantro to a salad and then throw a little Atlantic dulse on top, and mix spirulina and barley grass juice powder into water or coconut water (that's not pink or red). See the Heavy Metal Detox Smoothie recipe for recommended amounts of each of the five components. And remember, try to incorporate them all (or at least three) within 24 hours.

(In *Cleanse to Heal*, you'll find the Medical Medium Heavy Metal Detox Cleanse, which offers a more detailed protocol, further insights into how proper heavy metal detoxification works, and more answers about how to deal with missing ingredients.)

There is no more effective way on earth to remove toxic heavy metals than this process. If you stick religiously to this heavy metal detox protocol over a long-term period, you can see a radical improvement. I've seen people make miraculous recoveries by removing generations of mercury from their systems. There's almost nothing better you can do for your health than to get heavy metals out of your body.

Note that there are other foods and herbs out there, such as chlorella, advertised as being beneficial for removing heavy metals. Beware. Although chlorella is trendy in the supplement world, it does not move toxic heavy metals properly and is vastly different in its effectiveness from the items listed above. Chlorella is irresponsible when it comes down to protecting you from the hazards of mercury.

WATER POLLUTION

In this modern era, even with everything we've learned about environmental damage, our water supply is continually being polluted.

There isn't much you can do to avoid air and earth pollution (other than move to an ecologically cleaner area). There *is* a whole lot you can do about your water.

You can entirely bypass local pollutants by buying bottled water. If you do this, make sure the plastic bottles storing the water are free of *bisphenol A* (BPA), an industrial chemical that's poisonous. Although plastics have their faults, they are easily detoxifiable, and bottled water is safer than tap water, which has a much higher elevation of plastic byproducts. (I don't recommend man-made alkaline bottled water with added minerals or other additives.)

You can also buy a high-quality water purifier to remove all toxins from your tap water. If you choose this option, buy a system that removes heavy metals, chlorine, and fluoride. (Many communities add fluoride to water in the mistaken belief that it's good for you. That's far from the truth. It's actually a byproduct of aluminum—and a neurotoxin.)

Some purifiers sit on your countertop, some are set up at an individual faucet, some are whole-house filtration systems. There are other water purification systems that use a reverse osmosis process, and yet others that produce distilled water. Keep in mind that if you use a distilled water option, it does remove minerals that are good for you, along with some toxins. To remedy this, add a squeeze of lemon when you drink the water.

A great thing to add to *any* water that has been purified or filtered is a squeeze of juice from a freshly cut lemon or lime. Most water has lost its living factor due to filtering and processing. This tends to deaden water, while adding juice from a fresh lemon or lime reactivates and reawakens it, because the water that resides in the lemon or lime is alive. The water is then better able to latch on to toxins in your body and flush them out. The lemon or lime also adds trace minerals back into the water.

I do *not* recommend alkaline ionized water machines. They are not water purifiers, and they denature and contaminate the water, making it foreign to our bodies.

Anti-Chlorine/Anti-Fluoride Tea

For a powerful detox of recent chlorine and fluoride exposure, blend equal parts of blackberry leaf, raspberry leaf, hibiscus flower, and rose hips. Steep 1 tablespoon of this herb mixture per cup of hot water for tea. To address chlorine and fluoride in your organs from past exposure, turn to any of the Medical Medium cleanses.

PESTICIDES, HERBICIDES, AND FUNGICIDES

We're frequently at risk for exposure to pesticides, herbicides, and fungicides.

One avenue is conventional produce. Non-organic tomatoes, for example, are often sprayed at unregulated, off-the-chart levels. We can get a high dosage of herbicide in our systems just from ingesting conventional tomatoes, as well as other non-organic fruits, leafy greens, herbs, and vegetables. At minimum, you should wash any conventionally farmed produce you buy to get rid of as much of its surface toxins as you can. (Don't get scared away from conventional produce altogether if this is all you have access to—its nutrients are key to health.) Buy organic produce as often as possible.

If you eat animal products, they need to be at least organic, if not also grass-fed or free-range. Although these products will still have radiation from the fallout of Fukushima's nuclear power plant disaster in 2011 and toxic heavy metals and other chemicals from chemtrails, they will at least have lower concentrations of pesticides, herbicides, and fungicides than non-organic animal products, because non-organic animal products are extremely high in these chemicals, more so than any conventional sprayed fruit or vegetable. (More on radiation soon.)

Parks are also sprayed heavily with herbicides and pesticides. Take precautions, such as using a blanket (that you'll wash afterward) if you plan to sit in public green areas. Also avoid spraying toxic chemicals on your own lawn, and try to refrain from using insecticides inside your home. Getting lawn treatments and using pesticides, herbicides, and insecticides is much more exposure than eating conventional produce.

Anti-Pesticide/Anti-Herbicide/Anti-Fungicide Tea

If you think you've just been exposed to a pesticide, herbicide, or fungicide spray from a park, golf course, neighbor's yard, or treatment at your own home, this tea is an option: blend equal parts of burdock root, red clover, lemon verbena, and ginger. Make a tea by steeping 1 tablespoon of the herb mixture per cup of hot water. Do this protocol once daily for two weeks after exposure. Additionally, bring in the Heavy Metal Detox Smoothie from Chapter 23. You're welcome to turn to any Medical Medium cleanse as well, whether for recent exposure or to address deep-seated pesticides, herbicides, and fungicides.

PLASTIC

We surround our world with plastic. If it were up to plastic manufacturers, we would come out of the womb wrapped in plastic.

We use plastic bags to hold the food and drink we buy until we get them home, plastic containers to organize and store our food and drink, plastic wraps to keep our food and drink covered, and more plastic bags to throw away the remains. Pharmaceuticals, too, are extremely high in plastics. As a result, plastic inevitably gets into our bodies one way or another.

Some types of plastic are relatively benign. However, others have properties that promote inflammation, disrupt your brain's neurons and neurotransmitters, confuse the body's hormones, and burden the liver, because these plastics have additional chemicals added that may even contain toxic heavy metals. These more harmful plastics are not ones we use for food and beverage.

It's still a good idea to use cloth bags to carry your food when that's an option. Favor glass containers for your food over plastic ones. And when you can't avoid plastic—for example, when buying most bottled water, or a food processor—try to make sure the manufacturer is using BPA-free and human-friendly plastic. As you saw in "Water Pollution," in some cases, plastic is better than the alternative.

Anti-Plastics Tea

To rid yourself of plastic and plastic byproducts floating in your bloodstream from fresh exposure, blend equal parts fenugreek, mullein leaf, olive leaf, and lemon balm. Steep 1 tablespoon of the herb mixture per cup of hot water for tea. If you're concerned about getting out deep-seated plastics from your organs, try to bring one of the Medical Medium cleanses into your life.

CLEANERS

Industrial cleaners are designed to destroy dirt and grime—without sufficient regard to the effect they have on the people breathing in their fumes. For example, traditional carpet cleaners use chemicals such as perchloroethylene, ammonium hydroxide, hydrofluoric acid, and nitrilotriacetate, which are hazardous to one's health, in cleaning agents and solvents. And many carpets have toxins in them, so the "cleaning" adds poisons on top of poisons. If

you spend a lot of time indoors, you'll breathe these toxic fumes for most of each day, which can both weaken your immune system and possibly trigger a health condition.

One solution is to eliminate carpets in favor of hardwood floors and area rugs (although beware of hardwood stains and sealants, which also have the potential to give off toxic fumes when applied). Alternatively, you can buy a "green" carpet, and hire an environmentally intelligent carpet cleaning service—or maintain the carpet yourself using organic cleaners. Also try to avoid mainstream home cleaning products. There are numerous organic cleaners available to use instead. Beware if cleaning products that are advertised as "organic" or "natural" have a very strong fragrance, or if an "eco" carpet cleaning service is not giving you the confidence that its product is nontoxic and chemical-free. Use your instincts, and steer clear of heavy scents and fragrances.

Another source of toxins worth keeping in mind is clothing. Mainstream dry cleaners use chemicals that seep into your skin and your lungs as you wear your clothes day after day. To avoid this, seek out "green" dry cleaners.

Along the same lines, be aware that when you buy new clothes they're often covered with fungicides and even formaldehyde or other cancer-causing chemicals to keep them from wrinkling or becoming infested with mildew (i.e., funguses). Make sure to wash new clothes before wearing them.

Anti–Cleaning Solvents Tea

To minimize the effects of recent solvent exposure, blend calendula, chamomile, bladderwrack, and borage in equal parts. For tea, steep 1 tablespoon of the herb mixture per cup of hot water. To cleanse your body of any of these stored chemicals, try to incorporate one of the Medical Medium cleanses into your life.

RADIATION

When a nuclear power plant releases radiation into the air—as the Fukushima Daiichi power plant did following a 2011 earthquake and tsunami in Japan—that radiation lingers forever, mildly irradiating food, water, and air around the world.

There's nothing you can do to avoid this type of floating radiation. One way to *limit* exposure to radiation caused by the Fukushima Daiichi plant disaster is to eat lower on the food chain whenever possible. At this point, all of our meat, dairy, and poultry supplies have high concentrations of radiation. These animals eat large amounts of feed or grass, all of which contain radiation from the nuclear fallout. That's one reason why, if you eat animal products, it's best to eat those animal products once a day instead of two or three times a day. It's a process called biomagnification that results in the toxic matter accumulating at greater concentrations in creatures higher up on the food chain.

I'm not trying to scare anyone with this. If you want to forget what you've read here, I understand.

You can also remove radiation from your body system and work to limit your exposure to all *other* radiation. For example, if you're getting X-rays at your dentist, insist that all areas of your body besides your mouth be covered with a lead apron or other protection. That includes your throat, which can develop

thyroid disease from radiation exposure. (Radiation accumulation in the thyroid, which can come from various sources, is behind a bit less than five percent of thyroid disorders.) Try to minimize dental X-rays if possible, even if your dentist uses a digital process. Also, with any doctor, don't automatically say yes to X-rays. If you aren't sure whether an X-ray is necessary, don't hesitate to ask questions. Sometimes an X-ray isn't required, but rather optional for a particular medical concern.

Along the same lines, ask a whole lot of questions about any medical treatment that involves radiation. For example, if you're a woman receiving a chest X-ray, make sure you get a lead apron to cover your reproductive system and throat. This isn't always offered, so you may have to ask.

Many times there are less aggressive treatment alternatives that hold lower risks. Women, for example, can consider a thermogram (which uses infrared imaging) or ultrasound for gathering more information on breast health if needed, instead of feeling pushed into having another mammogram shortly after having a mammogram where the results were clear and all was well.

The human body is more sensitive to radiation than doctors realize. As with any other major toxin, strive to avoid radiation or minimize radiation exposure whenever possible.

Sea vegetables are a great way to protect your organs and glands from radiation. The fear that seaweed itself is saturated with radiation or heavy metals and can therefore harm your health is a misconception. Sea vegetables only take in toxins—they don't release them. So for example, if you eat a handful of dulse that *has* collected any pollutants from the ocean, they won't get discharged into your system. Instead, the dulse will hold on to the radiation and heavy metals—and collect even more of these toxins as it moves through your digestive tract, eventually expelling them from your body when you expel the dulse. (By the way, any pollutants that dulse has already picked up from the ocean are on a micro level compared to the radiation and heavy metals that fish such as tuna can contain. Seaweed won't release any of that into your body. Tuna will.) Try to select seaweeds from the Atlantic Ocean rather than the Pacific. They'll have greater capacity to absorb toxins from your system.

Anti-Radiation Tea

For an antidote to recent radiation exposure, blend Atlantic kelp, Atlantic dulse, dandelion leaf, and nettle leaf in equal parts. Make a tea from the mixture by steeping 1 tablespoon per cup of hot water. To assist with deeper exposure, bring in any of the Medical Medium cleanses. The Heavy Metal Detox Cleanse in particular can be helpful for radiation.

MORE DETOX METHODS

Lemon Water

A highly effective way to detoxify the body is to drink 32 ounces of water on an empty stomach after you wake up, squeezing a freshly cut lemon into the water. The lemon juice activates the water, making it better able to latch on to toxins in your body and flush them out.

This is especially effective for cleansing your liver, which works all night while you're asleep to gather and purge toxins from your body. When you wake up, it's primed to be hydrated and flushed clean with activated lemon water. After you drink the lemon water, give your liver half an hour to clean up. You can then drink celery juice or eat breakfast. If you make this into a routine, your health will improve dramatically over time.

For an additional option, add a teaspoon of raw honey and a teaspoon of freshly grated ginger to the lemon water. Your liver will draw in the honey to restore its glucose reserves, purging deep toxins at the same time to make room.

Aloe Vera Leaf Juice

A great way to detox your liver and intestinal tract is to eat the fresh gel of an aloe vera leaf once a day. To prepare it, cut off a two-to-four-inch section of the aloe leaf. (That's if it's large, as store-bought aloe often is. If you're using a homegrown aloe plant, it will likely have smaller, skinnier leaves, so cut off more.) Fillet the leaf as if it were a fish, trimming away the green skin and spikes. Scoop out the clear gel, taking care not to include any from the bitter base of the leaf. Blend it into a smoothie, blend it with water, or eat as is.

Cleansing

If you're interested in cleansing, see Chapter 22, "Medical Medium 28-Day Healing Cleanse." Be sure to read the full chapter, because on top of cleanse information, it offers modification options and critical tips for transitioning out of the cleanse.

For more cleanse options and answers to all your cleansing questions, see the Medical Medium book *Cleanse to Heal*.

Rebounding

Another way to assist detoxing is to use a mini-trampoline called a *rebounder*, which you gently jump up and down on. Doing this for 10 minutes a day will forcefully promote circulation throughout your lymphatic system, and help detoxify your entire body, especially your liver. The liver is the foundation to a healthy lymphatic system, and the rebounder assists by increasing blood flow to your liver, which helps purge easy-to-reach toxic debris so that the liver can be less burdened (at least on a surface level), which allows heart rate to improve and blood flow to be less of a struggle, in turn allowing the lymphatic system to circulate with more ease. You still need to work on cleansing your liver with the information in this book—so that the liver doesn't stay stagnant and sluggish and you can get the most out of what the rebounder can do for the lymphatic system.

If you have a structural issue in your body or impediment of some kind that doesn't allow you to rebound, ease your mind. You can still cleanse your liver and improve your lymphatic system with Medical Medium tools.

Infrared Sauna

Another device that's surprisingly useful for detox is an *infrared sauna*, which emits infrared light and heat on your skin for the purpose of healing. Its heat deeply penetrates your body, providing benefits such as increased blood flow and oxygenation of the blood, removal of toxins from the skin, elimination of aches and pains, and an immune system boost.

Some people are too sensitive for infrared sauna, so it's not the best support for them. For others, it's an option you can try out. Try it for 15- to 20-minute sessions twice a week. If you're sensitive, keep the heat's temperature lower and keep your sessions shorter.

Massage

Since the beginning of humankind, loved ones have put a hand on each other for support. Massage is our oldest form of therapy, and it remains to this day one of the most powerful methods of healing. A quality 45-minute full-body massage will promote circulation throughout your body and help draw out toxins, especially from your liver. One reason this occurs is because for most people, getting a massage is enjoyable, so the body goes into a deep state of relaxation. This can relieve tension in the liver, allowing the organ to enter a state where it's peaceful rather than tense or in spasm. While massage doesn't help with deep-seated toxins in the liver, it can help with surface toxins or recent toxic exposure.

The massage is likely to boost your adrenal glands and kidneys, relax your heart, and ease tension.

Ideally, drink 32 ounces of fresh lemon or lime water directly following your massage. This will optimize the detoxing benefits of your session.

If massage doesn't feel like an option for you right now, you can still promote relaxation, tension release, and the benefits those can offer your liver through other means. See Chapter 24, "Soul-Healing Meditations and Techniques," for a number of calming options.

CASE HISTORY:
Alzheimer's Under Arrest
2006

It had long been a family joke that Whitney was forgetful. Over the years, she'd lost her purse and keys countless times, blanked on her husband James's work number, and even forgotten her children's birthdays a few times. Each time they left for soccer practice, Whitney's daughter Kendra would ask, "Mom, did you forget anything?" before they walked out the door. The kids thought of it all as normal, and even funny.

That changed one Christmas, when Whitney was 53 years old. Everyone gathered early to open presents in the living room—everyone but Whitney.

"Where's Mom?" her daughter Miley finally asked. Whitney was usually the first one up for the holiday.

James found Whitney upstairs in the bathroom, applying makeup as though it were a normal workday. He told her the kids were waiting for her downstairs. Whitney looked at James with a furrowed brow but followed him to the living room. When she spotted the lit-up tree and the pile of wrapped gifts beneath, she was shocked. She'd already forgotten it was Christmas.

James accompanied Whitney to their family doctor, followed by a neurologist and several specialists. In the end, the diagnosis was Alzheimer's. The entire family was devastated at the prognosis: only three to five years ahead—at best—of quality living for Whitney. The unthinkable was before them. Whitney's doctors told James to get the family affairs in order while Whitney was still of sound mind.

Timothy, age 17, Miley, age 14, and Kendra, age 12, were old enough to understand the gravity of the situation. Miley started spending hours looking up Alzheimer's online, reading about the devastation it causes. Between panic attacks, Kendra began writing out lists of daily reminders for Whitney. Timothy dropped out of high school so he could help his mother out as much as she would allow.

Whitney's sister Sharon whisked her off to multiple alternative doctors, looking for an answer to reverse the disease. In one waiting room, Sharon stumbled across an article from the local newspaper that mentioned my name in connection with helping people heal from mystery illnesses.

During my first appointment with Whitney, Spirit directed my attention to two large pockets of mercury in the left hemisphere of her brain. They'd been there since her childhood. The mercury pockets were now oxidizing rapidly, causing runoff that was spreading fast, damaging brain tissue and accelerating the disease.

Spirit advised an immediate heavy metal detox regimen (as described in this chapter), coupled with a diet of little to no fat. That's because a high-fat diet raises blood fat, which makes mercury oxidize rapidly. A diet high in antioxidant-rich fruits, leafy greens, herbs, wild foods, and vegetables and low in fat slows down and even stops oxidation, and allows for complete detoxification of mercury.

Whitney removed all animal proteins from her diet because of the fat they contain and only used plant-based fats such as avocados, nuts, seeds, and oils sparingly. She switched her diet over to all types of fruit, especially wild blueberries, along with large servings of greens such as spinach, kale, and cilantro. Whitney was also allowed to consume potatoes, sweet potatoes, and other starchy vegetables.

Over time, Whitney's healthy, detoxifying, glucose-supporting, antioxidant-plentiful diet stopped the oxidation in its tracks. Her Alzheimer's symptoms started to reverse.

Timothy reenrolled in high school and got a weekend job at a local organic market so he could bring home discounted cases of produce. Miley redirected her Internet skills to looking up recipes. And Kendra started to breathe again and joined her sister in the kitchen to experiment with smoothie concoctions.

Six months into the program, Whitney's memory abilities were back to where they'd been before the Christmas tree nightmare.

One year into the program, Whitney's memory was better than it had been since before Timothy was born.

Today's trendy diets never would have allowed the level of fruit and starchy vegetables that Whitney needed for a true win. A fad diet would have been geared to higher levels of protein, which translates to higher levels of fat. It would have caused the disease to progress rapidly—not reverse.

With Whitney's Alzheimer's disease now arrested, the family is at ease again. It's an infrequent occurrence that Whitney forgets her keys anymore, but when she does, she, James, and the kids just laugh.

"Never before in our history have we been exposed to so many poisonous substances."

— Anthony William, Medical Medium

CHAPTER 19

What Not to Eat

We all want full control over our health. We want freedom of choice.

We like to decide what clothes to put on in the morning, and what shoes to wear. We want the ability to move away from someone holding a cigarette so we don't have to inhale the secondhand smoke. We like to choose the foods we eat.

We want to say what goes onto our bodies, around our bodies, and into our bodies.

Unless, that is, you don't mind any of that. You're allowed to wear the wrong size clothes, breathe in cigarette smoke, eat junk food, and not care—but you know you're doing it. That's your choice, one you make consciously, and that needs to be respected.

What if you were *unaware* that what you were doing could possibly be hindering you, or harmful to your health, though? That would take all choice out of it.

And that's exactly what's happening. People consume foods, supplements, and additives that can be instigating and irritating to their health, and limiting to the quality of their lives—and they have no idea. It's one thing to indulge in chocolate cake knowing it might be adding a few pounds to your

waistline. It's something else entirely if that cake contains an ingredient that you don't know could harm your health, or could even take a year off your life.

Every day, people are tricked into consuming poisons, irritants, and other substances that deplete health. They have no say in it, because they don't know it's happening. It takes away choice, freedom, decision, and control.

Sure, you can have the attitude, "Well, it's just a little," or "What doesn't kill you makes you stronger," or "It'll put hair on your chest," or "Everyone else is doing it," or "It can't be *that* bad." If you're perfectly healthy and have zero complaints, if you're young and feel indestructible, maybe it's not so bad that certain toxic ingredients can enter your body without your knowledge.

But if you're at all concerned about your health—if you have any sensitivities or conditions, if you've struggled with illness, or if you're just concerned about prevention—then it's critical to avoid as many triggers and instigators as possible. Your body needs every possible level of support so it can heal and then maintain optimal health.

There's no such thing as "What doesn't kill you makes you stronger" when it comes to your health. This has been a popular misconception for ages. Truth is, ingesting poisons doesn't make you immune to them. Quite the opposite: the more poisons in your body, the weaker and more vulnerable you become.

By now, we've all heard of preservatives and artificial flavors—we know to avoid those, for very good reason. There are other problematic ingredients, though, which you should know to avoid. These ingredients can feed existing viral, bacterial, and fungal conditions, which can lead to inflammation—and can also wreak havoc with your digestive system, compromise your immune system, strain your adrenal glands and liver, hinder cells anywhere in your body, disrupt or destroy your brain's neurons and neurotransmitters, make you anxious and/or depressed, set you up for strokes or heart attacks, and more.

Health professionals are unlikely to warn you about most of these foods, additives, and supplements, because it's not common knowledge that they can substantially worsen already-existing illnesses, nor that they can trigger new health conditions.

You deserve to have full knowledge of what you consume, and what effects it all has on your body. By reading this chapter, you will start to protect yourself. You're *worth* protecting. It's time you had control and informed choice over what enters your body—it's a powerful step toward recovering your health.

THE TROUBLEMAKER FOODS LIST

Here's an overview of the foods that can make healing harder—and in some cases, work against cleansing and healing. If you're struggling with any kind of symptom or condition, or if you're concerned about prevention, it's critical to begin the process of removing at least one or two of the top-level foods here. To take yourself even further, acclimate yourself to removing more of these foods from your daily life.

Level 1

- Eggs
- Dairy (including milk, cheese, butter, yogurt, cream, and kefir)
- Gluten
- Soft drinks
- Be mindful of salt consumption

Level 2

All of the above PLUS:

- Pork
- Tuna
- Corn

Level 3

All of the above PLUS:

- Industrial food oils (vegetable oil, palm oil, canola oil, corn oil, safflower oil, soybean oil)
- Soy
- Lamb
- Fish and seafood (other than salmon, trout, sardines, mackerel, halibut, and haddock)

Level 4

All of the above PLUS:

- Vinegar (including apple cider vinegar, or ACV)
- Fermented foods (including kombucha, sauerkraut, and coconut aminos)
- Caffeine (including coffee, matcha, and chocolate)

Level 5

All of the above PLUS:

- Grains (other than millet and oats)
- All oils (including healthier ones such as olive, walnut, sunflower, coconut, sesame, avocado, grapeseed, almond, macadamia, peanut, and flaxseed)

Bonus

For even better, faster results:

- Cut out salt and seasonings entirely (pure spices are okay)
- Avoid radical fats entirely for a period

And also limit or remove:

- Alcohol
- Natural/artificial flavors
- Nutritional yeast
- Citric acid
- Aspartame
- Other artificial sweeteners
- Monosodium glutamate (MSG)
- Formaldehyde
- Preservatives

What follows are insights about selected troublemaker foods, to give you an understanding of how and why these foods can stand in the way of your healing. If you'd like to learn more, see my book *Cleanse to Heal*.

CORN

Corn used to be one of the fundamental sources of nourishment on earth.

Unfortunately, the technology of *genetically modified organisms* (GMO) has destroyed it as a viable food.

Corn products and byproducts create substantial inflammation because it's a food that can feed viruses, bacteria, mold, and fungus. Even if you see corn advertised as being non-GMO, the chances are high that it can still feed a pathogen, which could trigger many kinds of health conditions—and that it may still be GMO.

Try to avoid *all* corn and *all* products that have corn as an ingredient. These include foods such as corn chips, taco shells, popcorn, corn cereal, and anything that clearly incorporates corn syrup or corn oil. They also include less obvious products, such as soda, gum, high fructose corn syrup (HFCS), some toothpaste, gluten-free foods that use corn in place of wheat, and herbal tinctures that employ alcohol as a preservative. (It's most likely corn grain alcohol. Buy the alcohol-free versions of tinctures instead.)

Try to read ingredient labels carefully . . . and do the best you can.

Staying away from corn products and byproducts can be a lot of work. For a treat in the summertime, it's okay to enjoy a fresh, organic corn on the cob. For the sake of your health, it's worth the effort of cutting out corn the rest of the time. It's best to keep corn out of your diet altogether when you're working on detoxing and healing.

SOY

Soy has suffered a similar GMO fate as corn.

Soy used to be a healthy food. However, you can now assume that any soy product you encounter could have some GMO contamination or contain added MSG. Be cautious when eating soybeans, edamame, miso, soy milk, soy nuts, soy pasta, soy sauce, textured vegetable protein (TVP), soy protein powder, artificial meat products made from soy, and much more.

Try to stay away from soy the best you can. If you really enjoy soy and feel deprived without it, stick to the safest options, and use it sparingly: plain, organic tofu or tempeh (made from sprouted soy if possible), or the highest-quality nama shoyu. If you have a health concern, symptom, or condition that's impeding your life, it's best to avoid soy altogether.

CANOLA OIL

Canola oil is mostly GMO at this point in time. And regardless, canola oil creates a great deal of inflammation, because the oil can create a barrier around *Streptococcus*, *E. coli*, and many other unproductive bacteria that can live in our gut. That barrier can allow the unproductive bacteria to stay alive and even potentially grow, eventually causing an irritated, inflamed gut lining. Long-term use in high quantities of canola oil can be especially compromising to your digestive system, potentially scarring the linings of both your small and large intestines, and is a major contributor to irritable bowel syndrome if bacteria such as strep or *E. coli* are present. Because canola oil can feed bacteria, fungus, and mold, it can accelerate chronic illness.

Canola oil is used in many restaurants and in thousands of products, often as a low-cost alternative to olive oil. Even reputable health food chains and restaurants use canola oil to keep prices down, sometimes advertising canola as a health food. Unfortunately, if canola oil is even a tiny part of an otherwise perfectly healthy dish of organic and all-natural ingredients, you should probably avoid that dish because of how irritating canola oil is.

If you're dealing with a mystery illness or a health condition, try to avoid canola oil at all costs.

PROCESSED BEET SUGAR

So far, GMO beets are mostly reserved for making processed beet sugar. You should therefore avoid products that contain processed beet sugar, because those products normally have gluten, dairy, or eggs in them, which feed cancers, viruses, and bacteria.

This is different from grating fresh, organic beets over your salad, or juicing fresh beets. If you stick to organic, most whole beets that you buy in the produce section at your local natural market or at the farmers' market are safe to consume.

EGGS

Humans have eaten eggs for thousands of years. They were once an amazing survival food for us to eat in areas of the planet where there were no other food options at certain times of year. That changed with the epidemic of chronic illness. Eggs were weaponized in the early 20th century. Private (not public) medical research and science used eggs to farm viruses and bacteria that were released into our environment throughout the decades, which led to our explosion of chronic illness today.

The average person eats over 350 eggs a year. That includes whole eggs and also all the foods with hidden egg ingredients.

If you're struggling with any illness, such as Lyme disease, lupus, chronic fatigue syndrome, migraines, or fibromyalgia, avoiding eggs can give your body the support it needs to get better.

The biggest issue with eggs is that they're a prime food for cancer and other cysts, fibroids, tumors, and nodules. Women with polycystic ovary syndrome (PCOS), breast cancer, or other cysts and tumors should avoid eggs altogether. Also, if you're trying to prevent cancer, fight an existing cancer, or avoid a cancer relapse, steer clear. Removing eggs from your diet completely will give you a powerful fighting chance to reverse disease and heal.

Eggs also cause inflammation and allergies because they feed viruses, bacteria, yeast, mold, and unproductive fungus, which can trigger edema in the lymphatic system.

People who are diagnosed with *Candida* or mycotoxins are often told that eggs are a good, safe protein that will starve the *Candida* and mycotoxins. Nothing could be further from the truth. In reality, eggs feed pathogens that the beneficial fungus *Candida* must then clean up, often leading *Candida* to proliferate in the process.

I know how popular eggs are. There's a growing trend that promotes them as a major health food. Plus they're a comfort food that's delicious and fun to eat. If eggs were good for us in the current day and age, though, I'd be promoting them as such.

DAIRY

Milk, cheese, butter, cream, yogurt, and other such products contain a substantial amount of fat, which is a strain for your digestive system—and especially your liver—to process.

Dairy contains lactose, and the combination of fat and sugar has negative effects on health, especially if you're diabetic. Further, dairy fat in your bloodstream helps viruses and bacteria proliferate, because the fat in the blood doesn't allow the immune system to easily seek out, find, and destroy the pathogens. Viruses and bacteria also feed on the lactose and proteins in dairy.

The reason why dairy is mucus producing is because the viruses and bacteria feeding on the lactose and proteins cause inflammation and allergies.

Those are the issues that have *always* held true for dairy, even when it's organic and free-range. And now, conventional, mainstream practice has made a problematic food into a more problematic one by creating farm industry pressure to give hormones, antibiotics, GMO corn and soy, and gluten to cows, goats, and sheep.

If you want a smooth healing process, it's best not to eat dairy at all.

PORK

Avoid all forms of pork, including ham, bacon, processed pork products, lard, and so on. It's difficult to heal any chronic illness while consuming any kind of pig product, due to these foods' high fat content, which puts an extreme burden on the liver and even the pancreas.

FARMED FISH

Farmed fish are often raised in small, enclosed spaces. This breeds toxic algae, parasites, bacterial infections, and other diseases—so the breeders often give the fish antibiotics and treat the water with toxic chemicals such as antifungals. This makes consuming farmed fish risky.

The safest fish you can eat are wild ones, such as sardines (which are the best and safest), salmon, trout, mackerel, halibut, and haddock. No matter what type you select, beware of mercury—especially with larger fish such as swordfish and tuna. Sardines are the safest to consume because they tend to have the least amount of mercury.

GLUTEN

Gluten is a protein found in many grains. The forms of gluten to which people are especially sensitive are in wheat, barley, rye, and spelt (a type of wheat). (When it comes to oats, be aware that growing and processing sometimes cross-contaminates them with grains that contain gluten. Oats can be a very good food for people who are less sensitive, though. Look for those that are labeled gluten-free.) Grains that contain gluten can trigger many conditions by feeding viruses and bacteria that cause those symptoms and conditions—and that truth of *why* gluten can be problematic is unknown to medical research and science. Gluten fueling pathogens creates disruption and inflammation, especially in your intestinal tract and bowels, where bacteria and some viruses can live and thrive. Chronic, low-grade viral and bacterial infections that gluten feeds then challenge your immune system—and often trigger celiac disease, Crohn's, colitis, and IBS. To be abundantly clear, gluten does not cause or create these conditions; it feeds the viruses and bacteria that cause the conditions.

Eating these grains makes it very difficult for your body to heal. If you'd like to recover from your illness as quickly as possible, minimize grains of any kind. Millet is your best option for a grain.

MSG

Monosodium glutamate (MSG) is a food additive that's used in tens of thousands of products and restaurant dishes. MSG is a salt that occurs naturally in glutamic acid (a non-essential amino acid). But there's nothing natural about the damage it can do to you in its additive form.

MSG typically builds up in your brain, going deep into your brain tissue. It can then cause inflammation and swelling, kill thousands of your brain cells, disrupt electrical impulses, weaken neurotransmitters, burn out neurons, make you feel confused and anxious, and even lead to micro-strokes. It also weakens and injures your central nervous system.

MSG is especially harmful if you have an illness that involves your brain or central nervous system. However, there are no circumstances under which it's good for you. As a result, this is an additive you should *always* avoid.

Because MSG is included in countless products, it's essential to read food labels carefully. It's also important to know what to look for. MSG is often "hidden" on labels because of its deservedly bad reputation. The following terms usually mean that MSG is an ingredient: *glutamate, hydrolyzed, autolyzed, protease, carrageenan, maltodextrin, sodium caseinate, balsamic vinegar, barley malt, malt extract, yeast extract, brewer's yeast, corn starch, wheat starch, modified food starch, gelatin, textured protein, whey protein, soy protein, soy sauce, broth, bouillon, stock,* and *seasoning.*

NUTRITIONAL YEAST

The specific glutamic acid that's only in nutritional yeast is highly irritating to the intestinal tract lining. It can contribute to intestinal tract disorders such as IBS and even worsen conditions such as celiac. This is true even with the purest forms of nutritional yeast.

Yeast is not an ingredient that the body sees as a helpful food. Nutritional yeast is not an immune system enhancer. It puts stress upon the immune system, because the human body views yeast as an unproductive invader.

So it's a situation where any possible benefits of even pure nutritional yeast don't outweigh the downsides when you're sick or susceptible to chronic symptoms or conditions. When someone has no problems to be concerned about, sparing use of nutritional yeast could be an option. If you have any symptoms or conditions, you want to steer clear.

NATURAL FLAVORS

Any ingredient with a name like *natural flavoring* is hidden MSG.

Natural cherry flavor, natural orange flavor, natural lemon flavor, natural fruit flavor . . . they're not just fruit extracts, and they're not your friends. The same goes for *smoke flavor, turkey flavor, beef flavor, natural peppermint flavor, natural maple flavor, natural chocolate flavor, natural vanilla flavor,* and all their "natural" and "flavor"-ful cousins. Be cautious—even with the term *organic* in front of a flavoring ingredient, it doesn't mean it's free of MSG. (Although pure vanilla extract is safe to use.)

Each type of natural flavor potentially contains multiple biohazards and chemical compounds. Natural flavoring has slipped under the radar and been allowed into thousands of health food store products that are advertised as good, safe, and healthy for you and your children.

Moms, take heed. Natural flavors are one of the newest and stealthiest now-you-see-it-now-you-don't tricks for hiding MSG. Take care reading labels so you and your family can avoid this hidden ingredient.

ARTIFICIAL FLAVORS

Artificial flavors can represent any of thousands of chemicals that were birthed in a lab. Don't take risks by consuming them. As much as possible, the best you can, stay away from chemical additives.

ARTIFICIAL SWEETENERS

Most artificial sweeteners act as neurotoxins because they contain aspartame. This can disrupt your neurons and your central nervous system. Long term, artificial sweeteners can cause neurological breakdowns and strokes in your brain.

If you crave sweets, eat as much fruit as you like. Fruit fights disease and has powerful healing properties.

CITRIC ACID

Citric acid is very irritating to the linings of the stomach and the intestinal tract, so it can create a lot of inflammation and discomfort if you're sensitive to it.

Citric acid (the additive) is not the same thing as naturally occurring acid in the citrus fruit family. Try not to confuse the two. Citrus itself is a healing food. The isolated ingredient citric acid, however, is often corn derived, which could feed viruses and bacteria.

Especially if you're experiencing any kind of stomach pain, keep an eye out for citric acid on ingredient labels and consider skipping foods that include it.

SUPPLEMENTS TO AVOID

Many over-the-counter supplements are wonderful. However, this section covers supplements that—depending on your condition—may not be appropriate for you.

When you're working on cleansing and healing, it's important to reevaluate any supplements you may be taking. If you stay on a supplement that's not Medical Medium–recommended while you're trying to heal, particularly a supplement from this list, you may not see the benefits you want to see:

- Whey protein powder
- Fish oil
- Collagen
- Chlorella
- Multivitamins
- Hair-nail-skin supplements
- Glandular supplements
- L-carnitine
- Gut powder blends
- Iron supplments (that are not plant based; see iron-rich foods below)
- Hydrochloric acid supplements
- Sodium bicarbonate (baking soda) taken internally
- Diatomaceous earth

Keep reading for explanations of why some of these supplements can work against healing.

(For more on this subject, see the entire section devoted to supplement protocols in *Cleanse to Heal*.)

L-Carnitine

The amino acid called *carnitine* is a top fuel for all herpes viruses. The same goes for a variety of viruses beyond herpes. *L-carnitine* is not helpful with cancers, either.

You need to beware of L-carnitine. Always stay away from this amino acid in a concentrated supplement form.

Glandular Supplements

Glandular supplements made from animals are prime foods for viruses, bacteria, and cancers, which all thrive on concentrated animal hormones.

Be cautious when taking supplements containing concentrations, however small, of bovine or other animal organs or glands. These are low-grade steroid compounds, and they're often prescribed by doctors for adrenals and other endocrine glands and organs. Glandular supplements suppress the immune system, which can hinder the immune system as it seeks out viruses and bacteria.

Whey Protein

Whey protein is a dairy byproduct that does nothing notable for you except create inflammation by feeding viruses and bacteria. Plus it usually includes MSG.

However, if you're into protein powders, you're generally safe with a high-quality organic hemp protein powder. Check the ingredients label before buying to ensure the powder contains nothing that's cautioned against in this chapter. Be mindful that if you have intestinal tract sensitivities or conditions such as Crohn's or colitis, hemp protein powder (along with other protein powders) can be irritating to the digestive linings.

Fish Oil Supplements

The fish oil trend is unstoppable at this point. Yet it's important that people understand what they're putting in their bodies. While it's okay to eat wild fish sparingly if you're someone who loves fish, fish oil supplements are another matter. You would think it's all the same, but it's actually very different.

The primary issue is mercury and dioxins, which are present in most of the fish used to make these supplements. When you eat fish with mercury in its flesh, the mercury has a tendency to stay mostly in your intestinal tract, liver, and stomach area. It's another, more dangerous story when you consume fish oil supplements. Although manufacturers say that the physical mercury is removed from their supplements, it's an impossible and unrealistic claim.

In fish, mercury concentrates itself mostly in the volatile omega oils. So when millions of fish are processed for their oil, mercury levels are at an unparalleled level. The process that supplement manufacturers then use to try to lower the mercury content actually destabilizes the toxic heavy metal. It becomes a highly absorbable, homeopathic version of itself. (For those who are into homeopathy: the more the substance is diluted, the more its frequency increases, and the more power and influence it has over the body.)

This concentrated mercury that ends up in fish oil supplements has the ability to cross the blood-brain barrier and quite easily enter sensitive organs, bypassing and disrupting the body's systems. It can also strengthen and feed viruses and bacteria. Fish oil supplements put you on the fast track for Alzheimer's, dementia, and chronic inflammatory diseases of the brain.

Unfortunately, the fish oil trend train is barreling down the tracks, fueled by misinformation. It is powerful, popular—and harmful. Do your best to stay out of its way. Instead of fish oil supplements, look for fish-free, plant-based, algae-derived omega supplements.

Whenever you start to feel persuaded by the arguments in fish oil's favor, remember: fish oil is the snake oil of today! Treat it warily. It will not fulfill its promises.

I'm not trying to stir the pot with information that goes against the mainstream. I just can't bear to choose the path of least resistance and repeat the misinformation that's out there, as if popularity makes it accurate. This is about you getting better with the truth.

Iron Supplements

Even though iron in the right amounts is good for you, viruses love to feed on this metal. Almost all cases of anemia are caused by a low-grade viral infection. You should therefore avoid iron supplements that are not plant based.

Increase your iron naturally by eating spinach, barley grass, parsley, wild blueberries, grapes (black, purple, or red), blackberries, cilantro, burdock root (juiced), potatoes (with skins), kale, sprouts, squash, pumpkin seeds (in small amounts), asparagus, sulfur-free dried apricots, and other fruits, leafy greens, herbs, wild foods, and vegetables with relatively high amounts of iron. Viruses are unlikely to consume iron from these sources because fruits, leafy greens, herbs, wild foods, and vegetables contain natural antiviral properties.

"You deserve to have full knowledge of what you consume, and what effects it all has on your body. You're worth protecting. It's time you had control and informed choice over what enters your body—it's a powerful step toward recovering your health."

— Anthony William, Medical Medium

CHAPTER 20

Fruit Fear

Everyone is unique—that's well established by now. I think we'd all agree that each person is different, and each person's soul is, too. No one would argue that Hitler's soul was the same as a saint's.

And think about rocks. There are sedimentary, metamorphic, and igneous—and so many types within each classification. There's a different story behind what went into forming each one, just like the experiences we go through that shape who we are. Rocks look different, weather differently, and behave differently. You'd be cautious, for example, climbing up a rock face of shale, because of its tendency to splinter—you wouldn't want to lose your grip and fall to the ground.

And let's look at water: Do all the bottled water companies think their offerings are the same? No; that's why high-end bottlers spend fortunes advertising their brands' singular benefits. And what if you compare a glass of drinking water to the water in the toilet bowl? Or to a puddle on the New Jersey Turnpike. Or to a freshly melted snowcap on a pristine mountain. Or to the water in an aquarium or bathtub or swimming pool. They're all H_2O. But are they the same? Not a chance.

That's how it works with sugar. You can't lump together all the different types and say they're all bad. You can't say, "Sugar is sugar."

Yet that's what's happened in our culture. In recent years, an important theory came to light about how processed foods feed obesity, and how many of these processed foods contain a form of corn syrup. Suddenly a fire started in the collective health-care consciousness about *all* sugar. Natural and conventional doctors alike declared a well-intentioned war on it. As you read in the previous chapter, "What Not to Eat," it's true that high fructose corn syrup is not beneficial. That said, the theory that HFCS is solely and directly responsible for obesity is flawed. What's really going on is that most of the time that processed food contains corn syrup, it also contains lard, processed oils, eggs, dairy, and/or gluten—and it seems that these were ignored while HFCS got the spotlight. Besides which, just because HFCS can be a contributor to health issues does not mean all forms of sugar are automatically bad.

The innocent casualty of the war on sugar was fruit.

Fruit has almost become a dirty word.

So much so that it's a little risky for me to even write this chapter. It sounds silly, but it's true. Because what I reveal about fruit in the pages to come goes against current thinking. It goes against the conditioning of fruit fear.

FRUIT IS NOT THE PROBLEM

There's a rapidly developing trend: millions of people who are struggling with their health all over the world visit doctors, practitioners, nutritionists, or healers and hear right off the bat, "Eliminate fruit from your diet." It started here in the U.S. and then found its way to countries around the globe.

Doctors who practice Eastern medicine will say fruit creates dampness in the body. Doctors who practice Western medicine will say fruit worsens *Candida*, gut problems, and even cancer. Dietitians and nutritionists will say fruit contributes to diabetes and energy issues or energy loss. And physical trainers will say fruit will make you overweight, or even obese.

This was not done by accident. Fairly recently in history, there was a deliberate attack to hinder and slow down fruit consumption. Starting in the U.S., a very small handful of health professionals were given direction to sabotage fruit. New appointees are picked to this day and given their marching orders to shun fruit from a higher order within the health industry.

At this point, most health professionals and medical communities don't know why they associate fruit sugar with health problems. There's no evidence, there's no data, there are no studies. They just do. How high fructose corn syrup got all the blame and how that led to blaming problems on fruit sugar is another

mystery, because HFCS is a processed food incorporated into other processed foods—and whole fruit is not a processed food. Without knowing why they're really doing it, health professionals and medical communities have gotten into the rhythm—the habit—of telling people that fruit is contributing to all their problems, including with *Candida,* mold, weight, cancer, diabetes, cardiovascular systems, and even their teeth.

In truth, who eats that much fruit? In mainstream diets, it's become a novelty. While people may still have the occasional banana or lunchbox apple, more often fruit is an accompaniment to something else: the strawberries on strawberry shortcake, for instance, or a few glazed blueberries swimming in the butter, cane sugar, and lard of blueberry pie.

So are the millions of people around the world who are sick with various illnesses unwell because of the occasional Granny Smith? Are millions of people with rotting teeth climbing into the dentist's chair for a root canal because of the clementine they ate at a holiday party? The reality is that even the average person who's concerned about sugar intake still consumes well over 100 pounds of *refined* sugar a year.

(By the way, people aren't even climbing into the dentist's chair because of refined sugar. They're experiencing dental issues because of trace mineral deficiencies, toxic heavy metals, chronic low-grade viral and bacterial infections, stagnant and sluggish livers, inability to produce the proper amount of bile, weakened stomach glands, low hydrochloric acid production to digest and break down food properly, nutritional deficiencies passed down from parents, and high-fat diets.)

The sugar in fruit is not to blame for illness. It is not the same as HFCS or the sugar cubes at the diner.

Fruit is not making people sick.

I'm not saying that fructose that's been processed and separated from its fruit source is an ideal source of food. Pure fructose is still harmless. But fruit in its whole form, full of living water, trace minerals, antiviral and antibacterial compounds, enzymes, and fiber-rich pulp, is the real deal for your health.

Fruit consumption around the world has substantially declined in recent years, and it's only growing worse as each year comes and goes. This path is going to continue as time goes on—not because fruit is causing any problems but because some leaders in health are chosen purposely to hinder people's trust regarding fruit.

Do not get a pound of fruit confused with a pound of sugar. A pound of *sugar* is a pound of sugar. A pound of fruit is a unique blend of life-creating, life-saving, life-sustaining phytonutrients and other phytochemicals that stop disease and promote long life.

Fruit does not have that much sugar in it. Fruits are made up of living water, minerals, vitamins, protein, fat, other nutrients, pulp, fiber, antioxidants, pectin—and just a fraction of sugar. If we wanted to compare 100 pounds of refined sugar to the equivalent amount of sugar you'd consume in fruit, we'd be looking at thousands of pounds of fruit.

Fruit fear propaganda started to really take hold in 2012. While some distrust of fruit had been present several years before this, 2012 is when fruit fear really started to get its grip. That's when "Fruit is bad" became more of a household term. Since then, the fruit-hating trend has been increasing every year.

That's not supposed to be the trend.

Don't get fooled by aisles of fruit stacked in the supermarkets. Most of it is thrown away on a weekly basis. Supermarkets stock fruit mostly for show. While yes, some people do buy and consume fruit, that's only a small percentage of the population. And for the people who do eat fruit, it only makes up a tiny percentage of their diet.

Before refined sugar production and trade became a major industry that turned products like table sugar and HFCS into dietary staples, we relied on a critical source of life. That source was fruit. Since humankind began, we've depended on fruit, in all its varieties, for our survival. The Tree of Life was an ancient symbol of interconnection, fertility, and eternal life—precisely because of this legendary tree's fruit. Fruit is part of our essence, a basic element of who we are. We cannot survive without fruit on this planet. It outweighs the nutrition of any other food.

Yet the current "health" movement toward low-carb, high-fat diets (such as keto) has put fruit—aside from a few berries—on the endangered species list, with the goal of making it extinct.

Is this denial? Ignorance? Foolishness? We're not talking about uneducated people who are driving the trend. We're talking about smart, highly intelligent professionals with advanced degrees in medicine and nutrition. If they're advising clients and patients to shun fruit, it must be because of their training, the misinformation out there, or their own selective interests.

Have you heard of book burning? If the anti-sugar war keeps up its momentum, fruit trees will be next to go up in flames. If fruit consumption halts, all of our ancient fruit orchards and groves worldwide will eventually be burned down so the land can be used for something else. This will shape our environment in destructive ways. Bees, migrating birds, and wildlife will suffer greatly, because they rely upon the fruits and fruit blossoms for survival.

FRUIT AND FERTILITY

It's critical that medical communities start distinguishing between fruit sugars and all the rest. Otherwise, the war could be more dangerous than anyone realizes; it could result in other innocent casualties: womankind, and the future of humankind.

That's because without fruit, fertility is at risk. Women are already up against enough infertility issues, and well-meaning doctors, nutritionists, dieticians, and health coaches have no idea that when they tell women patients to shun fruit, they're contributing to women's struggles to conceive. A woman's reproductive system is like a flowering tree that requires the proper nutrients to bear fruit. And those nutrients come from, well, fruit.

Fertility—and overall health—depends specifically on the fructose and glucose that occur naturally in fruit, as well as the phytochemicals bonded to those sugars. A woman's reproductive system also relies on the dozens of undiscovered antitumor, anticancer, antiviral, antibacterial compounds (and so many more components yet to be discovered by medical science) available only in fruit, as well as fruit's essential polyphenols, bioflavonoids, disease-stopping pectin, vitamins, and minerals. These elements help to stop polycystic ovary syndrome (PCOS), pelvic inflammatory disease (PID), fibroids, and an overextended reproductive system—examples of conditions that cause mysterious infertility.

FRUITFUL LANGUAGE

It's for good reason that the Bible mentions fruit over 300 times: because fruit is vital to the essence of who we are. Humankind exists because of the fruit we picked off trees since our species' beginning. It is what has allowed us to thrive on this planet.

Fruit is the divine word of wisdom. For thousands of years, we have used fruit in our language to express powerful truths. To this day, we use phrases such as "fruits of our labors" and "a tree is known by its fruit."

We talk about fruit in terms of prosperity. In business, we talk about "fruitful" collaboration and projects coming to "fruition." Motivational gurus who teach about achieving financial freedom refer to "fruit-bearing" processes. We call children "fruit of the womb" and "fruit of the loins." We warn against the dangers of "forbidden fruit" and settling for the "low-hanging fruit."

All this fruit in our daily language shows that we connect on some level with fruit's significance. When we only connect to fruit's meaning, though, it's like extracting the sugar. It's like getting only the sweet buzz of a hit of processed fructose and none of the benefits of the fruit in its whole form.

For true mind-body-spirit-soul-heart wisdom, we need to incorporate real, unadulterated fruit into our diets. Only then do we start to walk the talk of all those phrases we throw around. When fruit literally becomes part of who we are, our lives become that much more fruitful.

Why avoid the food we were most meant to eat? Eating whole fruit can make *us* whole again.

FRUIT'S ANCIENT ROOTS

Humans have been cultivating fruit for thousands of years, all over the globe. In Asia, peaches and citrus had historical significance. In Africa, oranges, dates, and figs were meaningful. In Russia, apples and pears were central. In England, it was berries and grapes. In the Middle East, figs, dates, and mangoes held (and still hold) an important place. And in South America, bananas and papayas have always had a vital role in health and culture.

Going all the way back to the Garden of Eden, fruit was a mainstay of the human diet. Once agriculture began and civilization and trade routes became established, it was the ones fortunate enough to have fruit delivered to them—emperors, kings, queens, dukes, earls, counts, barons, knights, and pharaohs— who lived the longest.

With access to fruit all year long, disease was not the problem for royalty that it was for the people of lower status. Peasants and other common people had to live off grains, porridge, scraps of dehydrated meats, and some vegetables. They went much of the year without a single piece of fruit. As a result, they were plagued by nutritional deficiencies.

Scurvy, a disease that research has pegged as a vitamin C deficiency but is also a deficiency in other critical nutrients found in fruit (as yet undiscovered by science), was rampant in these lower classes. Many people also died

of rickets eating away at their muscles and bones. Simple infections were life-threatening, too, and noncancerous tumors that thrived off protein, fat, and grain were responsible for a great many people's suffering at this time in history—all because they didn't have access to enough fruit.

Meanwhile, the fortunate kings of the planet led longer and healthier lives because of the sacrifices those below them made to bring fruit from all over the world. They'd order up oranges like we can call for pizza delivery, and lo, the oranges would appear.

(By the way, there's more sugar in pizza than you'll ever find in fruit.)

These rulers were constantly eating out of season, enjoying the best that other regions had to offer, and taking in hundreds of critical life-protecting nutrients.

SEASONAL EATING . . . AND EATING OUT OF SEASON

Which leads me to another topic: the seasonal eating trend.

It has its pluses. The popularity of seasonal eating has people visiting their farmers' markets for fresh fruits and vegetables—and of course that's wonderful. There's nothing like enjoying the local bounty that each season brings.

The downside is that out-of-season fruit (i.e., fruit transported from other parts of the country or globe) is getting a bad rap. Some people have started to walk past the grocery store offerings of blackberries in winter or oranges in summer because they don't line up with the growing season where they live. That's a crime for their health. This mentality robs people of disease-protecting nutrients, because they turn to other fillers in their diet instead. The truth is, those fruits *are* in season . . . in the places where they were grown.

If you took an autumn vacation from Michigan to southern Spain, wouldn't you eat the fresh mangoes there, even though they weren't available from the local vendors at home? Wouldn't you recognize that different parts of the world have different growing seasons and different varieties of produce, and let yourself enjoy the delicacy?

Just because you're not on vacation doesn't mean you're meant to ignore the fruits shipped in from out of town. It's how the ruling classes survived and thrived for thousands of years—and now their health secret is available to the masses.

Some people are less concerned about being out of tune with the seasons than they are about the environmental impact of transporting produce from other regions. That's understandable—though if the pollution from shipping is what's stopping you from buying Ecuadorian bananas, then you'll have to rethink using a car, a washing machine, a computer, a cell phone, or cloud storage, visiting the salon, wearing almost all modern-day clothes, ordering anything that's delivered to your door . . . the list goes on. You'd be much better off cutting back in one of those areas and letting yourself buy pears from New Zealand or honeydew from Mexico. The benefits that fruit will have for your health are worth it.

That said, if you prefer to eliminate all modern practices from your life, I'm not here to stop you. Just know that limiting fruit in your diet will increase your chances of illness and shorten your expected life span.

THE TRUTH ABOUT RIPENING

Another popular misconception about fruit is that it's not worth eating if it was picked early and unripe so it can withstand shipping and last on the grocery store shelf.

Truth is, if a fruit were truly picked too early to have nutritional value, it would never ripen at all, and you'd find it inedible.

Fruit trees and plants have a built-in database of information connected to the heavens. Once they log enough hours in the season and the growing conditions are right, the Higher Source delivers the signal, and the fruits enter their ripening phase. At this point, they can get picked at any time and still ripen and nourish your body.

It's true that it doesn't work to pick some fruits, such as berries, before they've ripened on the plant. With other fruits, though, such as mangoes, tomatoes, and bananas, they just have to cross that specific growing threshold, to which farmers are often well attuned.

HYBRIDIZATION

Don't get confused or concerned about hybridization or crossbreeding—not to be mistaken for genetic modification and the creation of GMOs. Grafting and hand-pollination are safe techniques that humans have used for thousands of years to create new varieties of fruit. It's a healthy adaptation and evolution of the cultivation process. While it's true that some heirloom varieties of fruits can be more nutritious, don't shy away from hybridized varieties— because some hybridized fruit varieties are more nutritious than heirlooms. Hybridized fruits are still preventative wonders that are antiviral and fight cancer and other diseases.

MAKING FRUIT A HABIT

Fruit has properties that help restore your adrenal glands, strengthen your entire endocrine system, repair your vascular system, restore and cleanse your liver, help purge your lymphatic system, and revitalize your brain and stop it from atrophying. There is no other food—and no pill—that enhances so many of your bodily functions as fruit.

Fruit keeps your body going in ways that science hasn't even begun to fully understand. It's an absolute necessity.

You can't function as a human being without glucose, the simple sugar into which your body breaks down foods. Glucose fuels your brain, your liver, your nervous system, and the cells throughout your body.

If you're an athlete—or a mom holding down multiple jobs between home and the office—then eating animal protein, nuts, and vegetables alone won't allow you to perform. You also need foods with sugar in them, and the highest-quality source of sugar is fruit. If you try to cut out all sugar from your diet, sooner or later your body will force you to "cheat"—because every muscle in your body functions on glucose—and eat something that provides the sugar you need. The chances are you'll binge on something that's not a nutritional plus for you, such as pastries or pasta or chocolate bars.

You'll be much better off if you make a habit of eating fruit every day. It will help curb sugar cravings—and make a huge difference in your health.

Fruit is best eaten by itself or paired with raw vegetables, herbs, wild foods, and leafy greens. That's because your stomach digests fruit and some other raw plant foods quickly and easily. Some fruits are even predigested. In contrast, protein and fat are harder to process, so they take a relatively long time to digest. Most people already have digestion problems and compromises. Even if they don't realize it, the food they're eating is not digesting well. So when you put a food like fruit that's very easy to digest on top of a food that's stuck at the top of your stomach waiting its turn, conflict can occur. The fruit is going to want to do the right thing—gently run its course, cleanse the intestinal tract, and break down and assimilate quickly. Protein and fat get in the way. For some people, the result can be some slight discomfort and a little extra gas. This is only because the protein and fat are not digesting well, and fruit is highlighting that as it tries to push the protein and fat through your stomach and intestinal tract—essentially, to fast-track digestion. While this does no serious harm, the bit of gas and other discomfort this process can create might discourage you from eating fruit—and *that* would be terrible. So consider consuming fruit on its own, in smoothies, or with raw, leafy greens or other veggies, and waiting to consume any other type of food a bit of time after you've enjoyed your fruit.

FRUIT IS ANTI-DISEASE

Almost all health professionals and medical practitioners advise their patients to avoid processed sugar because they believe sugar causes obesity. And then there are some medical professionals who believe processed sugar can potentially feed cancer.

The trouble is, these health-care professionals often go on to point to fruit as a source of harm, too, because of the sugars it contains.

Fruit does not feed cancer. It's *anti-cancerous*. Fruit fights cancer *more effectively than any other food*. Almost all cancers are caused by viruses and toxins combined, and fruit is antiviral and detoxifying. Any cancer patient removing fruit from her diet is giving up one of her most powerful natural weapons against the disease.

Vegetables combat cancer, too, but only about a quarter as well. If doctors insist you remove all fruit from your diet, you'd better quadruple your vegetable intake to compensate. Adding in leafy greens and herbs will also help make up the difference.

When doctors advise cancer patients against fruit, the irony is that cancer (and other disease) feeds on every food that is *not* a fruit, leafy green, herb, wild food, or vegetable.

In the 1960s, there was a trend among cocaine addicts to double one's intake of vitamin C to protect the body from the damage done by the illegal stimulant. The more vitamin C they took, the more cocaine people thought they could ingest.

What I'm getting at is, the more chocolate cake, soda, animal protein, milk, cheese, fried, greasy, non-fruit, non–leafy green, non-herb, non-wild, and non-vegetable foods you eat, the more you'd better counterbalance this fare with extra apples, berries, mangoes, papayas, grapes, melons, kiwis, oranges, vegetables, herbs, leafy greens, and the like to protect yourself.

If you keep eating foods other than fruits, leafy greens, herbs, wild foods, and vegetables, there's no guarantee that you'll become disease resistant. However, incorporating an abundance of fruit into your diet will be a positive, proactive step toward countering and preventing cancer's effects.

Cancer *cannot* feed off the sugar in fruit, which possesses critical components such as antiviral, antibacterial compounds and polyphenols (including resveratrol) and other antioxidants. These cancer killers cannot be separated from the sugar in fruit; they travel together as a team.

What little (and flawed) research that's been attempted on the link between sugar and cancer has been on sucrose and high fructose corn syrup. There was no true confirmation of the outcome. The appropriate studies have yet to be performed with an actual piece of fruit, or with most of the foods that truly do feed cancer. When those studies are performed—conducted ethically and reported accurately—they'll find that fruit is not to blame. Yet the rumor mill is going strong, and fruit fear is in danger of stopping countless people from preventing cancers and other health issues.

Cancer is already climbing at an alarming rate. With low fruit consumption taking a further nosedive, I hate to imagine where this is headed. It's another blunder for which our children and our children's children will have to pay. Some things are out of our control. It's in our control, though, to make sure that the generations to come know how to stay healthy and don't fall into the trend traps.

Not only does fruit fight cancer, it kills all types of viruses and bacteria. Certain fruits, such as bananas, wild blueberries, apples, papayas, oranges, mangoes, and red pitaya (dragon fruit), are the most powerful natural destroyers of viruses on earth.

Fruit is also vital to gut health—which is essential to a healthy immune system, because any pathogens, such as viruses and unproductive bacteria, that live inside the gut can't thrive when you're eating enough fruit. For example, the pectin in apples, and the skin, pulp, and fiber in figs and dates, are exceptionally effective at killing and/or clearing out anything that doesn't belong in your intestinal tract, including funguses, worms, and other parasites.

If you're worried that the sugar in fruit causes *Candida*, turn to Chapter 9. You'll find that, first, the sugar in most fruit is digested by your stomach so rapidly that within a short amount of time, it travels straight into your bloodstream, meaning the sugar never even reaches the majority of your intestinal tract. And second, fruit *kills* bacteria, unproductive fungus, and viruses so that *Candida* reduces, because fruit is helping resolve the threat of problematic pathogens. (*Candida* is not a problem of its own; an elevated level of it is an indicator that something else in the body is amiss.)

Another misconception is that fruit sugar hinders the liver. That couldn't be more misunderstood. This trend only goes to show that something is amiss with our medical systems, both alternative and conventional.

Does the term *fatty liver* sound like a condition that comes from fruit sugar? No. The occasional piece of fruit that most Americans eat is *not* why liver disease and disorders of the liver are rampant and on the rise.

As the name implies, a fatty liver comes from consuming fat. Almost all liver diseases are protein and fat related, because viruses thrive in an environment with lots of protein and fat. It's just that so many fatty foods are also high in bad sugars. And it's not always the obvious foods, like cupcakes and ice cream, but also whole milk (which combines butterfat and lactose), a hamburger in a bun (fat and carbohydrates), and french fries (drenched in oil) with ketchup (full of added sugar). So somewhere along the line, health professionals came under the misimpression that fruit hurts the liver because it has natural sugars.

The best way to get someone better from liver disease and/or hepatitis C is to feed them solely fruits, leafy greens, herbs, wild foods, and vegetables. It's the answer to their suffering.

Speaking of the liver, hypoglycemia often starts because of a dysfunctional liver that's lost its store of glucose due to a diet too high in fat and protein. Sugar isn't the bad guy here, especially sugar from apples, berries, oranges, melons, bananas, mangoes, papayas, kiwis, and other sweet and delicious fruits. Fruit *protects* the liver by providing the organ with the glucose reserve it needs in order to function and stave off illness, and to stabilize blood sugar.

Why am I championing fruit? Who cares if health-care professionals tell their patients to avoid it, and the practice of eating fruit vanishes altogether?

We *all* have to care and we *all* have to champion it, because it is critical to everyone's health.

It's imperative that women eat enough fruit so they can avoid fatigue, cancers, tumors, viruses, PID, PCOS, endometriosis, fibroids, and other illnesses. It's important to the future of our children, who currently get the message not to eat fruit.

If you're in the business of wanting your liver, kidneys, and pancreas to break down, then go ahead and listen to advice to eat a high-fat, high-protein diet and shun fruit. I don't side with any particular food program, diet, or nutritional belief system. I'm not against animal foods or plant-based fats and proteins. It's just that if animal products and/or plant-based fats and proteins completely take the place of fruit in your diet, you won't get enough nutrients to protect you for the long haul.

Fruit is a critical part of how you overcome illness. I have witnessed this in people for over 30 years.

(Don't feel stuck if fruit isn't an option for you right now. There are other ways of healing—consider potatoes as your next best option for a glucose-producing food. Winter squash and tomatoes, which are actually fruits, are options, too. Sweet potatoes and raw honey are also supportive. If you're in a critical state and need an alternative to fruit, whether because fruit isn't accessible or for any other reason, the potato mono eating protocol in *Cleanse to Heal* may be your answer. Read more in that book.)

Take comfort. Fruit is your friend. It does not cause sickness. Rather, it's one of the most effective foods at preventing disease, killing pathogens, and repairing the body.

THE FRUIT FOUNTAIN OF YOUTH

Consider this: We're eating less fruit as a society than ever before, and more protein and fat. Life expectancy and fruit consumption are dropping at the same time. That's not a coincidence.

Longevity is a popular term right now. Everybody wants to know the secret to living longer. Yet so many people are blinded by an anti-sugar mentality that they can't see the truth: fruit has the ability to grant us longer life.

Alzheimer's disease, dementia, memory loss, and neurological diseases such as Parkinson's and ALS can all be prevented by fruit.

That's because not only does fruit prevent these diseases, it prevents *oxidation*—which is the process that ages us. It's the same process that makes the flesh of a pound of chopped meat turn brown after prolonged exposure to oxygen, just like our muscles break down from aging and oxidization. Essentially, we oxidize a little more every day—unless we take action against it. The best way to do that is to eat foods rich in *antioxidants,* which you'll find most plentiful, by a wide margin, in fruit. Antioxidants from fruit can even *reverse* aging.

The most powerful fruit on the planet is the wild blueberry. Science hasn't yet fully tapped into the healing, adaptogenic properties that wild blueberries possess. They're the most antioxidant-rich food available. They can prevent and reverse disease. They are the most powerful brain food in existence. The wild blueberry plant grows like an herb, and the wild blueberry fruit has the strength of herbal medicine.

You can usually find wild blueberries in the frozen fruit case at your local grocery store. You're welcome to seek out any variety of edible wild blueberry in your area of the world (and don't shun other edible native berries that are local to you). If you can't find fresh or frozen wild blueberries, pure wild blueberry powder can be an option.

And don't confuse wild blueberries with their cultivated cousins. While cultivated (highbush) blueberries are a nutritious food, they're not the superfood that wild (lowbush) blueberries are. Every single wild blueberry contains thousands of years of survival information. Each one you consume allows this wisdom into your body, helping you adapt in today's changing times.

Wild blueberries bring up another critical point. People who are anti-fruit tend to claim that over time, we've made fruit too sweet and that therefore, fruit has been ruined. They claim that in ancient times, fruit wasn't sweet. Well, in the wild blueberry, we have a prehistoric record of fruit's sweetness. A taste of wild blueberry is an instant debunk of the theory that fruit didn't used to be sweet—because wild blueberries are sweeter than cultivated blueberries. From this fruit that is thousands of years old, we have living proof and can draw a proper conclusion: that ancient fruits were sweeter than fruits we cultivate now. And from all you've read in this chapter, you know that sweetness is an asset.

One reason people actually avoid fruit today is that it's not sweet enough. Some fruit's low sweetness even makes it "yucky" to a lot of people—because much of the fruit readily available today is tart, astringent, watery, bland, and grainy, as certain varieties are chosen to sit on a shelf for long stretches of time since so few people buy it. That lack of sweetness is also why a cup or two of sugar has to be added to apple pie, or to any number of other fruit desserts. While there's an illusion that fruit is sweet, it's not as sweet as people wish it to be. That's the opposite of what fruit haters in the health industry preach. A handful of ripe wild blueberries picked and placed in your mouth are sweet as candy, and again, those plants are thousands of years old.

If you're someone who believes in a carnivorous diet and you're told not to eat fruit, know that when your diet is defined by meat, you're going to get more sugar from that meat than from bland, non-sweet fruits that you eat once in a while. That's right; animal meat actually tends to be sweeter than some fruits at this point because of the glucose in the animal blood that resides in the meat. And then when you cook the meat, the sugars caramelize in combination with the fats. With fruit, you don't have to cook it; you can eat fruit fresh and raw. (Note that the glucose in meat is not the antiviral, antibacterial form of glucose you'll find in fruit. The glucose in meat is not filled with antioxidants and anti-aging compounds, plus meat's high fat blocks you from accessing usefulness from its glucose.)

People are so accustomed to sweets in different forms that fruit may not seem immediately appealing. The fruit varieties we're used to don't tend to be as sweet as the treats people often turn to for comfort. For some people, it takes backing down on those sweet treats to acclimate to the subtle, sweet flavors of fruit. Another key to helping yourself gravitate to fruit is to start paying attention to it. Once you learn what's available, you'll likely find some delightful, sweeter varieties.

We only have so many meals to eat in a lifetime. For the average person with an average life span (which is shorter than it used to be), that's roughly 80,000 meals. Since fruit is becoming less popular, it may account for about 10,000 of those meals—15,000 if you're lucky. Unless vegetables, leafy greens, and herbs make up most of the difference, that's a lot of missed opportunity for nutrition.

If it's well-being and longevity you're after, you want every meal to count for something. One of the best ways to do that is to eat more fruit—and not to get sucked into the antisugar game.

Fruit is the true fountain of youth.

BEFRIEND FRUIT

That old saying, "An apple a day keeps the doctor away," names a piece of fruit for a reason. It's not, "An egg a day keeps the doctor away," or "A cut of beef a day keeps the doctor away," or "A chicken breast a day keeps the doctor away."

Which is not to say that no one should eat chicken or beef. It's just that fruit is the foundation of health—and a long time ago, we used to know this.

For some people, it's more like an apple a month that they incorporate into their diet—and that one apple is the underlying structure of any wellness they maintain.

Many of us live in a world now where fresh fruit is available year-round—fruit that has the power to heal disease, prevent it, sweeten our days, give us energy, and give us back our lives. As I've said before: most health trends don't become popular because they work. The belief that all sugars are the same is one such powerful trend, and it's growing fast. It has turned so many health professionals against fruit.

Fruit fear creators and fruit haters in the health world don't understand fruit. They don't understand how to eat it when it's ripe, what it's supposed to taste like, and what it offers. They don't know how to incorporate fruit into someone's diet with other foods. They don't know how to use fruit as a healing tool. This lack of knowledge is part of why they discard fruit. They're afraid of it—because they don't understand it. Plus, not being able to understand fruit can hurt the ego of a fruit-hating professional. So they create fear around fruit. They cast it off as being bad and harmful rather than learning how to use fruit, even to benefit themselves. They spread their message of fruit fear propaganda to other health professionals, sometimes through paid-for campaigns in the industry, and never mention, "We don't know how to use fruit as a healing tool." In turn, those other health professionals don't learn how to use fruit as a healing tool, either. Because of this cycle, fruit gets thrown under the bus, along with the sick.

If it keeps going at this rate, there will be some kind of fruit prohibition. We'll be camouflaging our raspberry bushes so they're not confiscated and hiding in closets to snack on plums.

Unless fruit makes a comeback. If that happens, it's thanks to readers like you who took this information to heart and made change.

When you hear from a friend or practitioner that you should avoid fruit, remember what you've just read. It's not their fault that they're spreading misinformation; they've just gotten on board the fruit misinformation trend train. Keep your wits about you, and don't let the train take you away. You know the truth now.

CHAPTER 21

Critical Guide to Supplement Protocols

Before you leap into the supplement protocols in Part II and Part III, first make sure you read this chapter fully so you can interpret the lists correctly.

If you're wondering about whether supplementation is right for you, know that the supplements recommended in this book are an optional step. If you prefer to focus on foods for healing (both adding helpful foods to your life and removing troublemaker foods), you're more than welcome to do that. The 28-Day Healing Cleanse in Chapter 22 is also an option. You don't have to play in Supplement Land yet if you don't want to. Do stay open to supplements for the future if you're struggling with symptoms and conditions.

The supplement protocols in this book are for people looking for something more, looking for options because their situations are perplexing to them. If that's you, then delve into the treasure trove of options in the form of specialized supplement lists for the individual symptoms and conditions in this book. It's important to know that our deficiencies are a big part of why we're sick. Zinc, for example, is practically nonexistent in food today, and a zinc deficiency lowers the immune system, so we're always in need of it. We also have a lot of toxic heavy metals in us, and spirulina is critical for removing those metals.

The supplements in each list throughout Parts II and III are in alphabetical order, not necessarily order of importance. An exception is celery juice, which you'll see at the top of each list. Keep in mind that the extent of what these supplements do for your body and brain remains undiscovered by medical research and science. While a few are on their radar, many of them are completely unknown as health rescuers, and the benefits go far beyond what anyone realizes.

Spirit of Compassion has always said to me throughout the years of helping so many people heal that knowing the true cause of why you're sick is half the battle won. Knowing what to do, what to take, and how to apply those tools is the other half the battle won. Throughout this book, you've gained insights into the true causes of dozens of symptoms and conditions. You understand now why the population is up against this epidemic of chronic illness. You've also discovered what to do about it. The supplement options in this book are powerful tools to help you address the "why" and win the battle.

For any questions on supplementation that this chapter doesn't address—and for supplement protocols for over 200 symptoms and conditions—see this book's companion title, *Cleanse to Heal*.

CRITICAL TIPS FOR INTERPRETING SUPPLEMENT LISTS

These critical tips will help you interpret the supplement protocols in Parts II and III:

- When you see the term *dropperful*, that means as much liquid supplement as fills the bottle's eye dropper when you squeeze its rubber top. It may only fill up halfway; that's still considered a dropperful.

- There are also some supplements where dosages are given in drops. Make sure to check carefully whether it says drops or dropperfuls.

- Most of the liquid and powder supplements are meant to be taken in water. Check the directions on the supplement's label.

- When it comes to herbal tinctures, actively seek out alcohol-free versions (avoid the word *ethanol* too).

- When you see multiple herbal tinctures in a list, you're welcome to combine them into one ounce or more of water and take them together.

- Again, the same goes for teas. If multiple teas are listed for your symptom or condition, feel free to combine the herbs to make yourself a special tea blend or use a few different tea bags together.

- One cup of tea translates to either 1 tea bag or 1 to 2 teaspoons of loose leaf tea.

- Some of the dosages are listed in milligrams. If you can't find capsules that line up with the exact suggestions, try to get ones that are close.

- These chapters list adult dosages. Talk to a physician about what's right for a child.

- When you see the term *daily*, that means to take the given dosage of the supplement over the course of the day, and it's your choice how you do that. You're welcome to take the whole dose once a day. If you're sensitive, you may want to break it up into multiple servings. For example, if it says to take 2 teaspoons of barley grass juice powder daily, you may decide either to put both teaspoons together into a smoothie or have 1 teaspoon in a morning smoothie and 1 teaspoon in some water at night.

- When you see *twice a day*, that means two installments taken at any time of day, as long as they're at least four hours apart. If you miss one of the installments on any given day, try to start fresh the next day.

WHERE TO START?

Once you've found your symptom or condition in Part II or III, you don't need to take every supplement listed for it. If you're sensitive, you can try one supplement a day. If not, you can put them all together as your daily regimen. Or as a middle ground, you can choose a couple to start off with, and then take it from there. Celery juice is always a good place to begin. Beyond that, if vitamin B_{12}, zinc, vitamin C, and/or lemon balm are in your list, bring in those. Then, if you're ready to move forward and your list contains spirulina, curcumin, cat's claw, and/or L-lysine, add those as your next step. Later on, if you're not experiencing what you want from these supplements, you can add a few more from your list. And you can always take smaller amounts than the listed dosages if you feel you're sensitive.

You also have the option to intermix supplements from the different lists in this book. Any supplement from this book is an option to use, if your expert sense of what your body needs or your physician's recommendation tells you to do so. They're all helpful supplements for chronic health issues.

(When I mention tailoring a supplement protocol for yourself, I'm not talking about bringing in supplements outside of what I recommend in this book or its companion, *Cleanse to Heal*. More in a moment.)

If you're dealing with more than one symptom or condition at the same time and want one clear place to begin, pick the health struggle that looms largest in your life. For example, if you're plagued by chronic fatigue syndrome and that feels most pressing, you can focus on the supplements for CFS at the end of Chapter 3, "Epstein-Barr Virus, Chronic Fatigue

Syndrome, and Fibromyalgia." Over time, you may find that working on one issue takes care of another, or you can switch off after a little while and focus on a different supplements list in these pages.

DOSAGES

You're welcome to start at a much lower dose with any supplement listed in this book's protocols. Even with a smaller dose of one of these high-quality supplements, you will get more health benefits than a large amount of ingredients in a lower-quality supplement. If you're sensitive, use your own experience or healing intuition or talk to your physician about what dosage your body can handle.

CHILDREN

The dosages listed in each chapter's supplement protocols are for adults. If you're considering supplements for a child, consult with her or his physician about what's safe and appropriate.

For celery juice amounts for children, see the table later in this chapter.

QUALITY MATTERS

I'm continually asked, what is the most effective form of a given supplement, and does it really matter? Yes, it matters greatly. There are subtle and sometimes critical differences among the different supplement types available that can affect how quickly your viral or bacterial load dies off, if at all; whether your central nervous system repairs itself and how fast; how quickly your inflammation reduces; how long it takes for your symptoms and conditions to heal; and if you can safely remove toxic heavy metals or not. The supplement variety you choose can make or break your progress. To speed up healing, you need the right kinds of supplements. For these very important reasons, I offer a directory on my website (www.medicalmedium.com) of the best forms of each supplement listed in this book.

You'll notice that almost every one of the supplements listed in this book's protocols is a single herb or supplement. There's a reason for this—and you can learn more about why in *Cleanse to Heal.* Know that each one of the supplements in these lists holds God-given powers to help your body heal. Your liver, a processing center of your body, can understand each one of these and knows how to use it.

One powerful undiscovered tip is to consider taking your supplements with a piece of fruit such as a banana or even some potato, sweet potato, winter squash, raw honey, pure maple syrup, or coconut water (that's not pink or red). Natural sugar is what carries vitamins, minerals, and other nutrients through the bloodstream to help them find where they need to go, so taking your supplements with natural sugars ensures that your processing-center liver and other parts of your body can actually use them (The exception to this tip is celery juice, which you should drink alone.)

SUPPLEMENTS TO AVOID WHILE HEALING

Be very discerning about supplements not recommended in the Medical Medium book series. A lot of supplements have ingredients that work against you. As you read in Chapter 19, "What Not to Eat," some supplements such as fish oil and whey protein powder can work against your healing by feeding pathogens that create the symptoms and conditions you've read about throughout this book. That is, supplements other than what I recommend may be contributing to your problems in the first place. If you stay on a non-recommended supplement while working to cleanse and heal, you may not see the benefits you want to see.

HOW LONG?

The length of time to stay on these supplements depends on factors such as how deficient you are (in areas that blood work cannot even determine) and how viral you are (meaning what kind of low-grade, undetected, undiagnosed viral infections you're dealing with), as well as how many toxic heavy metals you may have in your brain and liver, how depleted your organs are of glucose and mineral salts, how much mystery inflammation you're experiencing from undiagnosed, low-grade viral and bacterial infections, and how weakened your overall body systems may be—all of it occurring beyond detection at the doctor's office. You may be someone who says, "My doctor checked me. I'm not deficient. They didn't say anything about heavy metals. Why should I be on supplements?" The point is that a doctor isn't given the training or tools to see all the factors behind chronic illness. Even if you checked out at the doctor's office, are your symptoms and conditions still persisting? That's a sign to stick with supplementation to address the underlying issues.

The other measures you're taking to care for yourself—that is, regularly turning to Medical Medium cleanse options and supporting yourself at other times by incorporating healing foods, lowering fats, and avoiding toxic troublemakers and troublemaker foods—will make a big difference to your healing timeline. How much your body was struggling and how long you'd been suffering when you started on your healing path will make a big difference, too. Everyone has a different healing process and time frame. You may have been ill for a long time, in which case supplements are great for maintaining critical progress after you heal. Even as you're feeling better and recovering, with your specific symptoms fading away, continuing with supplements is important.

PREGNANCY AND BREASTFEEDING

Every woman who is pregnant should check with her doctor about any type of supplements she's considering.

If you're a mom struggling with symptoms or conditions while breastfeeding, you're welcome to partake in any of the supplementation listed here. If you have any questions about using supplements in your particular situation, talk to your doctor.

CELERY JUICE AS A MEDICINAL

In every supplement list in Parts II and III, you'll find a recommended amount of fresh celery juice. As you got a glimpse of earlier in Part IV, celery juice is a powerful medicinal that elevates whatever you're doing right in your life.

The same guidelines apply for celery juice as always:

- Fresh, plain, unadulterated, straight celery juice. No added ice, water, lemon juice, apple cider vinegar, collagen, or other mix-ins. Also, as beneficial as green juice blends can be, they're not a substitute for pure celery juice.

- Juice means juice. Drinking blended celery without straining the pulp doesn't yield the same benefits. See "The Juicing versus Fiber Debate" in *Cleanse to Heal* for more on why.

- Fresh means fresh. Making a drink from reconstituted celery powder won't deliver the right benefits, nor will drinking pasteurized or HPP (high-pressure pasteurization) celery juice. Any kind of juicer is okay for celery juice, and you can also choose to purchase your fresh celery juice from a juice bar rather than making your own. For best results, drink it freshly made. If you can't drink it immediately after juicing—for example, if you're having a second serving in the day—that's okay. Store it chilled in an airtight container. Read more in Chapter 17, "Gut Health."

- Drink your fresh celery juice on an empty stomach. If you drank some water or lemon water beforehand, wait at least 15 to 20 and ideally 30 minutes before drinking your celery juice. After finishing your celery juice, wait at least 15 to 20 minutes and ideally 30 minutes before consuming anything else.

- If you're drinking celery juice later in the day, give any food you've eaten plenty of time to digest first. If your last snack or meal was high in fat/protein, it's best to wait a minimum of two hours and ideally three hours before having your celery juice. If you last ate something lighter such as fruit, vegetables, potatoes, or a fruit smoothie, you can drink your celery juice 60 minutes after eating.

- If you are on a doctor-prescribed medication, it's okay to take it either before or after your celery juice, depending on whether it's supposed to be taken on an empty stomach or with food. (Please note that if your medication is supposed to be taken with food, celery juice does not count as a food.) If you take the medication first, try to wait at least 15 to 20 minutes and ideally 30 minutes before you drink your celery juice. If you drink your celery juice first, try to wait at least 15 to 20 minutes and ideally 30 minutes before you take your medication. For any further questions or concerns, consult your physician.

- When it comes to the other supplements in this book, please hold off on taking them with your celery juice. While the supplements will do fine with the celery juice, the celery juice is better without most supplements. It's best to wait to take your supplements until at least 15 to 20 minutes and ideally 30 minutes after you've finished your celery juice.

- If you have any further questions about bringing celery juice into your life, the Medical Medium title *Celery Juice* is an entire book of answers waiting for you.

Celery Juice Amounts for Children

When selecting celery juice amounts for children, you can refer to this table. These are recommended daily minimums. It can be less if that feels right for your child, or more. You don't need to worry that going over these minimums is harmful.

AGE	AMOUNT
6 months old	1 ounce or more
1 year old	2 ounces or more
18 months old	3 ounces or more
2 years old	4 ounces or more
3 years old	5 ounces or more
4 to 6 years old	6 to 7 ounces or more
7 to 10 years old	8 to 10 ounces or more
11 years old and up	12 to 16 ounces

MEDICAL MEDIUM SHOCK THERAPIES

You'll also find that some of the supplement protocols in Parts II and III call for optional Medical Medium Zinc Shock Therapy and

Medical Medium Vitamin C Shock Therapy. These are powerful healing tools to rebuild your immune system by fueling it with what it needs to fight an infection, whether you're dealing with a condition that's occurring for the first time or you're experiencing a relapse.

These supplement therapies can be particularly useful for cold and flu, UTIs, sties, cold sores (herpes simplex 1), herpes simplex 2, shingles, rash, cough, sore throat, sinus infection, lung infection, canker sores, and mono.

Medical Medium Zinc Shock Therapy

Medical Medium Zinc Shock Therapy is a useful technique because most everyone is zinc deficient. It's a mineral that left our soils long ago due to a reaction that occurs when toxic heavy metals enter our soils, including our organic farm soils, and create dead soil over time by destroying the soil's immune system. Trace mineral zinc in foods at this point is minuscule and only becoming rarer as passing-by pollutants (such as pesticides, herbicides, car exhaust, old asbestos from car brakes in decades past, and DDT and toxic heavy metals falling from the sky) continue to enter our soil and deplete the soil's immune system. Zinc is supposed to be our own immune system's number one defense, and because we're deficient, we're in dire need of it.

If we don't have enough zinc in the body, our immune system may overreact to an invader such as a flu strain or underreact to a chronic viral infection such as Epstein-Barr. Overreaction could mean higher fever and other more advanced, severe symptoms. Underreaction could mean prolonged low-grade symptoms that become chronic over time. When our immune system is well supplied with an abundant amount of zinc, this overreaction or underreaction doesn't take place. Zinc also slows down viruses and unproductive, aggressive bacteria on its own merit. Viruses and unproductive bacteria are allergic to zinc; the mineral repels and weakens them, even making pathogens docile, which allows the immune system to kill off and eliminate the pathogens more quickly.

Medical Medium Zinc Shock Therapy Directions

- **If you think you're coming down with a bug, you're already sick with the flu, or you have one of the infections listed above, then for an adult, squirt 2 dropperfuls of high-quality liquid zinc sulfate into your throat every three hours. Let it sit for one minute before swallowing. If the flu isn't making you nauseated and you can palate the zinc, you can do this up to five or six times a day (that is, two squirts of zinc every three hours for a total of 10 to 12 dropperfuls a day) for two days.**

- If your palate is more sensitive, you're welcome to try a milder Medical Medium Zinc Shock Therapy: 1 dropperful every three hours up to five times a day or 2 dropperfuls three times a day.

- In any version of Medical Medium Zinc Shock Therapy, after the two days, bring the zinc dosage down to what your supplement list says.

For children, here are the adjusted amounts of liquid zinc sulfate for this supplement therapy:

- **Ages 1 to 2:** 2 tiny drops (not dropperfuls) in juice, water, or directly in the mouth every three hours during waking hours

- **Ages 3 to 4:** 3 tiny drops (not dropperfuls) in juice, water, or directly in the mouth every three hours during waking hours

- **Ages 5 to 8:** 4 small drops (not dropperfuls) in juice, water, or directly in the mouth every three hours during waking hours

- **Ages 9 to 12:** 10 small drops (not dropperfuls) in juice, water, or directly in the mouth every three hours during waking hours

- **Ages 13 and up:** 1 dropperful directly in the mouth every four hours during waking hours

Because of children's special sensitive nature, it's especially important to get the right kind of liquid zinc sulfate, which you can find on my directory online at medicalmedium.com. Almost all companies make zinc that's aggressive in taste and hard to palate, often with harsh additives too.

Medical Medium Vitamin C Shock Therapy

Why does Medical Medium Vitamin C Shock Therapy bring healing to a new level? Because it takes a specific type of glucose that you'll find mainly in raw honey, pure maple syrup, and fresh-squeezed citrus to bind onto the right type of vitamin C to drive it into cells and organs. The raw honey and the squeezed orange combined attach themselves directly to the vitamin C, allowing this powerful delivery of antiviral, antibacterial healing nutrients to occur within the body.

Medical Medium Vitamin C Shock Therapy Directions

- **For Medical Medium Vitamin C Shock Therapy for adults, the ingredients are 2 500-milligram capsules of Micro-C, 1 cup of water (preferably warm), 2 teaspoons of raw honey, and the freshly squeezed juice from one orange.**

- **Here's how to prepare it: Open the Micro-C capsules and pour their powder into the warm water. Stir until dissolved. Add the raw honey and orange juice and stir well. Starting at the first sign of cold, flu, or any of the infections listed, drink this tonic every two hours during waking hours. You can do this for two days and then switch to the dosage in an individual supplement list, or you can use this technique throughout the duration of a cold or flu.**

- If you feel you need more vitamin C per drink, you can add more than 2 capsules of Micro-C to each. If you don't want to use raw honey, you can use 100 percent pure maple syrup (not maple-flavored syrup) in its place. If you don't like orange, you can substitute the juice of one lemon.

For children, here are the adjusted amounts of vitamin C for this supplement therapy:

- **Ages 1 to 2:** 1 500-milligram capsule Micro-C emptied and mixed with 1/2 cup water, 1 teaspoon raw honey, and the freshly squeezed juice from half an orange, every six hours during waking hours

- **Ages 3 to 4:** 1 500-milligram capsule Micro-C emptied and mixed with 1/2 cup water, 1 teaspoon raw honey, and the freshly squeezed juice from 1 orange, every five hours during waking hours

- **Ages 5 to 8:** 1 500-milligram capsule Micro-C emptied and mixed with 1 cup water, 2 teaspoons raw honey, and the freshly squeezed juice from 1 orange, every four hours during waking hours

- **Ages 9 to 12:** 1 500-milligram capsule Micro-C emptied and mixed with 1 cup water, 2 teaspoons raw honey, and the freshly squeezed juice from 1 orange, every two hours during waking hours

- **Ages 13 and up:** 2 500-milligram capsules Micro-C emptied and mixed with 1 cup water, 2 teaspoons raw honey, and the freshly squeezed juice from 1 orange, every three hours during waking hours

"When we become well, doubt melts away. We have energy to devote to our true purpose. We watch ourselves transform, and we believe in the good in life again. We get reacquainted with our path in this world. We find our way back home with peace in our heart and soul.

When we connect to our bodies, truly listen to them, and give them the nourishment they're yearning for, everything changes. True miracles happen."

— Anthony William, Medical Medium

CHAPTER 22

Medical Medium
28-Day Healing Cleanse

Our bodies love us unconditionally. They do not judge or blame or hold on to resentment. Day in and day out, all of our body systems—ones like the digestive, lymphatic, endocrine, and central nervous systems—are working for us without complaint. The immune system is constantly ready for battle, patrolling every part of the body looking for invaders.

We take all this for granted. We eat things our systems don't appreciate, indulge in foods to comfort our emotions rather than feed our bodies and souls. As we seek out snacks, meals, beverages, and desserts that temporarily keep emotions at bay, our bodies become the victims of our soul injuries. We get confused and misled and cross the line between what we think we like to eat and what our bodies need.

Eventually, the physical body begins to show wear and tear. It starts with small breakdowns (taking the form of first symptoms), then the larger breakdowns come (in the form of symptoms that lead to a label or diagnosis). Imagine a car running low on oil. For a while you can get by on the smallest amount of oil,

but at some point the oil will get too low. You'll turn on the car, the engine will heat up, cause friction, and *bang*—you'll blow a valve.

The human body is forever forgiving. Your body wants to heal. It *can* heal. Even after years of being ignored, mistreated, or misunderstood, your body will fight for you like nothing else and no one else can. When you tend to it in the right way, your body has the ability to rejuvenate and restore from the most extreme conditions and diseases.

You have to think of your body like an old friend in need. Imagine yourself reaching out a helping hand to this friend as she climbs out of a ravine. This is your commitment to use your free will and the power of your intention to give your body the support it's crying out for.

When we connect to our bodies, truly listen to them, and give them the nourishment they're yearning for, everything changes. True miracles happen.

When someone grows up with the pick of almost anything to eat, this can be a hard mind-set to change. Our food routines can feel like part of who we are. Hidden addictions and unproductive choices often go into them, though.

We all have cravings. It's important not to confuse these cravings with intuition. We may feel a strong desire to eat certain foods and mistake that desire for our bodies telling us we need that bacon cheeseburger, or that omelet.

Yet when people eat anything and everything under the sun, unknowingly subjecting the liver, pancreas, gallbladder, heart, and more to greasy, processed, fried-oil, and even dangerous gastronomic concoctions, it's because the soul and body are out of alignment—the bridge between the soul and the physical brain is tattered. That happens because the hardships we encounter on this earth can injure our souls. A gap is created, and within that gap, fear enters and takes its place. We search for ways to literally fill the gap that the fear resides in with food, or to push down other unpleasant emotions—except it doesn't last. Eating troublemaker foods, we get sicker. Our souls and physical bodies suffer more.

If you are struggling with your health in any way, the game has to change. Eating restorative foods—and eliminating foods that feed problems—is the most critical aspect of healing any illness or health condition.

The healing food plan I present in this chapter can move health mountains. It's like a restorative button for your body. Following these guidelines for four weeks will help reduce inflammation from illness—not just the conditions I cover in these chapters but also many more I didn't have room for in this book. It can make a huge difference in mental health. And the cleanse will help if you're healthy and just looking to lose weight, or if you want to maintain and maximize your potential.

I get that it's not just emotional desire that misleads people about the right foods to eat. It's social media, podcasts, articles, fads, advertisements, peer pressure, and health-care industry advice or trends that are supported by vast amounts of money and marketing promotion. There's always a new superfood in the news, a new story about this or that diet, a new rumor about what truly healthy food people mistakenly believe isn't good for you.

Now you get to tune out all the noise and guessing games. Focusing your food choices for 28 days on the options listed here will let you stop wasting your energy on the misinformation overload coming from sources that don't know why people are sick to begin with. It's not about deprivation in any way; it's about abundance. It's about repairing the bridge and sending fear away by restoring your physical body and mending your soul. This delicious, healing cleanse has brought profound results to countless people. It has changed people's lives. It can change yours.

If you follow the advice here to the letter, you'll find that your body will respond in untold ways. It has been waiting patiently for you to discover this information. It's ready to work with you. It's ready to reignite its healing powers. It's ready to heal.

THE PLAN

Here's the deal: for four weeks, eat only raw fruits, leafy greens, herbs, vegetables, and specific wild foods such as wild blueberries.

For best results, follow the plan below for the whole 28 days. While that's the best length of time, even just a week is likely to bring you significant results. Another alternative is one cleanse day per week. And if this doesn't feel like the right time for you to try the cleanse for any length of time, turn your attention to the other healing techniques throughout the book and come back to this chapter when you feel ready. On the other hand, if your health is in dire straits, or if you have a lot of weight to lose, you're welcome to extend the cleanse beyond the first month.

One reason this plan is so effective is that it maximizes the nutrition you get in every meal. Fruits, leafy greens, herbs, specific wild foods, and vegetables in their raw state contain the highest level of nutrients of any foods, in the form most readily available to your body. When you consume these nutrients in such a high quantity, you'll flood your body with the building blocks it craves. The vitamins, trace minerals, antiviral compounds, antibacterial compounds, antioxidants, minerals, phytochemical compounds, and other nourishing components will help cleanse and strengthen every system in your body.

Your liver and digestive system are some of those beneficiaries. Liver health and related digestive health have a major impact on immunity and overall health. Not to mention that normally, digestion takes up an enormous amount of your body's energy.

It's almost like your body has a daily to-do list. There are the things it *has* to attend to every day, like keeping your heart pumping and your lungs inflating and food moving through your intestinal tract. Then there are all the things it *wishes* it could get to—taking out the toxin trash, repairing critical tissue, and so much more—if only it had the time and support.

Imagine a wobbly doorknob in your home. One of these days, it's going to fall off, and you're going to have a real problem. Every day, you mean to fix it, but paying the bills and making food for your family and shoveling fresh snow outside take precedence—plus your screwdriver's gone missing. Same with the body. When it's overloaded with tough-to-digest foods and it's missing critical nutrients, those wish list items just keep getting put off.

The body processes uncooked fruits, leafy greens, herbs, some wild foods, and vegetables quickly and easily. These foods also have live enzymes, which makes digestion even smoother. When your body's not busy processing heavy fats and proteins, or additives and irritants, it frees up hours every day for your body to rebuild itself on a cellular level. It's as though someone appeared on the front step ready to snowblow your sidewalk for free, and handed you a full toolkit at the same time. Suddenly, nothing would be holding you back from fixing the doorknob—or the nails poking out of the floor, or the dripping faucet.

Note that while meat, fish, and grains can have helpful nutrients, they can also be tough for the body to break down when you may already have low hydrochloric acid and low bile reserves because your stomach glands and liver have been tattered or beaten down along the way from the stress of a high-fat diet. When our bodies are overloaded by illness or toxicity or even just sluggishness, we lose the ability to process these foods in an optimal way. The plan below gives us the reboot we need to come back to these foods with digestive vigor.

It also helps cleanse and rebuild the soul. As your body remineralizes, detoxifies, mends, and rejuvenates, your soul learns that powerhouse foods like fruit are the true sustenance that will bring it comfort. When you come out on the other side of the 28 days, foods that you know are detrimental to your health won't hold the same sway they once did.

Your soul, spirit, and body will also be operating on a new frequency. Each piece of fruit you eat, each raw spinach leaf, holds a living vibration. When you consume it, you assimilate that. The living food brings you back to life.

Are you ready to kick-start your healing process? Then for the next four weeks, eat the most healing foods on the planet—and nothing else.

In other words, consume raw (organic if possible) fruits, leafy greens, herbs, vegetables, and some recommended wild foods, with an emphasis on keeping fat intake low. Limit or remove salt intake, too—only add a sprinkle of high-quality sea salt or rock salt to a dish if you feel you need it to stay on course.

Stay hydrated with plenty of water, coconut water (that's not pink or red), herbal tea, and/or fresh juice from the recipes chapter to follow. (The hot water for tea doesn't destroy the nutrients in the herbs; it releases their medicinal properties.)

Over the course of the day, try to get in 1 liter of water (roughly equivalent to 32 ounces, or 4 cups). That's not counting the lemon or lime water you drink upon waking, or any lemon or lime water or tea you choose to drink just before bed—this liter of water is in addition to those, something you drink between meals and snacks as you go about your day. Any coconut water or fresh juice you choose to drink during the day is also in *addition* to that liter of water. Feel free to squeeze some lemon or lime into your drinking water. If a liter of water feels like too much, even spread out every few hours, don't force it all down. On the other hand, you're welcome to do more than 1 liter. If you feel you require more fluids at any point throughout the cleanse, don't hold back; allow yourself to improve your water levels.

(As ever, be mindful not to drink your water too close to celery juice—make sure to space them at least 15 to 30 minutes apart.)

If you're suffering from a condition for which this book lists a specific protocol of supplements and healing foods, then feel free to add those to the mix.

For all of your cleanse questions, I recommend *Medical Medium*'s companion book, *Cleanse to Heal*. There you'll find "The Insider Cleanse Guide," which includes insights about hunger and portions, cleansing while pregnant or breastfeeding, how to interpret possible healing reactions, and how to handle cleanse interruptions. *Cleanse to Heal* also offers additional recipes, information on supplementation while cleansing, and answers about symptom and condition complications (for example, if you're dealing with gastroparesis), plus it provides further cleanse options, whether you want to embark on more advanced cleansing or you'd like to start with a shorter cleanse.

Now let's get into what a day on the 28-Day Healing Cleanse looks like. Get ready for the healing to begin.

Early Morning

Start the day with 16 to 32 ounces of lemon or lime water. After at least 15 to 30 minutes, move on to 16 to 32 ounces of fresh celery juice. (Cucumber juice is an option if you're struggling to like celery juice. Although cucumber juice will not have the same benefits as celery juice, it's there for you if needed.) This routine will do wonders to maximize the dotox work your body performed overnight and hydrate you for the day ahead.

If you don't have any of these options for morning beverages, drinking 16 to 32 ounces of plain water instead is fine. At least try to squeeze lemon into it.

Once you've finished your celery juice (or cucumber juice or water), wait at least another 15 to 30 minutes before you move on to breakfast or cleanse beverage options such as herbal tea or coconut water.

Breakfast

Make a fruit smoothie for breakfast. A good baseline recipe is three bananas, two dates, and 1 cup of berries. If this doesn't fill you up, don't hesitate to add more bananas or berries. This can be switched out for the Medical Medium Heavy Metal Detox Smoothie or one of the other smoothies from the next chapter. Don't deprive yourself—this isn't about going hungry.

If a smoothie's not an option, try for fresh fruit. Papayas, pears, melons, and mangoes make delicious options.

Healthy smoothie add-ins are greens such as a handful of spinach or cilantro; two stalks of celery; or a teaspoon of barley grass juice powder. Just make sure that fruit remains the main ingredient. Do not deviate from these recommendations by bringing in protein powders and such.

Mid-morning

If you get hungry, make another fruit smoothie as described above (or make two servings first thing, and have your second serving now). Alternatively, you can snack on fresh fruit, cucumber slices, and/or celery sticks.

Lunch

At midday, make a salad using one of the recipes in the next chapter, or using this basic recipe: assemble spinach, lettuce, and cucumbers as the base, then toss in the fruits of your choice. Examples include berries, sliced mangoes, papaya chunks, grapes, and orange or grapefruit segments. For dressing, you can blend a handful of cilantro with the juice from two oranges (plus garlic and/or fresh ginger to taste, if you'd like). This is meant to be a large salad, so make sure you eat enough to feel full.

Optional additions include chopped cabbage, celery, or cauliflower; arugula or baby kale; sprouts; and scallions.

If you're opting for one of the salad recipes from the next chapter, look for an all-raw one, unless you're doing the modified version of the cleanse that includes steamed options. (Read more in "Modifications.")

If you have chewing complications or need a fast lunch option, feel free to blend your salad or chop it finely in the food processor. You can also make a food-processor grind-up of apples with cauliflower or apples with cabbage. Or you can select the Spinach Soup recipe from the next chapter.

Mid-afternoon

As you become hungry throughout the afternoon, snack on any fruits of your choice. Good examples include apple or pear slices, dates, oranges, and grapes. It's an option to munch on celery sticks alongside each serving of fruit. A spoonful of raw honey also makes a great pick-me-up.

Dinner

For a creamy suppertime Spinach Soup, turn to the recipes chapter. It can be a lot of fun to eat this dish served over cucumber noodles, which you can make with a kitchen gadget such as a julienne slicer or spiral slicer. These tools make it easy to turn vegetables into long, slim, crunchy strips. Keep in mind that while zucchini noodles have become popular (and are much healthier than wheat pasta), raw zucchini can be a bit uncomfortable to digest. If maximum healing and detoxification are your priorities, save the zucchini (and carrot and butternut squash) noodles for when you've completed this cleanse.

You're also welcome to eat the Spinach Soup ingredients as a salad instead of blended, or you're welcome to pick a different recipe from the next chapter for dinner. Preferably, look for a raw recipe, unless you're doing a cleanse modification and need a cooked option.

Evening

If you're still hungry after dinner, snack on an apple, orange, and/or one date. Evening beverage options are the herbal teas recommended in this book, lemon or lime water, plain water, or coconut water (that's not pink or red).

MODIFICATIONS

You don't have to eat the exact same menu every day. Try out different recipes from the next chapter. Cycle through different salad and soup greens if you'd like, too.

Pay no mind to the trend that says too much of a particular raw, leafy green such as spinach will cause you harm. That's misinformation. If you eat raw Spinach Soup every day for a month, it will be the best thing you've ever done for yourself. Don't be afraid to eat as many greens as you'd like.

It's also okay to mono eat an entire meal of just one fruit. For example, you can spend the morning eating only bananas if they're calling your name, as long as you've also had your celery juice. If not, you can balance them with a few celery sticks, or eating your bananas with lettuce is another option. If you find yourself eating a lot of one food in particular, many grocery stores, co-ops, and farmers will sell you cases of produce at a discount.

The recipes chapter will show you that you have options. Just remember your path: raw fruits, leafy greens, herbs, wild foods, and vegetables.

If your gut needs healing, remember this is one of the reasons you're starting the day with a glass of fresh, plain celery juice on an empty stomach. (For more information, see Chapter 17, "Gut Health.")

If blood sugar or energy levels are of particular concern, employ the grazing technique I describe in Chapter 8, "Adrenal Fatigue."

For quicker progress, try a week or more with no avocados or other radical fats. Also try cutting out added salt entirely.

And if, on the other hand, you're okay with a less rapid rate of cleansing and healing, add a half avocado two to three times a week at dinner.

You can also pull back the reins on this diet by swapping out the Spinach Soup dinner for a meal of simply steamed potatoes, vegetables, or one of the cooked recipes from the next chapter. This can be part of a less intense cleanse, and it can also be an excellent way to transition into or out of an all-raw cleanse.

And remember, *Cleanse to Heal* is there for you as a companion resource. That book offers more insights into cleanse modifications (including an entire chapter on adaptations and substitutions), plus more cleanse options and more recipes—as well as options for how to deal with symptom or condition complications.

TRANSITIONING

When you're adjusting to this way of eating, you may miss certain comfort foods. In their absence, one source of comfort is that this isn't forever. The cleanse is for a month. If you're 40, you've lived through 480 of those things. You've blinked before, and a month has gone by.

As you're venturing into your cleanse, your liver will start to do its work, releasing toxic troublemakers it's been storing for a long time—in some cases years, or even decades. These troublemakers include pesticides, herbicides, fungicides, toxic heavy metals (such as aluminum, mercury, and copper), petrochemicals (such as exhaust fumes from cars and gasoline fumes), plastics, colognes, perfume, scented candles, air fresheners, toxic byproduct and debris from pathogens (such as Epstein-Barr virus, shingles, herpes simplex, cytomegalovirus, and HHV-6), stored-up adrenaline from fight-or-flight or caffeine use, and stored up fats from a high-fat diet for years if not decades before your cleanse. It's natural to need extra rest during your cleanse, and extra sensitivity and caring from loved ones. (For spiritual support, turn to Chapter 24, "Soul-Healing Meditations and Techniques," and Chapter 25, "Essential Angels.")

For information on how we're exposed to these and more toxic troublemakers in our everyday lives, refer to *Cleanse to Heal*. That book also offers answers about your body's healing process as it releases these troublemakers, plus further emotional, spiritual, and soul-healing insights. Here's a peek into the emotional aspect of cleansing:

As your cells release old, stored-up adrenaline from emotional upsets and residues from troublemaker foods you ate during those difficult times in the past, cravings and memories may burst to the surface of your consciousness. Consider each of these mental twinges a gift. It means a pocket of toxins is leaving you, and even some emotions associated with them. If you give in to the craving, it may make you feel momentarily satisfied, but you'll cut off the detox process and seal remaining toxins in the liver until you can go back to cleansing.

This cleanse could also bliss you out. We don't just suppress challenging emotions stored in our cells—we also suppress joy. Sometimes we feel overburdened by the world's worries, so we feel we don't deserve to be happy. This detox plan will help reset that thinking. Cleansing is a spiritual experience when the information for the cleanse comes from above, as this does. As your body pushes out the toxic clutter, your brain will clear. You could find yourself experiencing realizations about who you truly are, and about the direction you want your life to go. Embrace that.

Listen to it. Your happiness matters to the good of humanity.

As for transitioning on the other end: Don't go out for a meat lover's pizza, mac and cheese, or cheeseburgers to celebrate the day you finish the cleanse. Don't order a chocolate ice-cream cake. Your liver and digestive system will become overloaded if you reintroduce large amounts of fat right away. Be patient with the process. Bit by bit, here and there, you have the option to start adding in some cooked vegetables and legumes; some healthy grains such as millet, oats, and quinoa; a little more fat (stick to healthy fats); or lean protein. If you want to enjoy your best health, then keep the foods listed in Chapter 19, "What Not to Eat," out of your diet for good.

And if you feel so great on the cleanse that you want to keep going, or keep going with minor modifications such as a bit more avocado, nuts, seeds, coconut, or cold-pressed olive oil, or a cooked meal here and there, then I'm not saying you should stop yourself from doing that. If you want to make the Medical Medium tools from the 28-Day Healing Cleanse—which means specific fruits, leafy greens, herbs, wild foods, and vegetables—your way of life, go for it.

Everyone's different. Everyone has different pathogens, such as viruses and bacteria, inside of their bodies. Some have one variety of Epstein-Barr virus, some have two EBV varieties, plus a variety of shingles and/or another pathogen, such as *Streptococcus*. Some people have more toxic heavy metals in their brain

or liver. And some people have more of one specific toxic heavy metal. Some people have more pesticides and herbicides, and some people have more air fresheners and gasoline inside their liver. Women's and men's immune systems work differently. And everyone has different emotional challenges and circumstances, different living and financial circumstances, and different health histories that can lead to lowered immune systems at different times in their lives and different ages. On a spiritual level, we all have different souls.

In practical terms, these differences in what each of us is up against mean that we'll make different choices in how to move forward after a cleanse. Some people, for example, need animal protein in their non-cleanse lives to feel all is right with the world. Some feel that a bowl of brown rice with salmon at lunch is what keeps them going. Others don't.

Feel it out for yourself by using the Medical Medium tools and protocols that work for where you are in your life. There are over a thousand combinations that you can create for yourself. Venture in a little at a time. Remember that your body is looking out for you. It wants to heal. Understanding the information here about how your body works and what it needs to overcome your symptoms and conditions—and rise out of the ashes—makes all the difference. If you start by giving your body a bit of what it needs at a time and take it day by day, you can bring yourself to a place of peace.

"If fruit makes a comeback, it's thanks to readers like you who took this information to heart and made change."

— Anthony William, Medical Medium

MEDICAL MEDIUM 28-DAY HEALING CLEANSE SAMPLE MENU PLAN

These sample menu plans offer ideas about how to structure your days and weeks on the 28-Day Healing Cleanse. For the recipes that it references, turn to the next chapter.

You'll notice a great deal of variety in these sample menus. That's in order to show you the range of options available for inspiration. If you prefer, you are more than welcome to keep it simple. Go back over the meal-by-meal guidelines in this chapter to ground yourself in the basics and take it from there. You could select a handful of meal options from these samples that appeal to you and create a menu that seems doable.

Feel free to customize your menus using the other suggestions in this chapter. For example, you could decide to drink the Heavy Metal Detox Smoothie for breakfast every morning if that's a priority. You could decide to graze for blood sugar support, snacking on cleanse options every hour and a half to two hours. In the evenings, you may decide to sip one of the tea recipes from Chapter 18, "Freeing Your Brain and Body of Toxins," for specific support.

The recipes in these menu plans are all raw options. If you're okay with a less rapid rate of cleansing, you'll find cooked options at the end of the next chapter that you can select at dinnertime. On the other hand, if you want a faster rate of cleansing, you're welcome to omit avocado from any of the raw dinner recipes in these menus.

This is about customizing your cleanse using the Medical Medium tools and information here in this book to make the cleanse work best in your life.

Week 1 Sample Menu Plan

	DAY 1	DAY 2	DAY 3
UPON WAKING	16 to 32 ounces Lemon or Lime Water	16 to 32 ounces Lemon or Lime Water	16 to 32 ounces Lemon or Lime Water
BEFORE BREAKFAST (at least 15 to 30 minutes later)	16 to 32 ounces Celery Juice	16 to 32 ounces Celery Juice	16 to 32 ounces Celery Juice
BREAKFAST (at least 15 to 30 minutes later)	Heavy Metal Detox Smoothie	Mojito Fruit Salad	½ Maradol Papaya with sliced Kiwis and Bananas
MORNING SNACK	Apples	Apple, Celery, and Cucumber Juice	Fresh Orange Juice
LUNCH	Cucumber Noodles with Bruschetta Topping	Banana Strawberry Salad	Apple Salad
AFTERNOON SNACK (as you become hungry)	Dates & Celery Sticks	Defrosted Wild Blueberries with 1 teaspoon of Raw Honey	Oranges and Cucumber Slices
DINNER	Mango Salad	Israeli Salad	Leafy Greens with Avocado Dressing
EVENING (optional)	Apple Slices with one Date Ginger Tea	Orange Thyme Tea	Apple Slices Coconut Water

Week 1 Sample Menu Plan

	DAY 4	DAY 5	DAY 6	DAY 7
UPON WAKING	16 to 32 ounces Lemon or Lime Water	16 to 32 ounces Lemon or Lime Water	16 to 32 ounces Lemon or Lime Water	16 to 32 ounces Lemon or Lime Water
BEFORE BREAKFAST (at least 15 to 30 minutes later)	16 to 32 ounces Celery Juice	16 to 32 ounces Celery Juice	16 to 32 ounces Celery Juice	16 to 32 ounces Celery Juice
BREAKFAST (at least 15 to 30 minutes later)	Heavy Metal Detox Smoothie	Watermelon, Canteloupe, or Honeydew	Honey Berry Bowl	Heavy Metal Detox Smoothie
MORNING SNACK	Sliced Peaches	Apple, Celery, and Cucumber Juice	Coconut Water with Spirulina and Barley Grass Juice Powder	Aloe Water, then wait 15 minutes and eat a Banana
LUNCH	Spinach Soup	Mango Salsa with Vegetable Crudités for dipping (e.g., Radishes, Cucumber, Celery, Bell Pepper, Asparagus	Banana Lettuce Boats	Nori Sheets filled with Butter Lettuce, Green Onions, Maradol Papaya or Mango, and Tomato. Dip in Raw Honey and Orange Juice Dressing (see Banana Salad recipe)
AFTERNOON SNACK (one to two hours after lunchtime)	Plums and Kiwis	Raspberries	Grapes with Celery Sticks	Cucumber Juice
DINNER	Chopped Salad	Sprout Salad with Orange Honey Dressing	Red Cabbage Tacos with Mango Ginger Sauce	Burrito Bowl
EVENING (optional)	Orange with one Date Lemon Water	Apple Slices Lemon Balm Tea	One Date Chaga Tea	Apple Slices with Orange Hibiscus Tea

Week 2 Sample Menu Plan

	DAY 1	DAY 2	DAY 3
UPON WAKING	16 to 32 ounces Lemon or Lime Water	16 to 32 ounces Lemon or Lime Water	16 to 32 ounces Lemon or Lime Water
BEFORE BREAKFAST (at least 15 to 30 minutes later)	16 to 32 ounces Celery Juice	16 to 32 ounces Celery Juice	16 to 32 ounces Celery Juice
BREAKFAST (at least 15 to 30 minutes later)	Heavy Metal Detox Smoothie	Vanilla and Cinnamon Cantaloupe Smoothie	½ to 1 Maradol Papaya blended smooth into a Pudding
MORNING SNACK	Oranges	Watermelon	Turmeric Ginger Shots and Strawberries dipped in Date Caramel Sauce (see Banana Lettuce Boats recipe)
LUNCH	Banana Nori Wraps	Israeli Salad	Apple Salad
AFTERNOON SNACK (as you become hungry)	Cauliflower Florets and Apple Slices	Honey Berry Bowl	Oranges
DINNER	Chopped Salad	Banana Lettuce Boats	Massaged Kale Salad
EVENING (optional)	Apple Slices with one Date Ginger Tea	Orange Thyme Tea	Apple Slices Coconut Water

Week 2 Sample Menu Plan

	DAY 4	DAY 5	DAY 6	DAY 7
UPON WAKING	16 to 32 ounces Lemon or Lime Water	16 to 32 ounces Lemon or Lime Water	16 to 32 ounces Lemon or Lime Water	16 to 32 ounces Lemon or Lime Water
BEFORE BREAKFAST (at least 15 to 30 minutes later)	16 to 32 ounces Celery Juice	16 to 32 ounces Celery Juice	16 to 32 ounces Celery Juice	16 to 32 ounces Celery Juice
BREAKFAST (at least 15 to 30 minutes later)	Heavy Metal Detox Smoothie	Nectarines, Peaches, and/or Apricots	Layered Fruit Salad	Heavy Metal Detox Smoothie
MORNING SNACK	Apples or Applesauce made by blending fresh Apples	Banana Berry Smoothie	Pear Slices with Cinnamon	Blackberries
LUNCH	Mojito Fruit Salad with Celery Sticks, Romaine or Butter Lettuce Leaves, and Cucumber Slices	Spinach, Arugula, Celery, and Cucumber Salad topped with Mango Salsa	Banana Salad	½ Maradol Papaya or more with defrosted Wild Blueberries and 1 teaspoon Raw Honey
AFTERNOON SNACK (one to two hours after lunchtime)	Chopped Tomato, Radishes, and Cucumber with Orange or Lemon Juice	Grapes	Apple and Greens Juice	Cherries
DINNER	Spinach Soup with side of apple slices	Red Cabbage Tacos with Mango Ginger Sauce	Burrito Bowl	Spinach Soup over Cucumber Noodles
EVENING (optional)	Orange with one Date Lemon Water	Apple Slices Lemon Balm Tea	One Date Chaga Tea	Apple Slices with Orange Hibiscus Tea

Week 3 Sample Menu Plan

	DAY 1	DAY 2	DAY 3
UPON WAKING	16 to 32 ounces Lemon or Lime Water	16 to 32 ounces Lemon or Lime Water	16 to 32 ounces Lemon or Lime Water
BEFORE BREAKFAST (at least 15 to 30 minutes later)	16 to 32 ounces Celery Juice	16 to 32 ounces Celery Juice	16 to 32 ounces Celery Juice
BREAKFAST (at least 15 to 30 minutes later)	Heavy Metal Detox Smoothie	Banana Berry Smoothie	Mojito Fruit Salad
MORNING SNACK	Tangerines	Cucumber Juice	Turmeric Ginger Shots and Apple Slices
LUNCH	Banana Salad	Spinach Soup	Honey Berry Bowl alongside or scooped into Butter Lettuce Leaves (Add Sliced Bananas or Mango if you prefer a heartier meal.)
AFTERNOON SNACK (as you become hungry)	Kiwis	Asparagus and Bell Pepper dipped into Honey Orange Juice Dressing (see Banana Salad recipe)	Radishes, Cucumbers, and Dates
DINNER	Sprout Salad with Tomato Mango Dressing	Banana Romaine Boats	Mango Salad
EVENING (optional)	Apple Slices with one Date Ginger Tea	Orange Thyme Tea	Apple Slices Coconut Water

Week 3 Sample Menu Plan

	DAY 4	DAY 5	DAY 6	DAY 7
UPON WAKING	16 to 32 ounces Lemon or Lime Water	16 to 32 ounces Lemon or Lime Water	16 to 32 ounces Lemon or Lime Water	16 to 32 ounces Lemon or Lime Water
BEFORE BREAKFAST (at least 15 to 30 minutes later)	16 to 32 ounces Celery Juice	16 to 32 ounces Celery Juice	16 to 32 ounces Celery Juice	16 to 32 ounces Celery Juice
BREAKFAST (at least 15 to 30 minutes later)	Heavy Metal Detox Smoothie	Grapes and Banana	Watermelon Aloe Slushy	Heavy Metal Detox Smoothie
MORNING SNACK	Bananas	Coconut Water with Spirulina and Barley Grass Juice Powder	Mango and Celery Sticks	Maradol Papaya
LUNCH	Israeli Salad	Mango Salsa Romaine Boats	Apple Salad	Spinach Soup with Vegetable Crudités to dip
AFTERNOON SNACK (one to two hours after lunchtime)	Fresh Figs and Celery Sticks	Bananas and Mâche	Apricots	Bell Pepper Halves topped with Tomato Slices and optional Sprouts
DINNER	Cucumber Noodles with Bruschetta Topping	Cherry "Ice Cream" made by processing Frozen Bananas or Mango and Frozen Cherries in the blender or food processor	Red Cabbage Tacos with Mango Ginger Sauce	Leafy Green Salad with Avocado Dressing
EVENING (optional)	Orange with one Date Lemon Water	Apple Slices Lemon Balm Tea	One Date Chaga Tea	Apple Slices with Orange Hibiscus Tea

Week 4 Sample Menu Plan

	DAY 1	DAY 2	DAY 3
UPON WAKING	16 to 32 ounces Lemon or Lime Water	16 to 32 ounces Lemon or Lime Water	16 to 32 ounces Lemon or Lime Water
BEFORE BREAKFAST (at least 15 to 30 minutes later)	16 to 32 ounces Celery Juice	16 to 32 ounces Celery Juice	16 to 32 ounces Celery Juice
BREAKFAST (at least 15 to 30 minutes later)	Heavy Metal Detox Smoothie	Apples and Greens Juice	Mangoes
MORNING SNACK	Fresh Berries (e.g., Mulberries, Raspberries, Blackberries, and/or Blueberries)	Vanilla and Cinnamon Cantaloupe Smoothie	Dates, Apples, and Celery Sticks
LUNCH	Banana Nori Wraps	Layered Fruit Salad	Apple Salad
AFTERNOON SNACK (as you become hungry)	Apple Slices with Cinnamon	Cherry Tomatoes, Celery Sticks, and Dates	Coconut Water with Spirulina and Barley Grass Juice Powder
DINNER	Cucumber Noodles with Bruschetta Topping	Massaged Kale Salad	Chopped Salad
EVENING (optional)	Apple Slices with one Date Ginger Tea	Orange Thyme Tea	Apple Slices Coconut Water

Week 4 Sample Menu Plan

	DAY 4	DAY 5	DAY 6	DAY 7
UPON WAKING	16 to 32 ounces Lemon or Lime Water	16 to 32 ounces Lemon or Lime Water	16 to 32 ounces Lemon or Lime Water	16 to 32 ounces Lemon or Lime Water
BEFORE BREAKFAST (at least 15 to 30 minutes later)	16 to 32 ounces Celery Juice	16 to 32 ounces Celery Juice	16 to 32 ounces Celery Juice	16 to 32 ounces Celery Juice
BREAKFAST (at least 15 to 30 minutes later)	Heavy Metal Detox Smoothie	Banana Cherry Smoothie	Honeydew Melon	Heavy Metal Detox Smoothie
MORNING SNACK	Raspberries and Cucumber Slices	Grapefruit	Maradol Papaya with Lime Juice	Pears and Apples
LUNCH	Banana Strawberry Salad	Tomato Mango Dressing (see Sprout Salad recipe) with Vegetable crudités (e.g., Celery, Cucumber, Bell Pepper, Cauliflower, Radish, Asparagus, Cabbage, Lettuce)	Spinach Soup over Cucumber Noodles	Israeli Salad
AFTERNOON SNACK (one to two hours after lunchtime)	Aloe Water, wait 15 minutes then Orange Wedges	Grapes	Mango	Apple, Celery, and Cucumber Juice
DINNER	Sprout Salad with Dressing of Choice from recipes chapter, wrapped in optional Nori Sheets, Lettuce, or Cabbage Leaves	Apple Salad	Burrito Bowl	Banana Salad
EVENING (optional)	Orange with one Date Lemon Water	Apple Slices Lemon Balm Tea	One Date Chaga Tea	Apple Slices with Orange Hibiscus Tea

"You have to think of your body like an old friend in need. Imagine yourself reaching out a helping hand to this friend as she climbs out of a ravine. This is your commitment to use your free will and the power of your intention to give your body the support it's crying out for.

When we connect to our bodies, truly listen to them, and give them the nourishment they're yearning for, everything changes. True miracles happen."

— Anthony William, Medical Medium

CHAPTER 23

Medical Medium
28-Day Healing Cleanse Recipes

When preparing juices and other recipes with apples, cucumbers, and other fruits and vegetables that have edible skins, you can keep the skins on if a recipe does not specify and the items are organic, or you're welcome to peel them. If they're conventional, peel and discard the skins—or if you can't peel the conventional fruit or vegetable for any reason, wash it with vigor before using.

LEMON OR LIME WATER

Makes 1 serving

While it sounds simple, don't overlook lemon or lime water as a powerful part of your daily routine. This easy hydration source takes only a moment to prepare, is extremely beneficial for everyone, and brings your water to life!

½ lemon or 2 limes, freshly cut

16 ounces (2 cups) water

Squeeze the juice from the freshly cut lemon or limes into the water, straining seeds if necessary.

Wait at least 15 to 20 minutes and ideally 30 minutes after you finish drinking your lemon or lime water before you consume your celery juice or anything else.

TIPS

- If you prefer 32 ounces (4 cups) of lemon or lime water upon rising, that's a great way to give yourself extra hydration and cleansing support. Simply double the recipe and enjoy.

- In your daily life, it's best to drink at least two or more 16-ounce lemon or lime waters over the course of a day. A great routine is to drink one upon rising, another in the afternoon, and another one hour before bed.

- Limes vary in size and juiciness. If your limes are dry, use two limes per 16 ounces of water, as the recipe calls for, to get enough juice. If your limes are big and juicy, you may only need half of a lime.

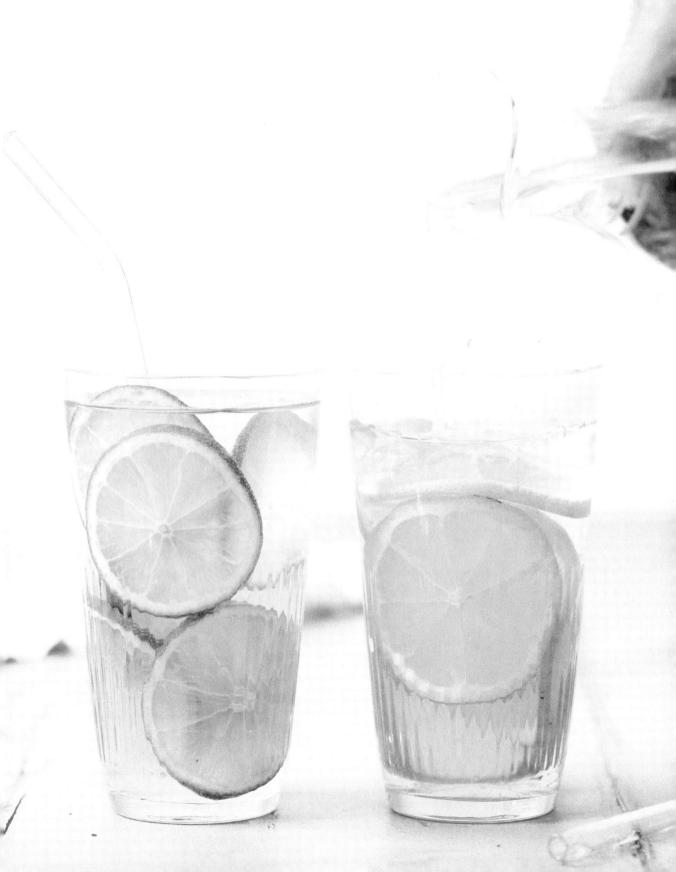

CELERY JUICE

Makes 1 serving

This simple herbal extraction has an incredible ability to create sweeping improvements for all kinds of health issues when consumed in the right way. That's why celery juice is an important component of the 28-Day Healing Cleanse and all the other cleanses in the Medical Medium book series. It's an ideal way to start your day even when you're not cleansing.

1 bunch of celery

Trim about a quarter inch off the base of the celery bunch, if desired, to break apart the stalks.

Rinse the celery.

Run the celery through the juicer of your choice. Strain the juice, if desired, to remove any grit or stray pieces of pulp. Drink immediately, on an empty stomach, for best results. Wait at least 15 to 30 minutes before consuming anything else.

If you don't have a juicer, you can make celery juice in a blender. Here's how:

Trim about a quarter inch off the base of the celery bunch, if desired, to break apart the stalks. Rinse the celery. Place the celery on a clean cutting board and chop into roughly 1-inch pieces. Place the chopped celery in a high-speed blender and blend until smooth. (Don't add water.) Use your blender's tamping tool if needed. Strain the liquefied celery well; a nut milk bag is handy for this. Drink immediately, on an empty stomach, for best results. Wait at least 15 to 30 minutes before consuming anything else.

TIPS

- Steer clear of putting additional ingredients such as lemon, apple, ginger, or leafy greens in your celery juice. While these are wonderful foods, celery juice only offers its full benefits when consumed alone.

- If you're not going to be able to drink your full batch of celery juice right away, the best way to store it is in a glass jar, with a sealed lid, in the fridge. Freshly juiced celery retains its healing benefits for about 24 hours. It does lose potency by the hour. If you have no choice but to keep it for longer than 24 hours, it's still worth juicing ahead and consuming it when you can.

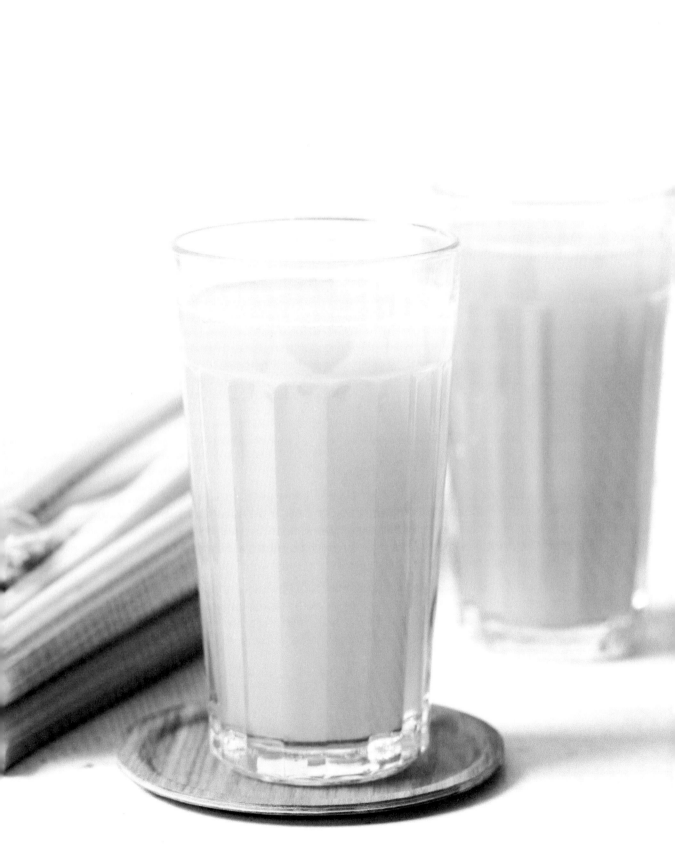

CUCUMBER JUICE

Fresh cucumber juice is an alternative rejuvenation tonic. Highly alkalizing and hydrating, cucumber juice has the ability to cleanse and detox the entire body. Its mildly sweet flavor makes it easy to drink.

2 large cucumbers

Rinse the cucumbers and run them through the juicer of your choice. Drink immediately, on an empty stomach, for best results.

If you don't have access to a juicer, here's how you can make it instead:

Rinse the cucumbers, chop them, and blend them in a high-speed blender until smooth. (Don't add water.) Strain the liquefied cucumber well; a nut milk bag is handy for this. Drink immediately, on an empty stomach, for best results.

TIPS

- Fresh cucumber juice is a good alternative to celery juice if you're not able to find celery or you really struggle with the flavor of celery juice. While cucumber juice is an incredible healing drink, it does not offer the same healing benefits as celery juice, though, so it's important to include celery juice daily as much as possible. For most people, the taste of celery juice becomes more enjoyable with consistent consumption.

- Steer clear of putting additional ingredients such as lemon, apple, ginger, or leafy greens in your cucumber juice. While these are wonderful foods, cucumber juice offers the most benefits when consumed alone. Instead, enjoy a mixed green juice at another time of day if you wish, such as the Apples and Greens Juice on page 306.

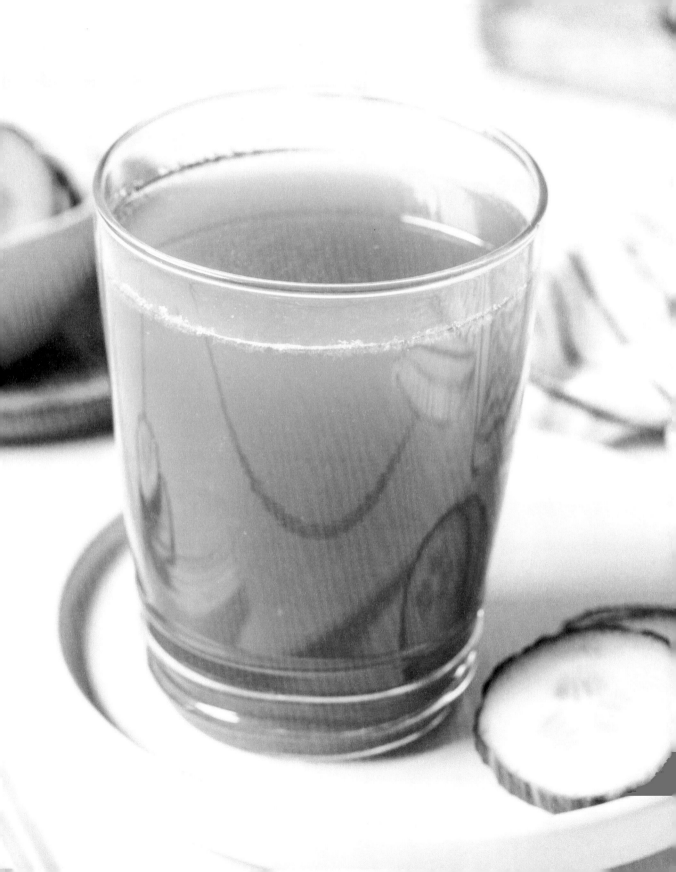

APPLES AND GREENS JUICE

A refreshing green juice can be an energizing start to the day or the perfect afternoon or pre-dinner pick-me-up. Packed full of healing nutrients and critical mineral salts, this juice makes it easy to consume a large amount of the precious leafy greens we all need.

½ cucumber

4 to 6 cups tightly packed leafy greens, such as spinach, romaine lettuce, or kale

2 medium-sized red apples

½ cup tightly packed fresh cilantro or parsley

½ lemon

1-inch piece of fresh ginger (optional)

Juice the cucumber, leafy greens, apples, cilantro or parsley, lemon, and ginger (if using) in a juicer. Serve immediately.

TIPS

- If you can't access cucumbers or don't favor them, you can swap in celery stalks for the cucumber.

- For a milder-tasting green juice, stick with spinach or romaine. If you are used to drinking green juices or like a stronger green flavor, you could try kale. Or feel free to use a blend of all three or experiment with other leafy greens you like.

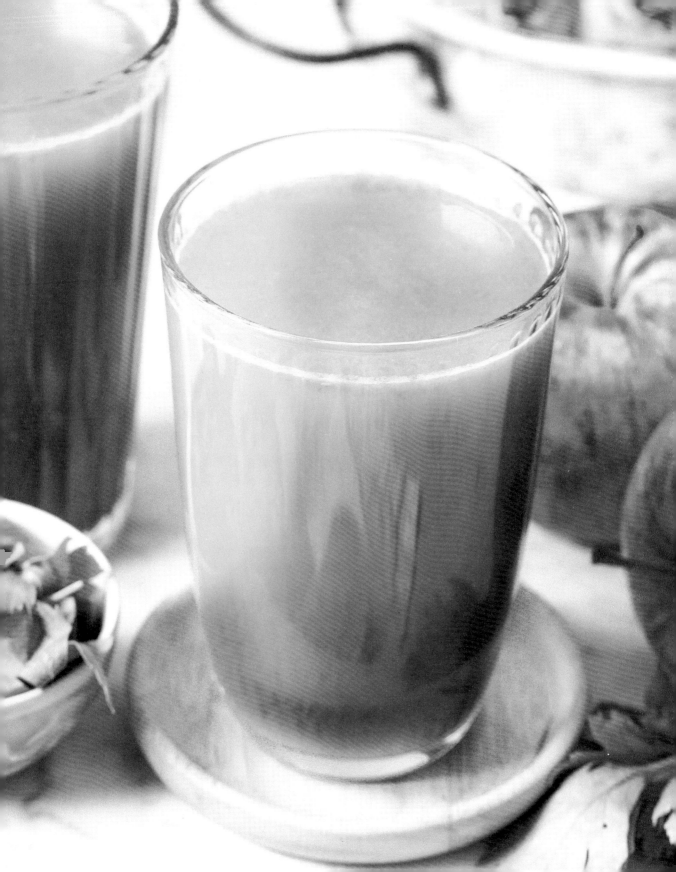

ALOE WATER

Makes 1 serving

While the taste of aloe may take some getting used to, it will be well worth the effort. As you drink your aloe water, think about all of the amazing benefits that your liver, your adrenals, and the rest of your body will reap from this amazing healing food.

2- to 4-inch piece of fresh aloe leaf

2 cups (16 ounces) water

This recipe is based on using a large, store-bought aloe leaf, which you can find in the produce section of many grocery stores. If you're using a homegrown aloe plant, it will likely have smaller, skinnier leaves, so cut off more. Either way, avoid using the bitter base of the leaf.

Carefully slice your section of aloe leaf open, filleting it as if it were a fish and trimming away the green skin and spikes. Scoop out the clear gel and place it in the blender.

Add the water to the blender and blend for 10 to 20 seconds, until the aloe is thoroughly liquefied.

Drink immediately, on an empty stomach, for best results.

TIPS

- Save the remainder of the aloe leaf by wrapping the cut end in a damp towel or plastic wrap and storing it in the refrigerator for up to two weeks.

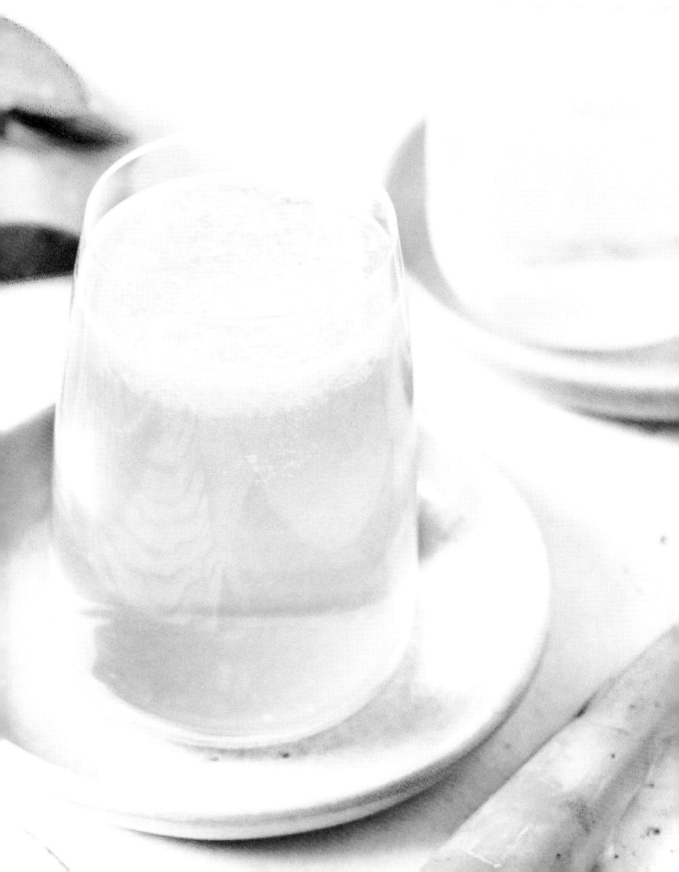

THYME TEA AND THYME WATER

Thyme Tea and Thyme Water are both powerful antiviral drinks you can incorporate daily or as often as possible to receive their healing benefits.

THYME TEA

Makes 1 serving

2 sprigs fresh thyme or 2 teaspoons dried thyme

1 cup hot filtered or spring water

Juice of ½ lemon and/ or 1 teaspoon raw honey (optional)

Place the thyme in a mug and pour hot water over the herb, allowing it to steep for 15 minutes or more. Remove the thyme sprigs or strain the tea, especially if you're using dried thyme. Sweeten with lemon juice and/or raw honey.

THYME WATER

Makes 4 to 8 cups

4 to 8 cups filtered or spring water

8 sprigs fresh thyme or 1 tablespoon dried thyme

Optional additions: fresh lemon slices or freshly squeezed lemon juice, raw honey, berries, cucumber slices, mint

Fill a jug or pitcher with room temperature water and add the thyme. Steep at room temperature on the counter overnight. In the morning, remove or strain out the thyme and add lemon juice or raw honey or any optional ingredients you'd like.

TIPS

- Fresh thyme can be found in the produce section of your local supermarket or health food store. Thyme is also very easy to grow and can produce abundantly in both containers and home gardens.

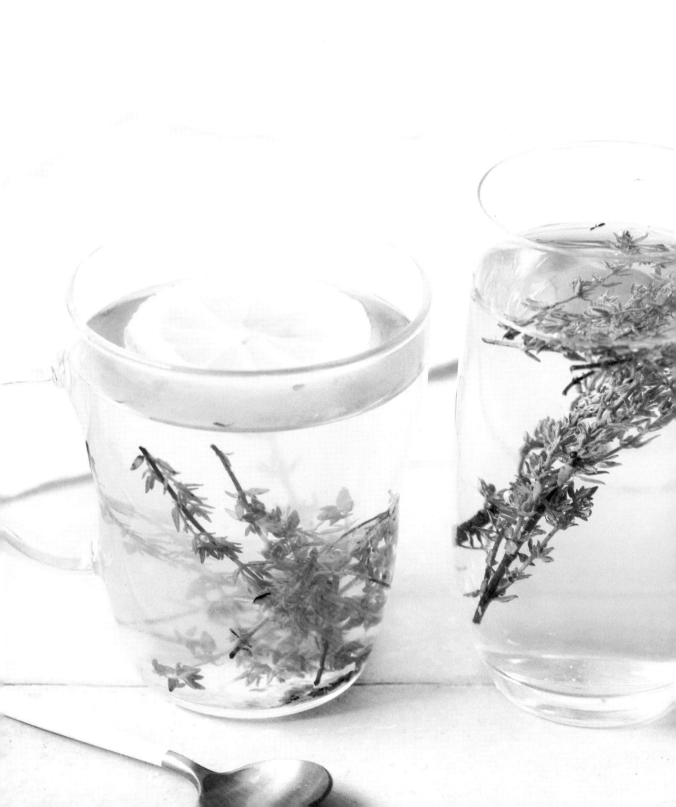

GINGER WATER

Whether it's hot ginger tea after dinner or a glass of ginger water mid-morning, this drink is easy to customize in a way that works for you!

1- to 2-inch piece of fresh ginger

2 cups water

Juice of ½ lemon (optional)

2 teaspoons raw honey (optional)

Grate the ginger into the water. Allow the water to steep for at least 15 minutes, ideally longer. You can even leave it steeping on the counter or in the fridge overnight. Strain the water. Add lemon and raw honey, if desired, and enjoy warm or cold throughout the day.

TIPS

- As an alternative to grating the ginger, try chopping it into a few small pieces and squeezing them in a garlic press—it will act like a mini juicer.

- It can be helpful to prepare a big batch of ginger water in advance to sip as desired. For best results, add the raw honey and lemon just prior to consuming.

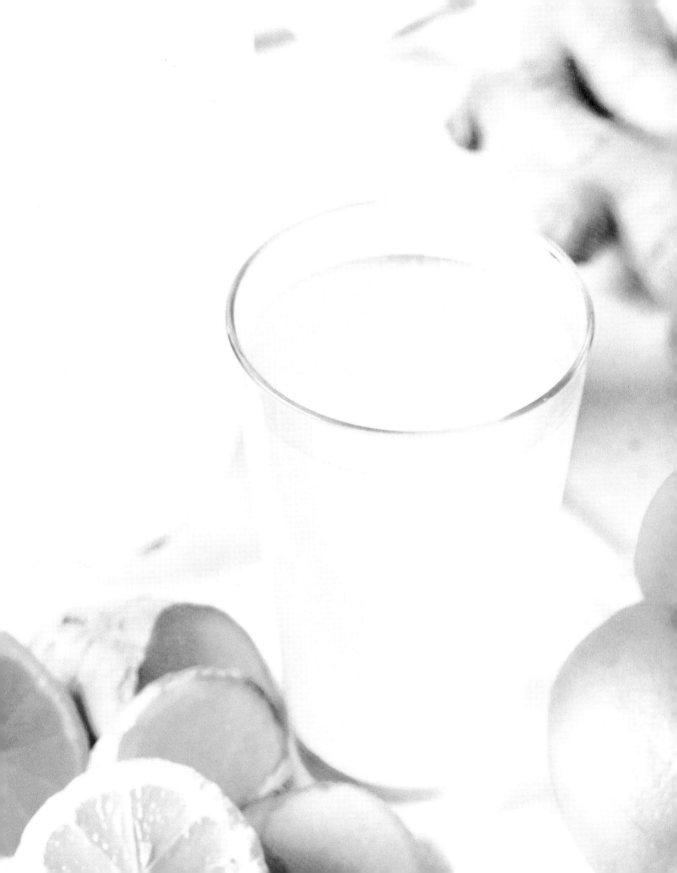

TURMERIC GINGER SHOTS

Makes 2 to 4 shots

These fiery, immune-boosting shots are a tasty go-to option at the first sign of a cold. These shots will help your body fight back against anything that tries to come against it!

4-inch piece of fresh turmeric

4-inch piece of fresh ginger

2 oranges, peeled and roughly chopped

4 garlic cloves, peeled

Juice the turmeric, ginger, oranges, and garlic using an electric juicer. Serve immediately.

Note: The amount of ingredients necessary will vary greatly based on the juicer that is used.

TIPS

- You can also make a simpler version of turmeric ginger shots by juicing just fresh turmeric and fresh ginger together. If you're dealing with congestion, cough, sore throat, cold, flu, and/or sinus problems, you can sip on this concentrated serum periodically throughout the day, taking tiny sips. The juice will act as an expectorant and help speed up the healing process.

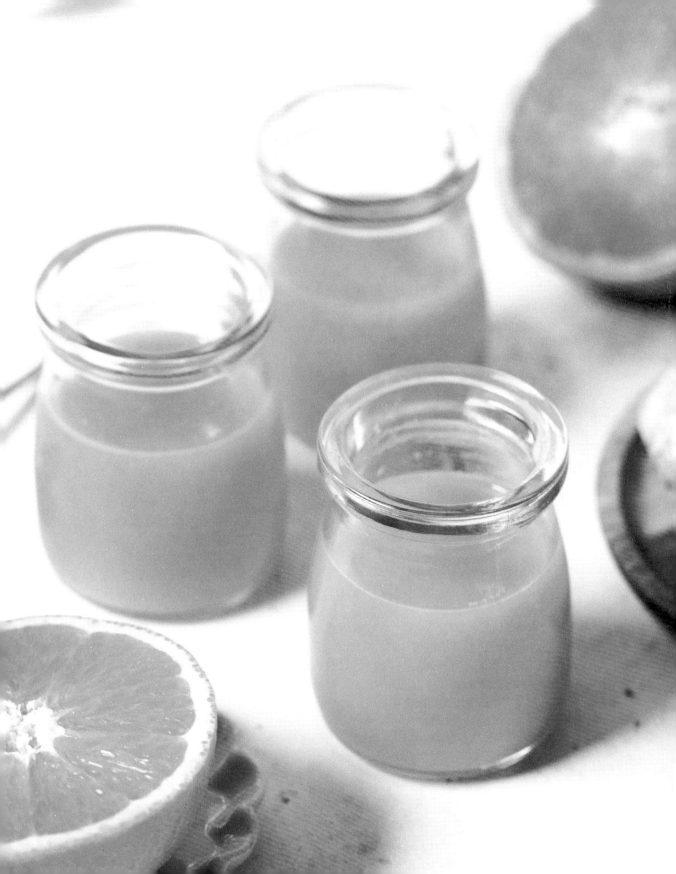

APPLE, CELERY, AND CUCUMBER JUICE

Makes 1 serving

The combination of equal parts celery, cucumber, and apple in this recipe provides the right balance of mineral salts, potassium, and sugar to stabilize your glucose levels and support your body in cleansing.

1 medium-sized cucumber, roughly chopped

4 celery sticks, roughly chopped

2 medium-sized apples, cored and chopped

Juice the cucumber, celery, and apples using an electric juicer. Serve immediately.

TIPS

- You can adjust how much of each ingredient you use based on the size of your produce. For example, if you only have small celery stalks or apples, you may need to use more to get equal parts celery juice, apple juice, and cucumber juice.

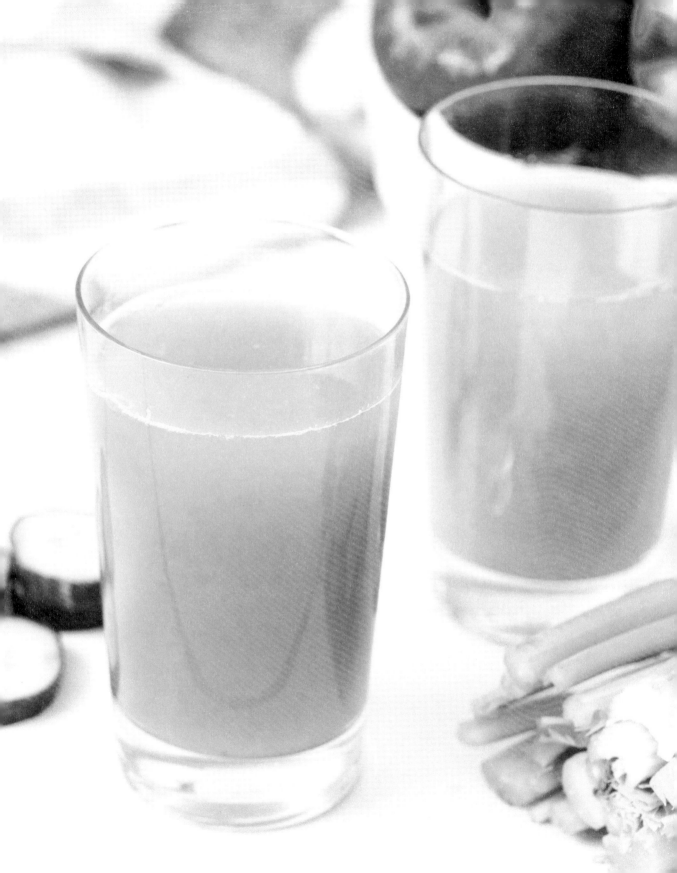

HEAVY METAL DETOX SMOOTHIE

Makes 1 serving

This Medical Medium smoothie recipe is helping people heal all over the globe. It contains a powerful combination of the five key ingredients for safely detoxifying toxic heavy metals from your brain and body. It's an honorable, life-giving blessing to help reverse so many symptoms.

2 bananas

2 cups frozen or fresh wild blueberries or 2 tablespoons powdered wild blueberries

1 cup fresh cilantro

1 teaspoon barley grass juice powder

1 teaspoon spirulina

1 tablespoon Atlantic dulse

1 orange

½ to 1 cup coconut water, fresh-squeezed orange juice, or water (optional)

Combine the bananas, wild blueberries, cilantro, barley grass juice powder, spirulina, and Atlantic dulse with the juice of 1 orange in a high-speed blender and blend until smooth. Add up to 1 cup of one of the additional optional liquids (coconut water, fresh orange juice, or water) if a thinner consistency is desired.

Serve and enjoy!

TIPS

- If you'd like to focus on removing toxic heavy metals from your brain and body, it's best to drink this smoothie every day.

- If the barley grass juice powder and spirulina make the taste too strong for you, start with a small amount of each and work your way up.

- If using coconut water in this smoothie, make sure the coconut water doesn't contain natural flavors and isn't pink or red.

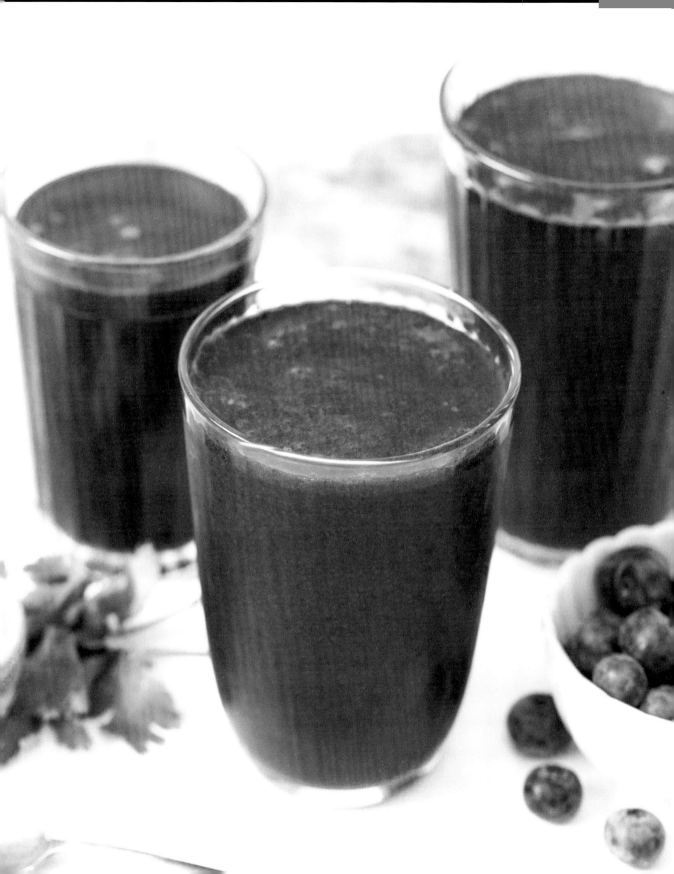

WATERMELON ALOE SLUSHY

Makes 1 serving

This delicious slushy is a fantastic way to sneak in the incredible healing benefits of aloe vera. It's refreshing and sweet and only takes a few minutes to prepare.

2 cups diced frozen watermelon (seeded or seedless)*

2 tablespoons aloe gel

½ cup fresh strawberries

1 tablespoon lime juice

Place all the ingredients in a blender and blend until smooth. Serve immediately.

*You can use fresh watermelon and frozen strawberries if you prefer.

TIPS

- Dice your watermelon before freezing—don't try to cut it up after it's been frozen.

- See the Aloe Water recipe on page 308 to read how to cut out the aloe gel from a fresh aloe vera leaf.

- For extra medicinal benefits, use double the amount of fresh aloe. Keep in mind it will make the aloe flavor of the slushy stronger.

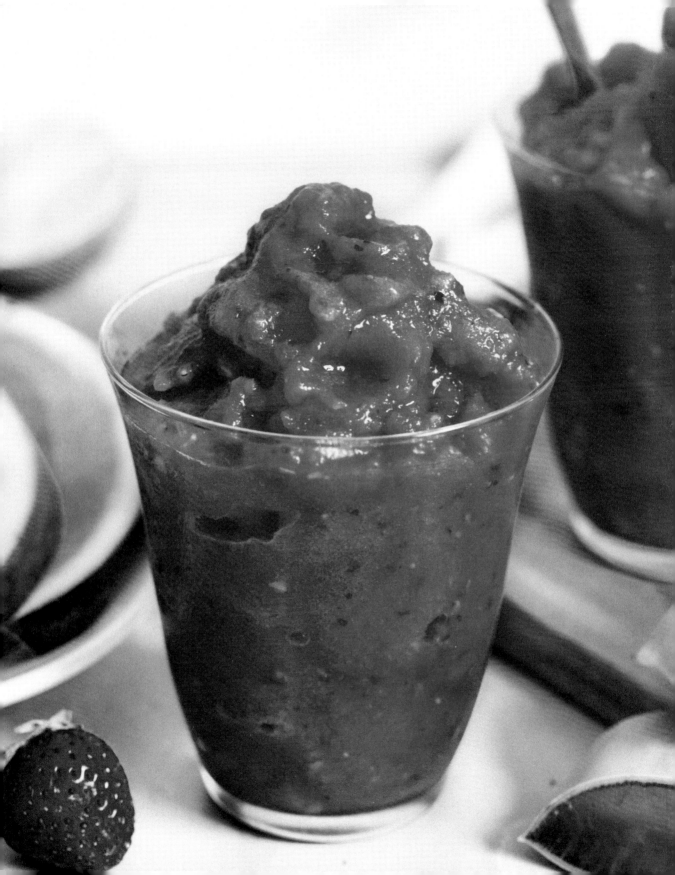

VANILLA AND CINNAMON CANTALOUPE SMOOTHIE

Makes 1 to 2 servings

While ripe cantaloupe (also known as rockmelon) is delicious all on its own, turn it into a creamy, frosty smoothie with a touch of vanilla and cinnamon, and you'll be delighted by how decadent it tastes!

1 cantaloupe, peeled, deseeded, and roughly chopped

Seeds from ½ vanilla pod or ½ teaspoon alcohol-free vanilla extract

½ teaspoon cinnamon

1 tablespoon raw honey (optional; recommended if your melon isn't very sweet)

1 cup ice

Place the cantaloupe, vanilla, cinnamon, raw honey (if using), and ice in a blender and blend until smooth. Serve immediately.

TIPS

- Using ripe cantaloupe is the key to this recipe. You will know your cantaloupe is ready to cut into when it emits a sweet and lightly floral aroma and yields slightly to gentle pressure applied to the skin. Feel free to double or triple this recipe according to your appetite.

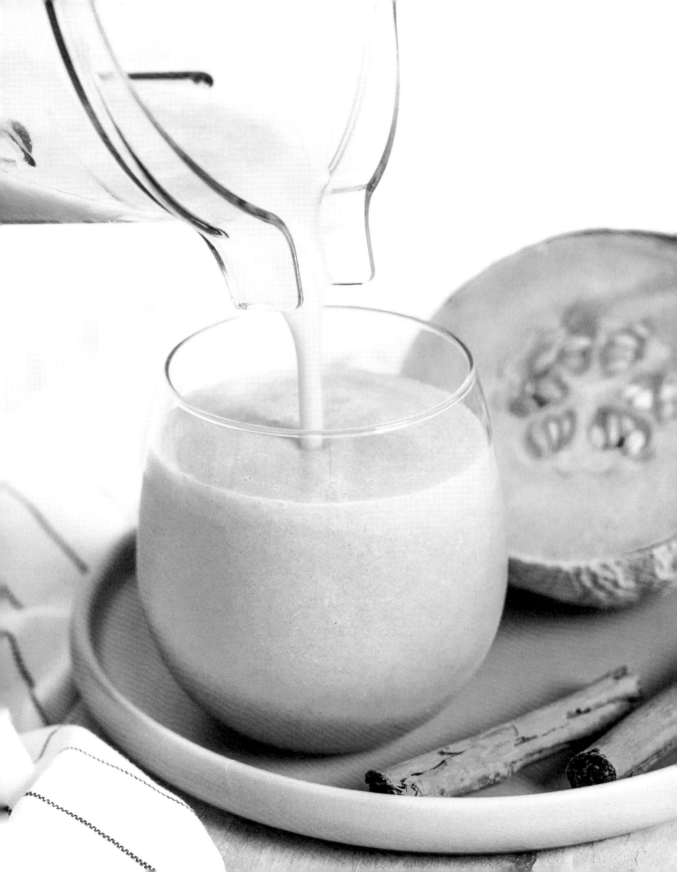

HONEY BERRY BOWL

Makes 1 serving

The simplicity of this recipe, along with its delicious flavor, may well make it a regular breakfast favorite. It's also one of the most nutrient-dense meals or snacks you can eat! Enjoy it for breakfast or a snack, or as a light lunch alongside or on top of a leafy green salad. Or serve up a big bowl of this recipe for the whole family to enjoy over the course of a day.

1 cup strawberries, hulled and halved

1 cup raspberries

1 cup wild blueberries or blueberries

1 cup blackberries

1 tablespoon raw honey

Place all the berries in a bowl, add the honey, and mix until coated. Serve immediately.

TIPS

- Feel free to have as many berries as you'd like in your Honey Berry Bowl. If you'd like to double the amount of berries to make it a sufficient meal or snack for you, that's more than okay.

- Also feel free to make your Honey Berry Bowl with one type of berry rather than a mix. And don't overlook local berry varieties available near you—you're welcome to substitute other types of berries for those listed in the recipe.

- If you'd like, you can also add other fruits such as fresh banana slices, kiwis, peaches, or apricots.

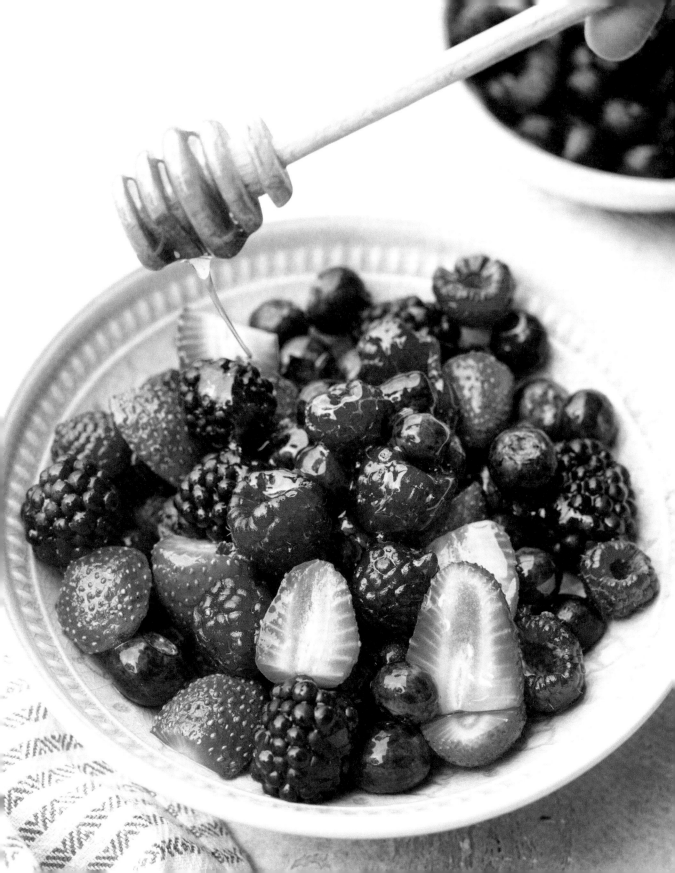

BANANA CHERRY SMOOTHIE

Whip up this easy and tasty smoothie in a matter of minutes. If you choose to include the barley grass juice powder, it will provide an extra boost of vital nutrients and mineral salts.

2 bananas, fresh or frozen

1 medjool date

1 cup frozen cherries

1 cup water or coconut water, to blend

1 teaspoon barley grass juice powder (optional)

Combine the bananas, date, cherries, water, and barley grass juice powder (if using) in a high-speed blender and blend until smooth. Serve and enjoy!

TIPS

- If you're using coconut water in this smoothie, make sure it doesn't contain natural flavors and isn't pink or red.

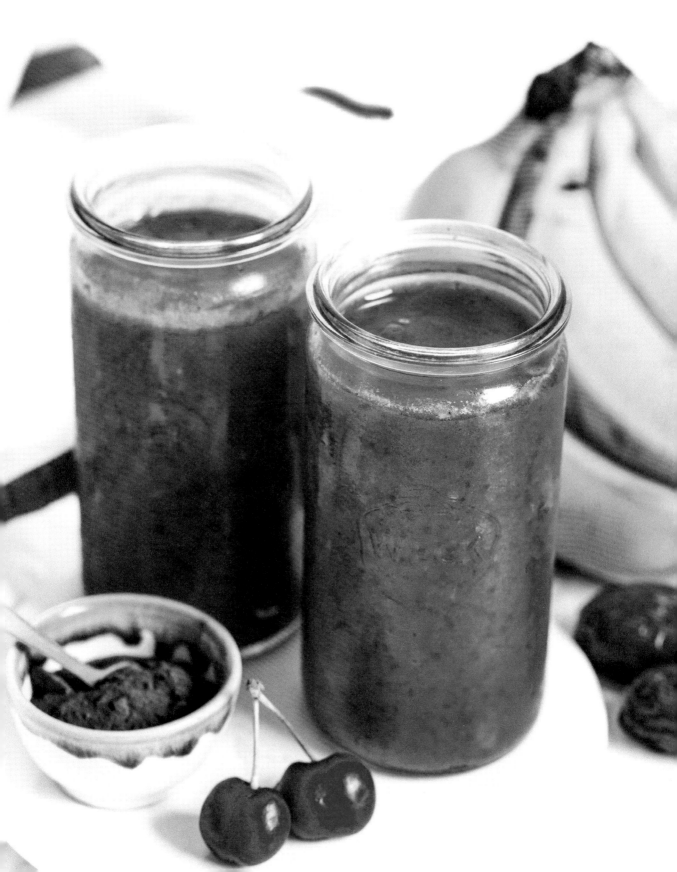

BANANA BERRY SMOOTHIE

This classic banana and berry fruit smoothie is one you can come back to over and over again. Try it with a variety of berries or choose one berry at a time and experience the different flavor options.

2 bananas, fresh or frozen

1 medjool date

1 cup frozen cherries

1 cup berries, fresh or frozen (such as wild blueberries, raspberries, strawberries, or blackberries)

1 cup water or coconut water to blend

Combine the bananas, date, cherries, berries, and water (or coconut water) in a high-speed blender and blend until smooth. Serve and enjoy!

TIPS

- If you're using coconut water in this smoothie, make sure it doesn't contain natural flavors and isn't pink or red.

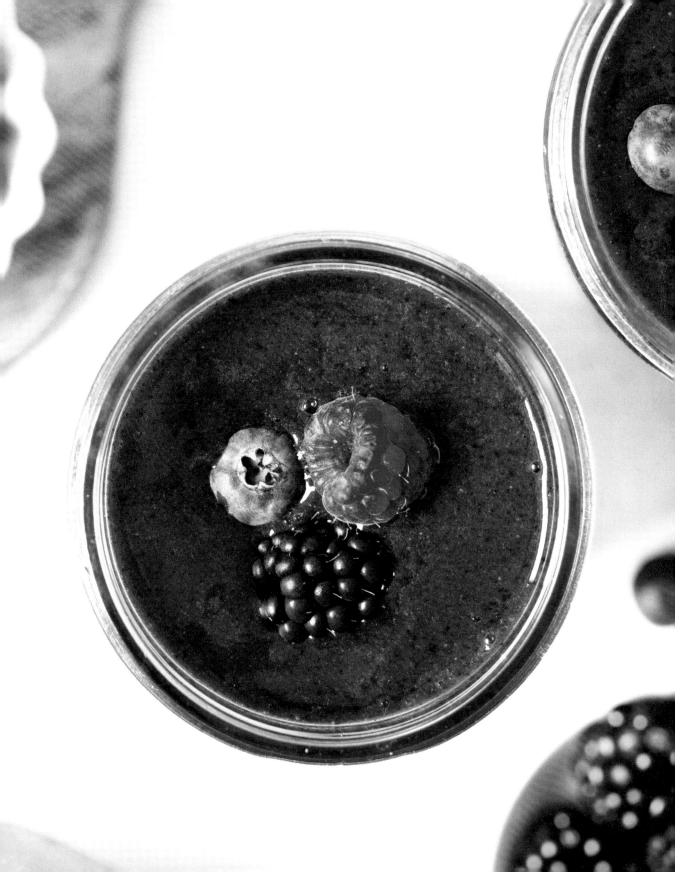

LAYERED FRUIT SALAD

Makes 2 to 3 servings

This gorgeous recipe lets the vibrant colors of the fruits speak for themselves. Any fresh fruits of your choice can be used; simply layer them on top of each other and dig in!

2½ cups chopped Maradol papaya

2 cups chopped strawberries

2 cups diced mango or pineapple

2 cups blueberries

2 cups chopped kiwi

Juice from ½ lime

Layer the chopped fruit in a medium-sized glass bowl. Squeeze lime juice over the top and serve.

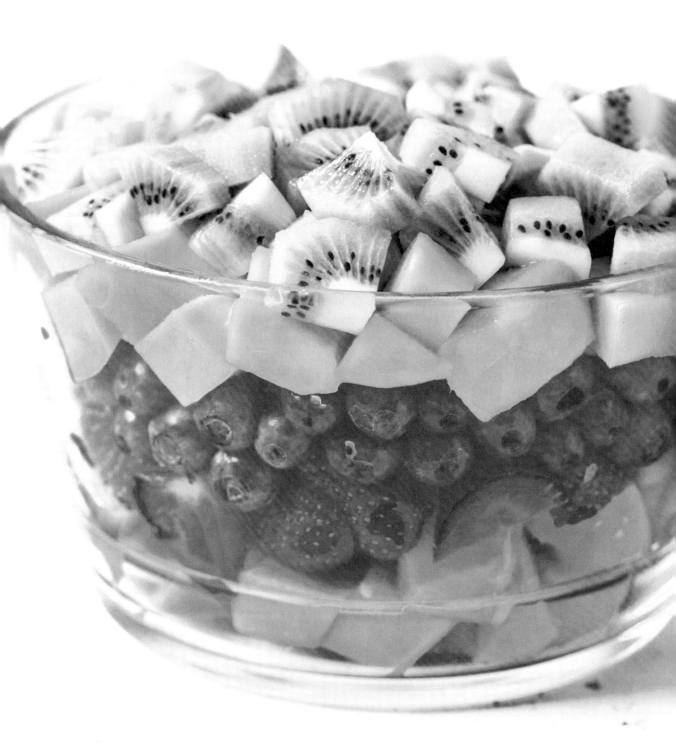

MOJITO FRUIT SALAD

Fresh lime juice and mint take this fruit salad to a new level! Enjoy this refreshing snack or meal any time the mood strikes.

2 tablespoons freshly squeezed lime juice

1 tablespoon raw honey

2 cups halved black, purple, or red grapes

2 cups strawberries, blackberries, and/or raspberries

2 cups chopped peaches, nectarines, and/or apricots

¼ cup loosely packed fresh mint, finely chopped

Place lime juice and raw honey in a medium-sized bowl and whisk until uniform. Add the grapes, berries, peaches, and mint. Gently stir until evenly mixed and serve.

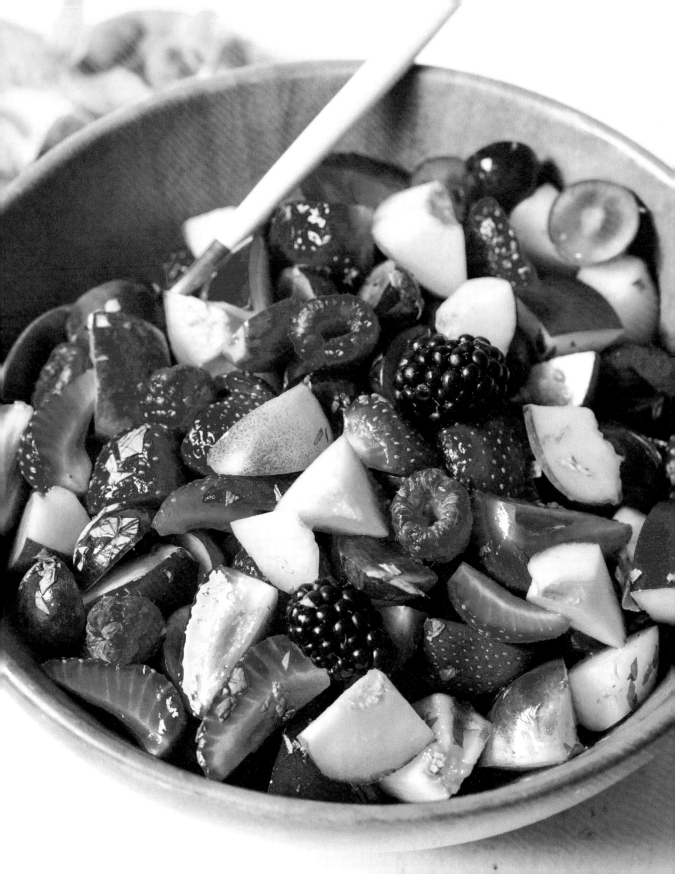

SPINACH SOUP

Makes 1 serving

One of the amazing things about incorporating more fruits and vegetables into our diet is the way our taste buds change, and we begin to crave more and more fresh ingredients over time. When you find yourself yearning for leafy greens and the benefits they provide, this easy-to-make, richly flavored soup is a great way to incorporate them into your day in an easily digestible form. With all of the minerals the spinach provides, you'll also help curb any cravings for the foods you know don't serve your health right now.

1½ cups grape tomatoes

1 stalk celery

1 garlic clove

1 orange, juiced

4 cups baby spinach

2 basil leaves or a few sprigs fresh cilantro

Place the tomatoes, celery, garlic, and fresh orange juice in a high-speed blender and blend until smooth.

Add the spinach by the handful and blend until completely incorporated.

Add the basil or cilantro and blend until creamy and smooth.

Pour the blended soup into a serving bowl and serve immediately.

TIPS

- If this soup doesn't have you singing "Hallelujah!" at the beginning of your journey, give it another try in a few weeks. As your palate begins to change, you may find that you wind up loving this soup so much that you make it a staple of your diet!

- If you can't use spinach, you can substitute butter leaf lettuce.

- If you can't use tomatoes, you can substitute ripe mango. If you can't get fresh, sweet mangoes, you can substitute thawed frozen mango.

- If neither tomato nor mango is an option, you can blend up banana with greens instead. Be sure not to include both banana and tomato in the recipe, as they don't digest well together. Use banana only for this substitution.

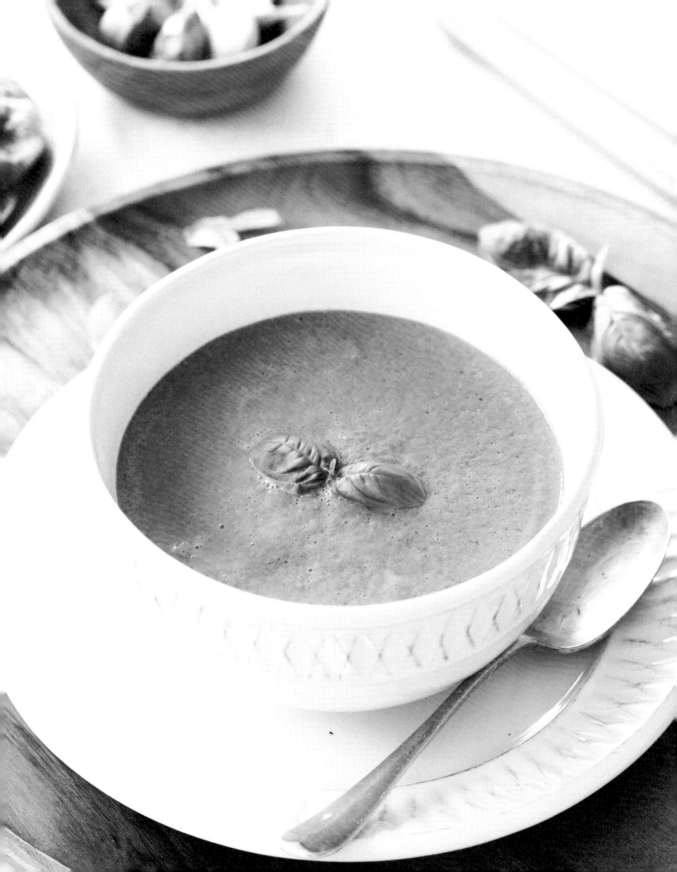

MANGO SALSA ROMAINE BOATS

Makes 1 serving

A wonderful blend of sweet and savory, this mango salsa is a versatile recipe during the 28-Day Healing Cleanse or at any other time. Make lettuce boats as per the recipe, or pile the salsa on top of salads, eat it on its own, or enjoy it as a dip with vegetable crudités.

5 to 6 romaine lettuce leaves or other lettuce leaves of choice

FOR THE SALSA

3 cups finely diced mango

⅓ cup finely chopped red onion

¼ cup finely chopped fresh cilantro

1 cup finely chopped red bell pepper or tomato

2 tablespoons lime juice

½ teaspoon cayenne (optional)

1 teaspoon ground cumin (optional)

In a large bowl, combine the mango, red onion, cilantro, red bell pepper or tomato, lime juice, cayenne (if using), and ground cumin (if using). Gently stir until evenly mixed.

Spoon the salsa into romaine leaves. Serve immediately.

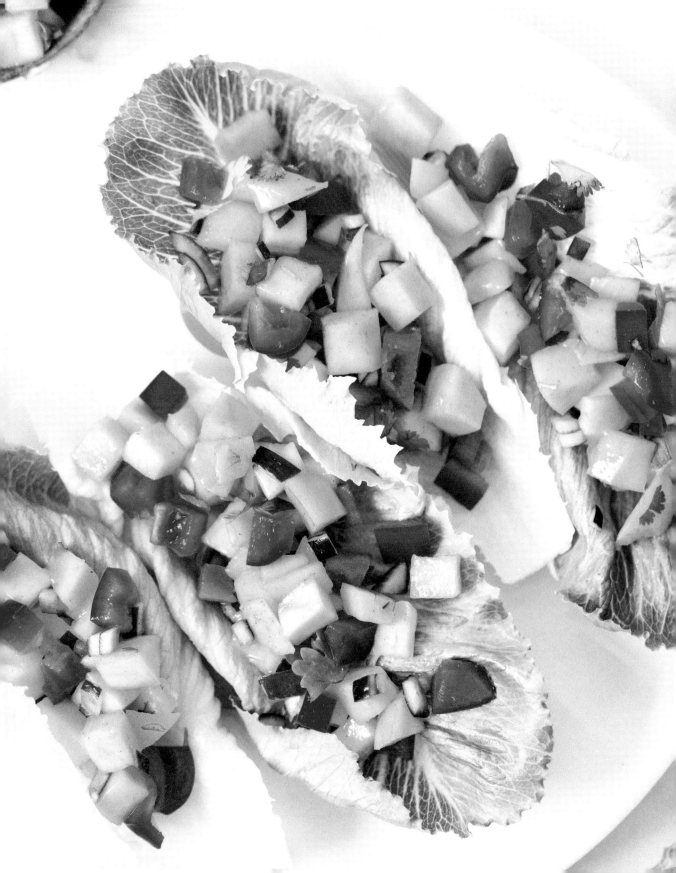

BANANA SALAD

While banana in a green salad may seem like an unusual combination at first, you may just find you come to love it. Include all the optional ingredients or make it as simple as bananas, lettuce, and Atlantic dulse. Either way, you'll support your adrenals and provide critical glucose and mineral salts to your body and brain.

½ cup thinly sliced onion (optional)

2 tablespoons to ¼ cup Atlantic dulse strips, quickly soaked in water, then chopped

4 to 6 bananas, chopped

1 cup chopped cucumber (optional)

2 to 3 sticks celery, chopped (optional)

4 to 6 cups leafy greens (such as butter lettuce, romaine, and/or red leaf lettuce)

FOR THE DRESSING

2 teaspoons raw honey

½ cup orange juice

Place the onion (if using), Atlantic dulse, bananas, cucumber (if using), celery (if using), and leafy greens in a medium-sized bowl. Toss until evenly combined.

Whisk together the raw honey and orange juice in a small bowl. Add to the salad and toss again. Serve immediately.

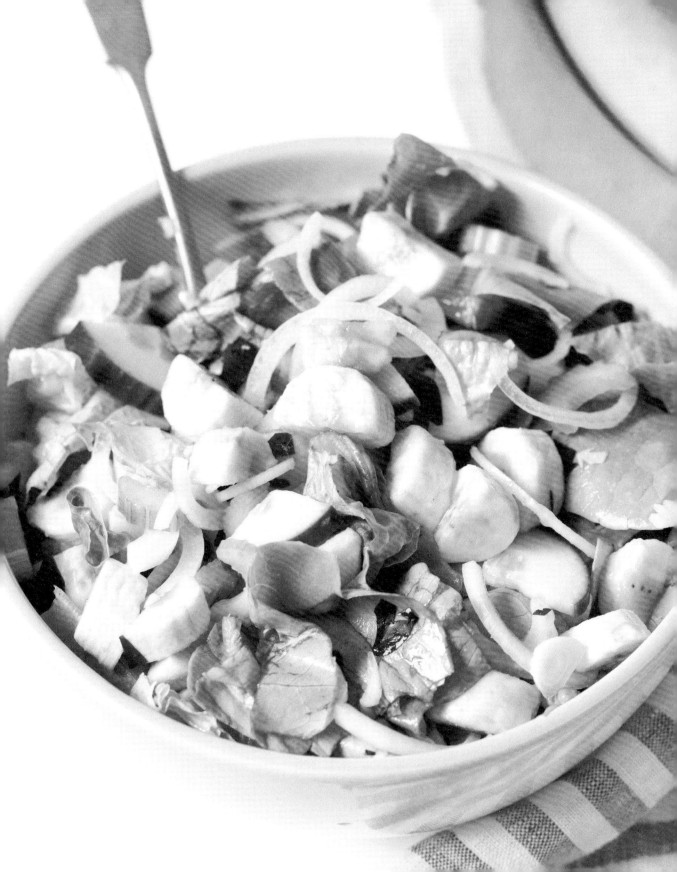

CUCUMBER NOODLES WITH BRUSCHETTA TOPPING

Makes 1 serving

A refreshing meal with Italian flavors, this simple dish is one you may find yourself turning to over and over again.

1 English cucumber, peeled

2 cups diced cherry or grape tomatoes

2 garlic cloves, finely chopped

¼ cup tightly packed basil leaves, finely chopped

2 tablespoons finely chopped red onion

¼ teaspoon red pepper flakes (optional)

1 tablespoon lemon juice

1 teaspoon raw honey

Make the cucumber into noodles using a spiralizer or vegetable peeler. Place in a bowl and set aside.

Combine the tomatoes, garlic, basil, red onion, red pepper flakes (if using), lemon juice, and raw honey in a bowl and mix well. Spoon on top of the cucumber noodles and serve immediately.

TIPS

- You're welcome to make cucumber noodles with any type of cucumber. English cucumbers are listed here because they're the easiest to spiralize.

- You can leave the skin on your cucumber or remove it—it comes down to personal preference. If you're using a regular cucumber instead of an English cucumber, peeling the hard skin off first will produce the best cucumber noodles.

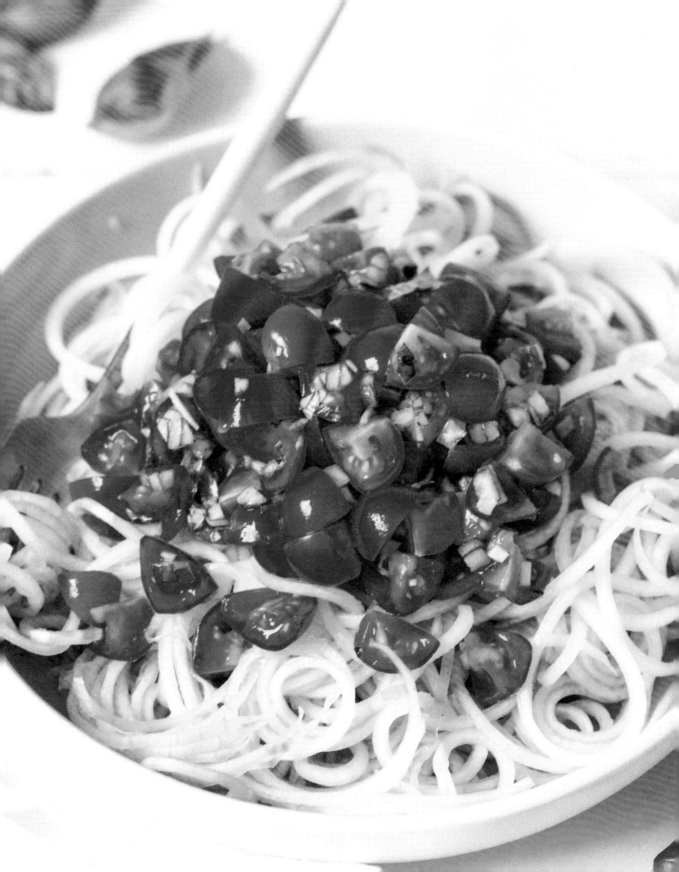

BANANA NORI WRAPS

Makes 2 servings

These quick and easy wraps are a perfect snack or meal for busy days or when you want a simple meal that will nourish you without requiring much time or energy to prepare. They're also a convenient option to take with you on the go.

4 nori sheets

2 cups alfalfa sprouts, divided

4 green onions

4 bananas (or 4 steamed potatoes, roughly chopped— see Tips)

Atlantic dulse flakes, to taste

½ cup fresh cilantro (optional)

Place a nori sheet shiny side down on a chopping board with a long edge close to you. Arrange ½ cup sprouts, 1 green onion, 1 banana (or 1 chopped potato), dulse flakes, and cilantro (if using) on one end of the sheet.

Brush water across the other end of the sheet, and then roll it up tightly. Cut in half and repeat with the remaining ingredients. Serve immediately.

TIPS

- If you'd prefer, you can make these nori wraps with steamed potatoes instead of bananas—just don't use both banana and steamed potatoes. Steamed potato nori wraps would be best consumed in the evening away from any fruit snacks or meals. They're also a good choice for an easy meal any time after the cleanse.

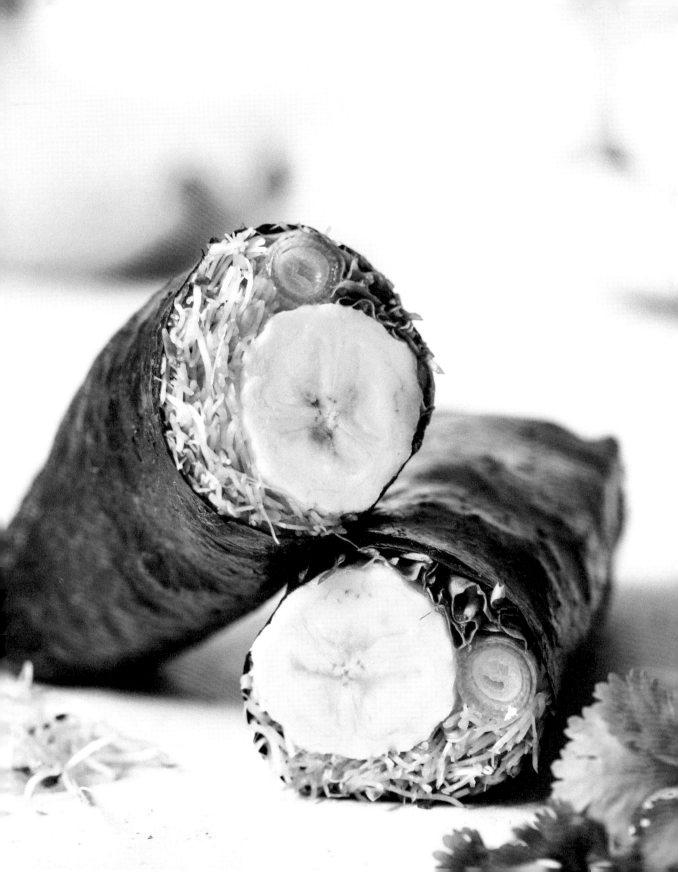

MANGO SALAD

Sweet mango, savory tomatoes, and the crunch of radishes and cauliflower over leafy greens make this a truly delicious and satisfying salad.

2 to 3 medium-sized tomatoes, roughly chopped

2 cups diced mango

1 to 2 green onions, chopped

3 to 4 cups leafy greens (such as spinach, butter lettuce, or green leaf lettuce)

1 to 3 radishes, thinly sliced

½ cup chopped cauliflower

FOR THE DRESSING

1 tablespoon lemon juice

1 tablespoon pure maple syrup (optional)

½ teaspoon mustard powder (optional)

Place the tomatoes, mango, green onions, leafy greens, radishes, and cauliflower in a medium-sized bowl. Toss until evenly mixed.

Whisk together the lemon juice, maple syrup (if using), and mustard powder (if using) in a small bowl. Add to the salad and toss again. Serve immediately.

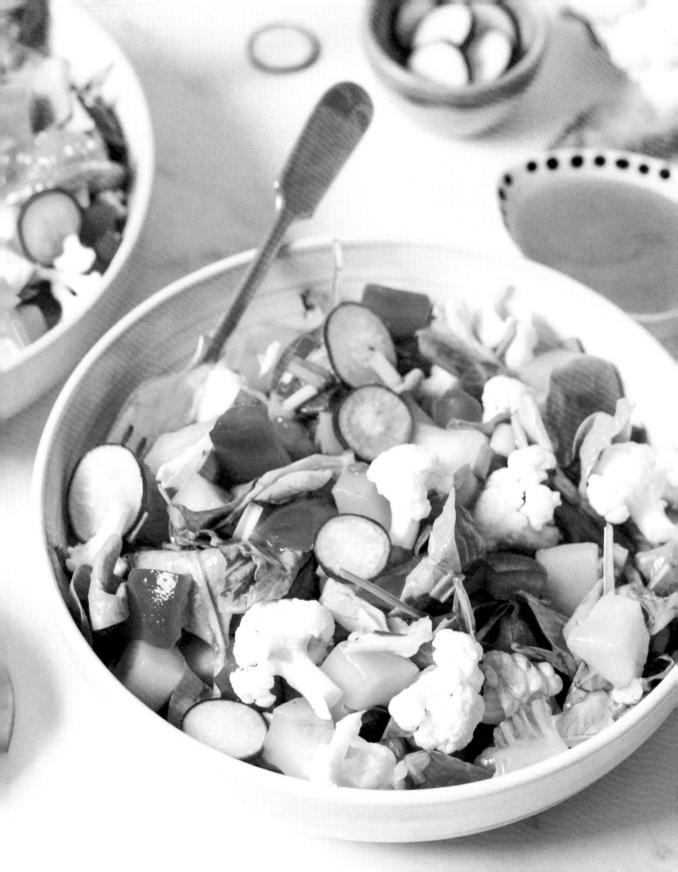

STRAWBERRY BANANA SALAD

Makes 2 servings

This fruit-focused salad is fresh, bright, and packed with flavor thanks to the herbs, fruit, and two different dressing options. Each dressing has its own unique taste and appeal, so try them both and pick your favorite, or alternate each time you make this pretty salad.

FOR THE SALAD

4 cups chopped strawberries

4 to 6 bananas, roughly chopped (about 4 to 6 cups)

4 cups leafy greens (such as spinach and/or butter leaf lettuce)

¼ cup finely chopped basil or sage (optional)

ORANGE HONEY DRESSING (OPTION 1)

½ cup orange juice

2 teaspoons raw honey

STRAWBERRY BANANA DRESSING (OPTION 2)

⅓ cup chopped strawberries

⅓ cup chopped banana

1 to 3 tablespoons water

1 teaspoon lemon juice (optional)

2 basil leaves (optional)

Place the strawberries, bananas, leafy greens, and basil or sage (if using) in a medium-sized bowl. Gently toss until evenly combined.

If you're using the first dressing option, whisk together the orange juice and raw honey in a small bowl. Add to the salad and gently toss again.

If you're using the second dressing option, combine the strawberries, banana, 1 tablespoon of water, lemon juice (if using), and basil (if using) in a blender and blend until very smooth. If you like a thinner consistency, add another 1 to 2 tablespoons of water. Add to the salad and gently toss again. Serve immediately.

TIPS

- If you're serving this salad with the Strawberry Banana Dressing to other people and want it to look as pretty as possible, it's best to include the lemon juice, as it will help the dressing retain a bright color.

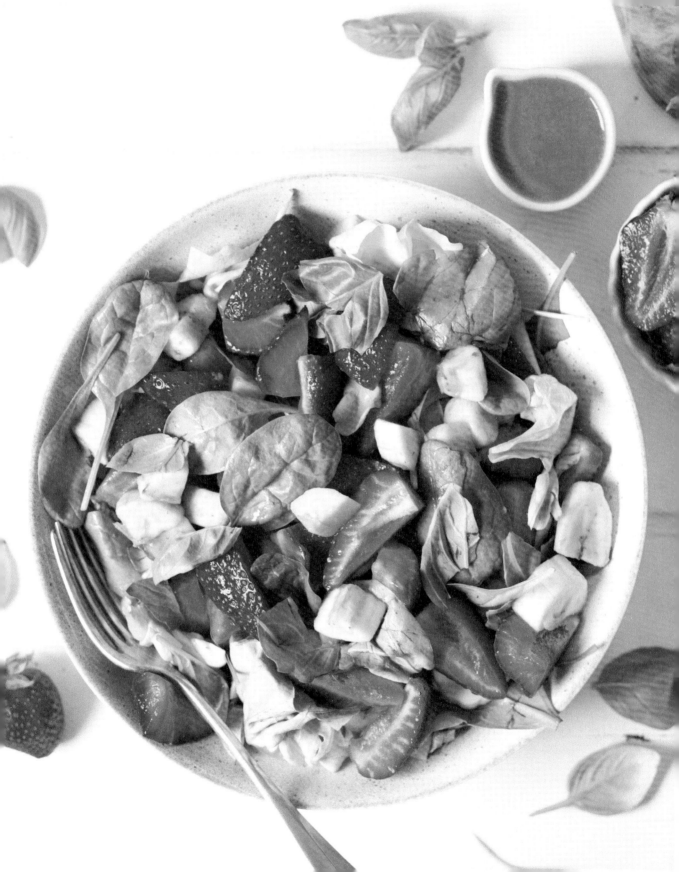

APPLE SALAD

This Apple Salad recipe offers you three different dressing options so you can pick your favorite or choose a different option each time for variety. No matter which one you choose, you will get an abundance of healing nutrients.

4 cups mixed leafy greens

2 apples, thinly sliced

¼ cup raisins

¼ cup thinly sliced red onion

DRESSING OPTION 1

1½ tablespoons pure maple syrup

2 tablespoons lemon juice

¼ teaspoon ground cinnamon

¼ teaspoon cayenne

DRESSING OPTION 2

1½ tablespoons pure maple syrup

2 tablespoons lemon juice

⅛ teaspoon ground nutmeg

¼ teaspoon ground cinnamon

¼ teaspoon ground ginger

DRESSING OPTION 3

1½ tablespoons pure maple syrup

2 tablespoons lemon juice

Arrange the leafy greens, apples, raisins, and red onion on a serving platter or in a bowl.

Whisk together all the dressing ingredients in a small bowl and pour on top of the salad. Toss gently and serve immediately.

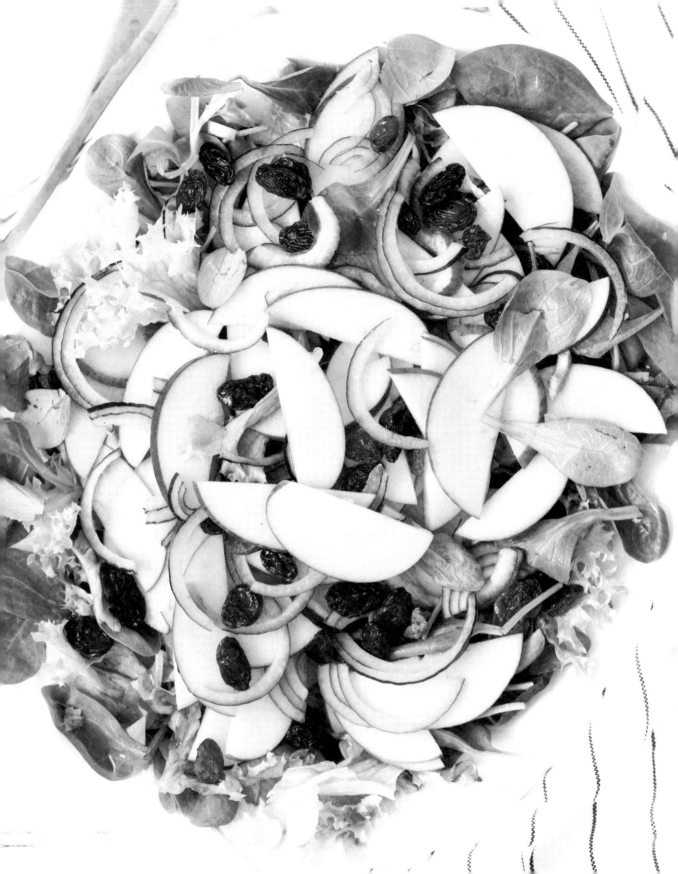

LEAFY GREENS WITH AVOCADO DRESSING

Makes 2 servings

A creamy dressing can transform a simple bowl or plate of leafy greens. The natural creaminess in avocado takes away the need for any of the oil you'd normally find in a dressing. Plus, it only takes a couple of minutes to prepare.

FOR THE SALAD

8 cups leafy greens (such as romaine, green leaf, or red leaf lettuce, spinach, or mâche)

FOR THE DRESSING

1 avocado

¼ to ⅓ cup water

5 to 6 sprigs fresh cilantro

1 tablespoon lemon or lime juice

½ clove fresh garlic (or more, to taste)

¼ teaspoon cayenne (optional)

Place the leafy greens in a medium-sized bowl. Combine the avocado, water, cilantro, lemon or lime juice, garlic, and cayenne (if using) in a blender and blend until very smooth. Add to the salad and toss until evenly coated. Serve immediately.

TIPS

- Enjoy this salad on its own or top with chopped cucumber, bell pepper, tomato, sprouts, and/or onion.

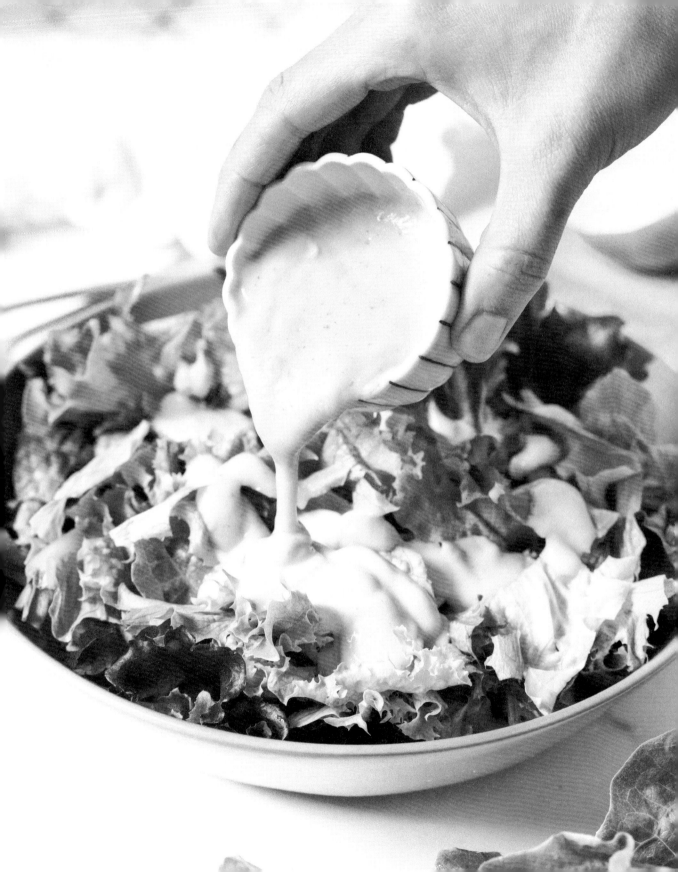

CHOPPED SALAD

Makes 1 to 2 servings

This pretty Chopped Salad looks beautiful and tastes delicious thanks to the brightly colored array of fresh fruits, leafy greens, herbs, and vegetables it showcases. It's also easy to customize with your own favorite fresh produce picks. A fun way to serve this salad to others is as a build-your-own salad bar so each person can create their own style of chopped salad.

4 to 6 cups chopped leafy greens (such as spring mix, arugula, lettuce, or kale)

2 cups chopped cucumber

½ cup chopped green onions

2 cups chopped tomatoes

1 teaspoon Atlantic dulse flakes (or more, to taste)

3 tablespoons freshly squeezed orange juice

2 medjool dates, finely chopped (optional)

½ avocado (optional)

1 cup chopped yellow, orange, and/or red bell peppers (optional)

¼ cup finely chopped dill, basil, cilantro, thyme, and/or parsley (optional)

Place the leafy greens, cucumber, green onions, tomatoes, Atlantic dulse flakes, orange juice, medjool dates (if using), avocado (if using), bell peppers (if using), and herbs (if using) in a large bowl. Toss until evenly combined and serve immediately.

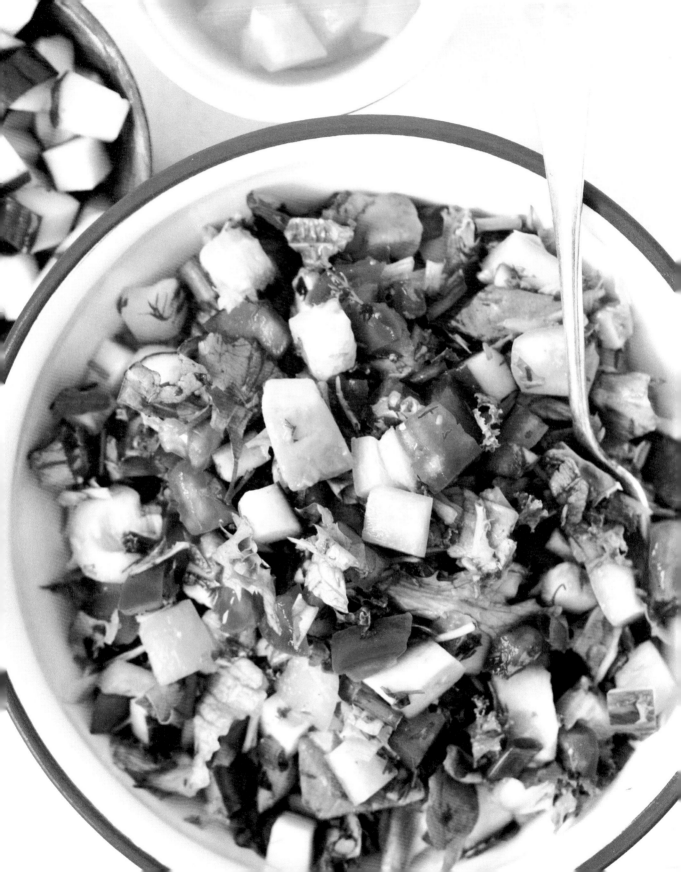

BURRITO BOWL

Makes 2 servings

Dig into this healing version of a popular favorite when you need a bowl of comfort. Alive with crunch and flavor, this is another great option for a group meal that lets everyone at the table assemble their own.

3 to 4 cups leafy greens (such as romaine, spinach, or green leaf lettuce)

1 to 2 tablespoons lime, lemon, or orange juice, to serve

Red pepper flakes, to serve (optional)

CAULIFLOWER RICE

1 medium-sized cauliflower, cut into florets

½ teaspoon ground cumin

½ teaspoon ground paprika

¼ to ½ teaspoon cayenne

2 tablespoons finely chopped fresh cilantro

SALSA

1½ cups diced tomato

1 clove garlic, finely minced

¼ cup loosely packed fresh cilantro, roughly chopped

¼ cup finely chopped red onion

2 tablespoons lime juice

GUACAMOLE (OPTION 1)

1 avocado

1 to 2 tablespoons lime juice

½ clove garlic, finely chopped

2 tablespoons finely chopped red onion

¼ cup diced tomatoes

SIMPLE MASHED AVOCADO (OPTION 2)

1 avocado

1 to 2 tablespoons lime juice

To make the cauliflower rice, place the cauliflower florets in a food processor and pulse until you get a coarse, rice-like texture. Add the spices and cilantro and mix.

To make the salsa, combine the tomato, garlic, cilantro, red onion, and lime juice in a small bowl and stir until evenly mixed. Set aside.

To make the guacamole, combine the avocado, lime juice, garlic, red onion, and tomatoes in a small bowl and stir until evenly mixed. Set aside.

Alternatively, if you prefer a simple mashed avocado instead of the guacamole, add the avocado to a small bowl and squeeze lime juice on top. Mash with a fork until uniform.

Divide the leafy greens, cauliflower rice, salsa, and guacamole or mashed avocado between serving bowls. Squeeze the lime (or lemon or orange) juice on top and sprinkle with red pepper flakes (if using). Serve immediately.

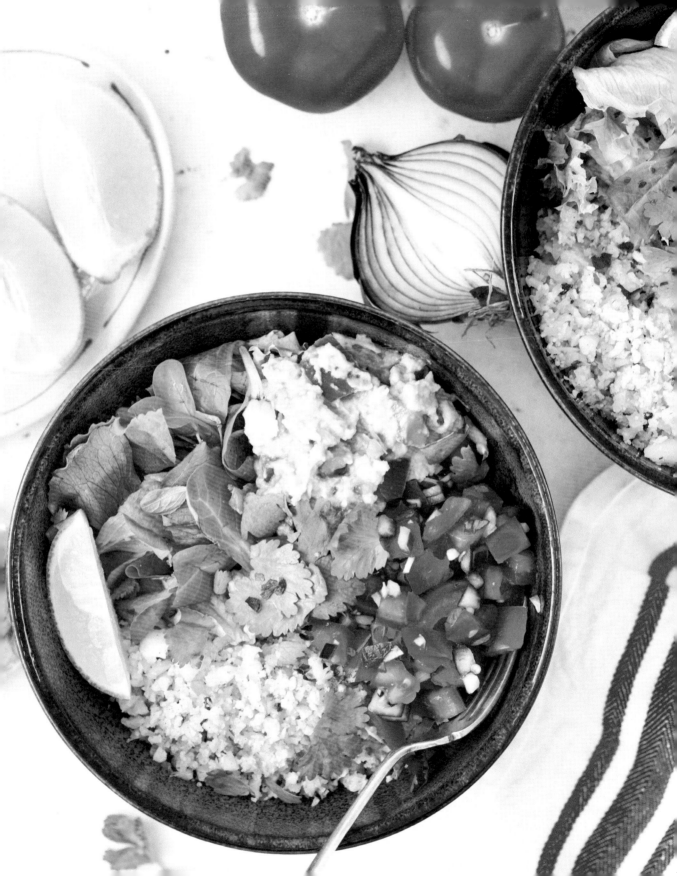

BANANA LETTUCE BOATS

Makes 1 to 2 servings

A sweet snack or meal that is easy to make and fun to eat for both adults and children, these Banana Lettuce Boats are delicious with or without the Date Caramel Sauce.

6 large leaves of butter leaf, red leaf, or romaine lettuce

3 bananas, sliced in half lengthwise

¼ cup raisins (optional)

½ teaspoon cayenne or cinnamon (optional)

DATE CARAMEL SAUCE (OPTIONAL)

6 medjool dates, pitted

5 tablespoons water

2 teaspoons lemon juice

Arrange the lettuce leaves on plates or on a platter. Top each with a banana half, raisins (if using), and an optional sprinkle of cayenne (or cinnamon). Set aside.

To make the caramel, add the dates, water, and lemon juice to a blender and blend until very smooth, scraping down the sides of the blender as needed. Spoon onto the Banana Lettuce Boats and serve immediately.

TIPS

- The Date Caramel Sauce is fantastic as a drizzle over other fruit-based snacks and meals, or use it as a dip for fruits such as apples, pears, strawberries, bananas, and more.

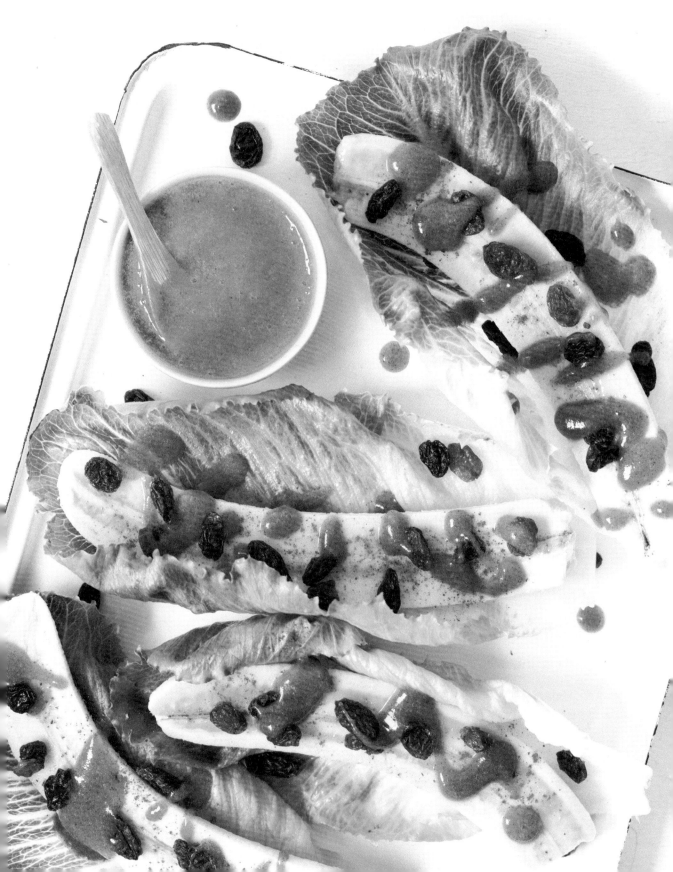

SPROUT SALAD

Makes 1 to 2 servings

Sprouts are a powerhouse food packed full of healing nutrients—the more of them you can get into your diet, the better. If you don't think you like sprouts, it's worth experimenting with different varieties to see if there are some you like more than others. Most people find there's at least one variety they enjoy, and usually the more you eat them, the more you'll love them! Topped with a delicious dressing, you may find this salad becomes a part of your regular meal rotation.

2 cups alfalfa sprouts or other sprouts of choice

½ cup clover sprouts or other sprouts of choice

1½ cups diced tomatoes

1½ cups diced cucumber

⅓ cup diced red onion

¼ cup loosely packed basil or cilantro, roughly chopped

2 to 3 cups arugula or green leaf lettuce

ORANGE HONEY DRESSING (OPTION 1)

¼ cup orange juice

2 tablespoons lemon juice

1 tablespoon raw honey

¼ to ½ teaspoon chili powder

½ teaspoon mustard powder

TOMATO MANGO DRESSING (OPTION 2)

¾ cup chopped tomatoes

1 cup diced mango

1 to 2 tablespoons lemon or lime juice

1 tablespoon chopped green onions

2 teaspoons raw honey (optional)

½-inch piece of fresh ginger

2 to 3 fresh cilantro sprigs

¼ to ½ teaspoon cayenne or red pepper flakes

Place the sprouts, tomatoes, cucumber, red onion, herbs, and leafy greens in a medium-sized bowl. Toss until evenly combined.

To make the Orange Honey Dressing, whisk together all the ingredients in a small bowl and pour on top of the salad. Toss again and serve.

To make the Tomato Mango Dressing, combine all the ingredients in a blender and blend until smooth. Top the salad with the dressing. Serve immediately.

TIPS

- While this recipe calls for alfalfa and clover sprouts, you can use any sprouts of your liking. There are dozens of other varieties to try, such as broccoli, sunflower, radish, onion, garlic, lentil, and mustard, or microgreens such as kale, basil, cilantro, and arugula.

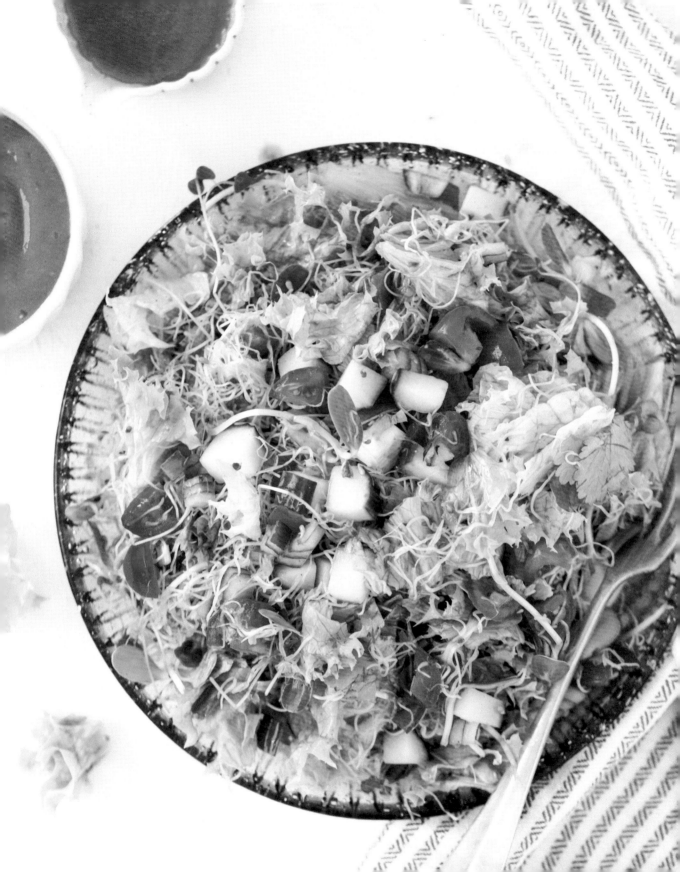

MASSAGED KALE SALAD

The kale in this salad is tenderized by massaging it with avocado, lemon or orange juice, and raw honey before adding the other ingredients to make a flavorful salad. This process softens the kale and makes it easy to chew. See Tips for a fat-free option, too.

½ pound (about 6 to 7 cups) kale, roughly chopped

1 avocado

1 tablespoon lemon or orange juice

1 tablespoon raw honey

½ cup thinly sliced radishes

1 cup diced red, yellow, or orange bell pepper

1 cup chopped cherry tomatoes

1 cup chopped cucumber

½ to 1 teaspoon red pepper flakes or cayenne

½ teaspoon ground cumin

½ teaspoon paprika (optional)

Massage the avocado into the kale leaves together with the lemon juice or orange juice and the raw honey until they become soft and tender, about 3 to 5 minutes.

Place in a large bowl and add the radishes, bell pepper, cherry tomatoes, cucumber, red pepper flakes or cayenne, ground cumin, and paprika (if using).

Toss until evenly combined. Serve immediately.

TIPS

- If you are omitting fat altogether, you can try this recipe without the avocado and massage the kale with just the orange or lemon juice and raw honey. You may wish to add a little extra fresh orange juice.

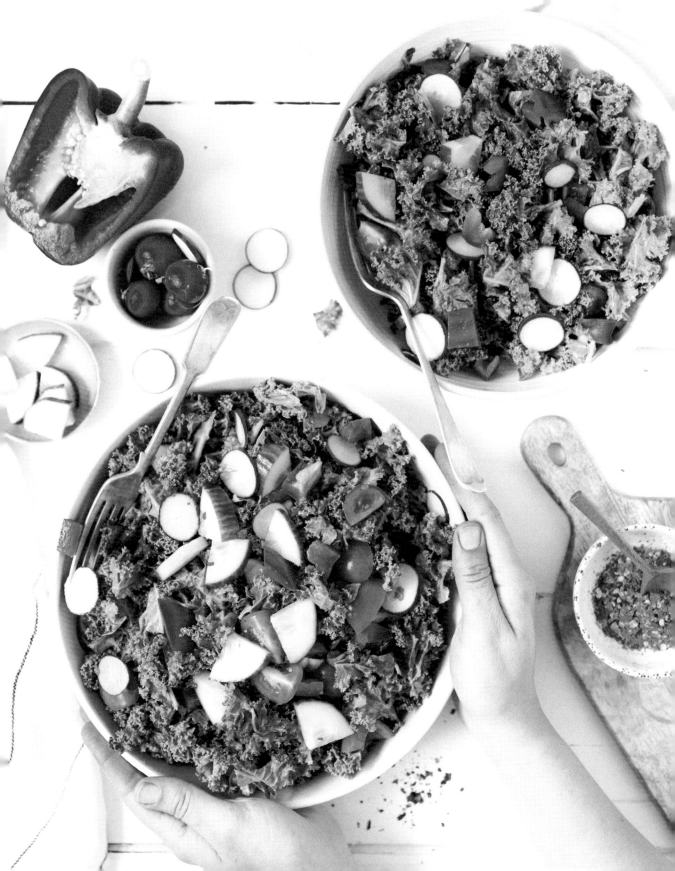

ISRAELI SALAD

Makes 1 to 2 servings

This salad is inspired by the delicious flavors of a traditional Israeli salad. It's refreshing, fragrant, and beautiful. Enjoy it alone or as a filling for lettuce cups.

2½ cups finely diced English cucumber

2 cups chopped tomatoes

1 cup diced red bell pepper

⅓ cup finely chopped red onion

1 cup chopped raw cauliflower

¼ cup roughly chopped parsley

¼ cup roughly chopped mint

2 tablespoons lemon juice

½ tablespoon raw honey

Place the cucumber, tomatoes, red bell pepper, red onion, cauliflower, and herbs in a medium-sized bowl. Toss until evenly combined.

Add the lemon juice and raw honey. Toss again and serve immediately.

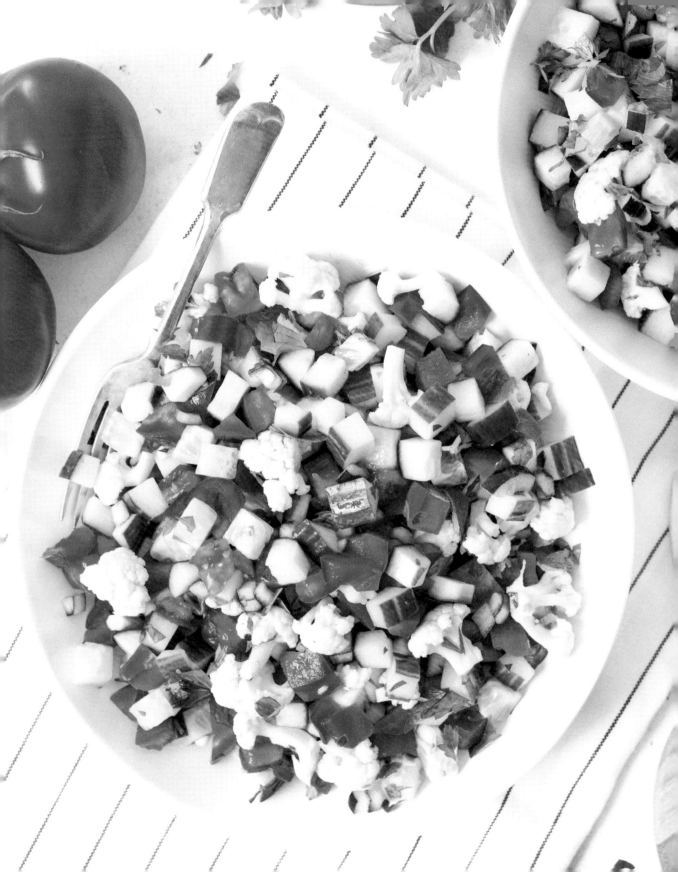

RED CABBAGE TACOS WITH MANGO GINGER SAUCE

Makes 2 servings

In this recipe, red cabbage leaves provide a sturdy taco-style shell that can hold the delicious fillings and sauce. Roll up your sleeves and dig into this fun meal!

FOR THE TACOS

1 small head of red cabbage, broken into leaves

1 to 2 medium-sized tomatoes, diced

¼ cup diced red onion

½ avocado, thinly sliced (optional)

1 red bell pepper, thinly sliced

¼ cup loosely packed fresh cilantro, to serve

MANGO GINGER SAUCE

1 cup diced mango

2 tablespoons lime juice

½-inch piece of fresh ginger

¼ to ½ teaspoon cayenne or red pepper flakes

2 medjool dates

3 tablespoons water

Arrange cabbage leaves on plates or a platter and top with diced tomatoes, red onion, avocado (if using), red bell pepper, and cilantro. Set aside.

Make the sauce by combining the mango, lime juice, ginger, cayenne or red pepper flakes, dates, and water in a blender. Blend until smooth.

Spoon sauce onto the Red Cabbage Tacos. Serve immediately.

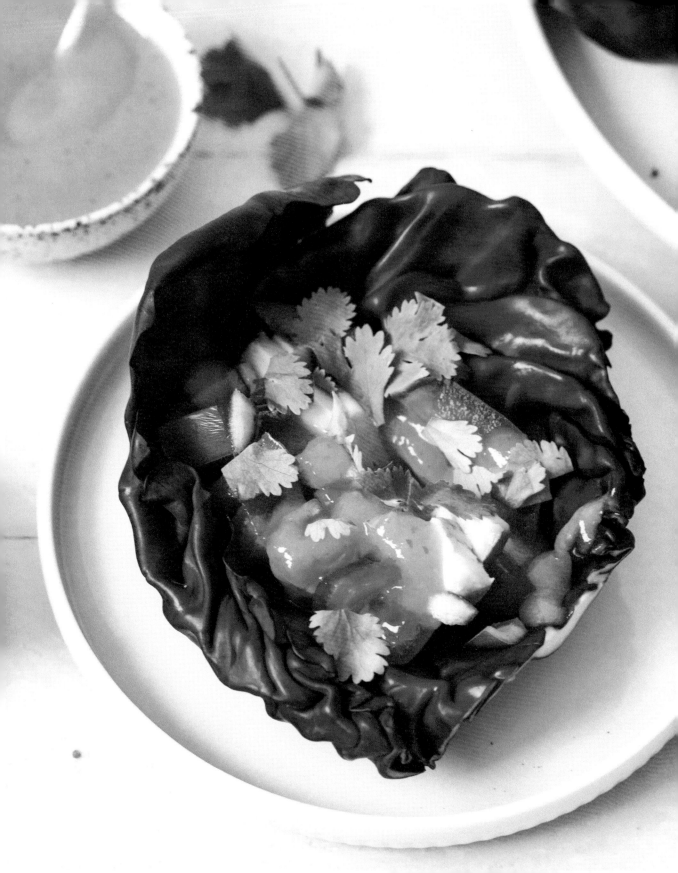

"The healing food plan I present here
can move health mountains.

This delicious, healing cleanse has brought profound
results to countless people. It has changed
people's lives. It can change yours."

— Anthony William, Medical Medium

The 28-Day Healing Cleanse is intended to consist of raw, living foods: specifically fruits, leafy greens, vegetables, and herbs. As you read earlier, a modification is to include some cooked vegetables during the cleanse. If you choose this modification, it's best to consume the cooked foods in the evening, away from any fruit-based snacks or meals. The best cooking methods to preserve nutrients are steaming and making broths, soups, or stews. Baking will result in more nutrient loss, although it's also a safe option—ideally oil-free—for some dinner meals during the cleanse. You can also use the recipes with cooked vegetables for ideas and inspiration for meals between or after rounds of the 28-Day Healing Cleanse.

HEALING BROTH

Makes 3 to 4 servings

Healing Broth is a powerful, mineral-rich liquid that carries the essence of vitally nutritious vegetables, herbs, and spices in a way that is easy for the body to digest, assimilate, and utilize. You will find this recipe as comforting as it is nourishing. The ingredients in this simple recipe provide tremendous healing benefits for both body and soul.

4 carrots, chopped, or 1 sweet potato, cubed

2 stalks celery, roughly chopped

2 onions, sliced

1 cup finely chopped parsley

1 cup shiitake mushrooms, fresh or dried (optional)

2 tomatoes, chopped (optional)

1 bulb garlic (about 8 cloves), minced

1-inch piece of fresh ginger, finely sliced, minced, or grated

1-inch piece of fresh turmeric, finely sliced, minced, or grated

8 cups water

1 hot chili pepper or ½ teaspoon red pepper flakes (or more, to taste; optional)

Place all the ingredients in a pot and bring to a gentle boil. Turn the heat down to low and allow to simmer for about an hour. Strain and sip for a mineral-rich, healing, and restorative broth.

TIPS

- As an alternative, you can blend the broth with the vegetables for a pureed soup.

- This recipe may also be enjoyed as a chunky vegetable soup by leaving the vegetables whole within the broth.

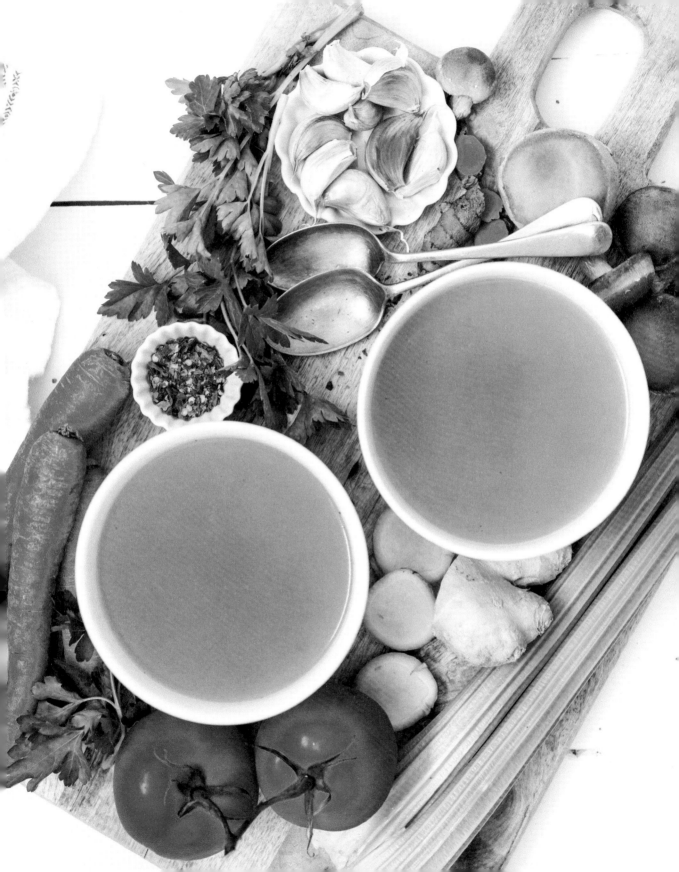

ARUGULA, POTATO, AND ASPARAGUS SALAD

Makes 2 servings

Warm, comforting, and satisfying, this salad brings together some of the most healing cooked vegetables—asparagus, brussels sprouts, and potatoes—with fresh leafy greens, herbs, onion, and a simple dressing. The result is a simple and delicious meal.

4 to 5 potatoes (about 3 cups roughly chopped)

1 cup chopped brussels sprouts

1 cup chopped asparagus

½ cup thinly sliced sweet onion

¼ cup loosely packed fresh parsley, roughly chopped

¼ cup roughly chopped fresh basil leaves

1 teaspoon dried thyme

2 tablespoons lemon juice

1 tablespoon pure maple syrup

4 cups arugula

2 cups chopped butter leaf, romaine, and/or green leaf lettuce

To prepare the potatoes, add 3 inches of water to a medium-sized pot, bring it to a boil, and add a steaming basket. Place the potatoes in the basket, cover, and steam for 15 to 20 minutes, until the potatoes are very tender.

To prepare the brussels sprouts, steam for 10 minutes, until tender.

To prepare the asparagus, steam for 5 minutes, until tender.

To streamline the above process, feel free to steam the potatoes, brussels sprouts, and asparagus together in one large basket. So that nothing gets overcooked, start by steaming the potatoes, then 5 to 10 minutes later, add the brussels sprouts. After another 5 minutes, add the asparagus. Steam for an additional 5 minutes, or until all contents of the steamer basket are tender.

Remove the potatoes, brussels sprouts, and asparagus and place them in a large bowl. Let them cool for 10 minutes, and then add the onion, parsley, basil, dried thyme, lemon juice, maple syrup, arugula, and lettuce. Toss until evenly mixed. Serve immediately.

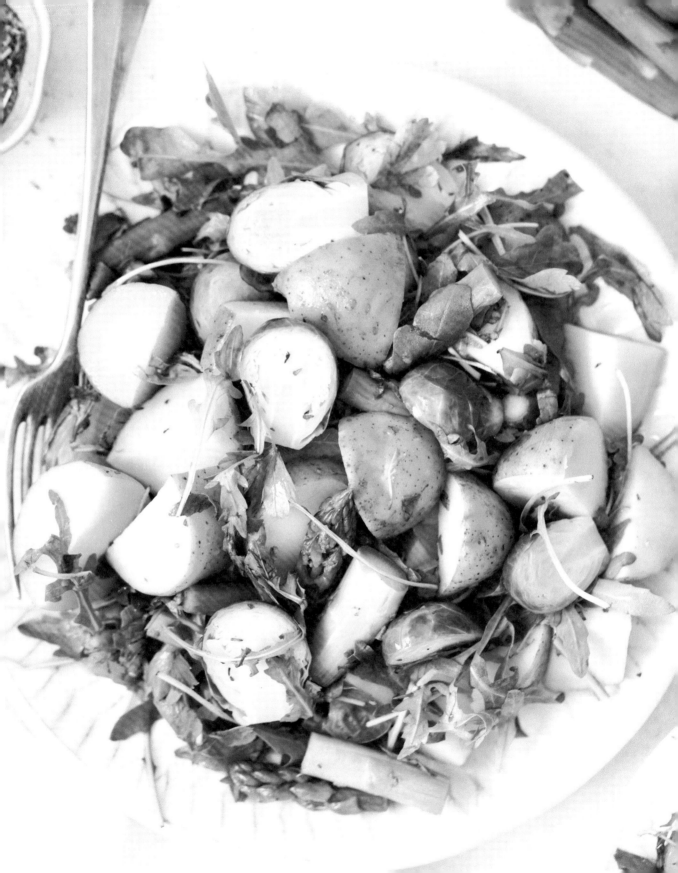

LOADED POTATO HASH

Makes 2 servings

This Potato Hash is great as a stand-alone meal or served with a fresh salad. However you enjoy it, you will be sure to receive an array of healing nutrients.

½ cup chopped onion

2 cups diced potato

1½ cups diced sweet potato

¼ cup water

1 cup chopped broccoli

1 cup chopped asparagus

1 cup diced bell peppers
(red, orange, and/or yellow)

1 teaspoon dried thyme

1 teaspoon garlic powder or
1 garlic clove, finely minced

½ teaspoon paprika
(optional)

½ teaspoon red pepper
flakes (optional)

¼ cup finely chopped fresh
parsley or cilantro, to serve

Add the onion, potato, and sweet potato to a large nonstick ceramic pan. Cook for 3 to 5 minutes, until the onion is translucent, adding a bit of water if needed to prevent sticking.

Pour ¼ cup water into the pan and cover with a lid. Cook for 10 to 15 minutes, until the potatoes are almost tender, stirring them every few minutes.

Add the broccoli, asparagus, bell peppers, thyme, garlic powder (or garlic), paprika (if using), and red pepper flakes (if using) to the pan. Cook for 5 to 10 minutes, until the potatoes and vegetables are all tender. Serve immediately with finely chopped fresh parsley (or cilantro).

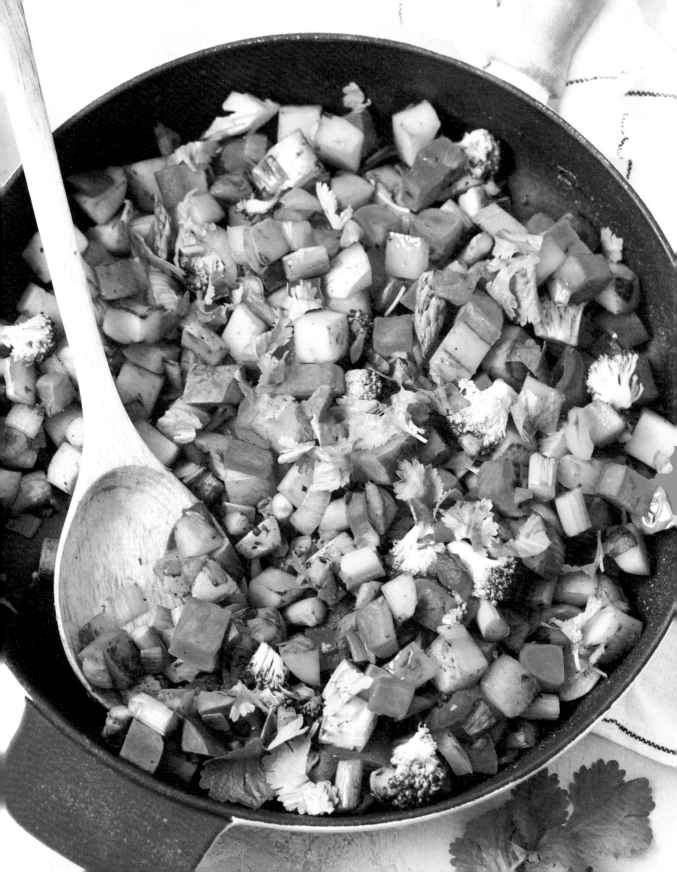

PIZZA POTATO WRAP
AND SALAD POTATO WRAP

Makes 2 wraps

Dig into one or both versions of these delicious and satisfying potato wraps. One comes stuffed with a pizza-inspired filling and the other a salad sandwich–style filling. You may want to make extra wraps and enjoy this recipe with family or friends.

FOR THE POTATO WRAPS

4 cups roughly chopped gold potatoes

1 teaspoon garlic powder

1 teaspoon onion powder

2 teaspoons pure maple syrup

PIZZA FILLING (OPTION 1)

PIZZA SAUCE

½ cup tomato paste

1 teaspoon dried oregano

½ teaspoon dried thyme

1 teaspoon raw honey

3 to 4 tablespoons water

VEGETABLES

⅓ cup thinly sliced mushrooms (optional)

¼ cup chopped red bell pepper

¼ cup chopped red onion

2 to 3 fresh basil leaves

SALAD FILLING (OPTION 2)

2 to 3 lettuce leaves

⅓ cup alfalfa sprouts

3 to 4 tomato slices

3 to 4 cucumber slices

2 tablespoons finely chopped red onion

1 to 2 tablespoons chopped basil or parsley

Preheat oven to 400°F/200°C.

To make the base, add 3 inches of water to a medium-sized pot and add a steaming basket. Cover the pot and steam the potatoes for 25 to 30 minutes, until soft. Remove and place the potatoes in a food processor with the garlic powder, onion powder, and maple syrup. Blend until smooth.

Line a baking tray with parchment paper and spread the mixture on top using a wet spatula, making 2 large tortilla wraps. Place them in the oven and bake for 15 to 20 minutes, until lightly browned. Remove the wraps and pat them down with a spatula. Cool them completely. Flip the wraps upside down onto a clean work surface or cutting board and gently peel off the parchment paper.

To make the Pizza Wrap, make the Pizza Sauce by mixing together the tomato paste, dried oregano, dried thyme, raw honey, and water. Set aside.

If you're using the mushrooms, add the slices to a small skillet and cook for 3 to 5 minutes, stirring occasionally, until browned, adding a bit of water if needed to prevent sticking. Remove from the heat and set them aside.

Spread the Pizza Sauce on the wraps and top with the mushrooms (if using), red bell pepper, red onion, and fresh basil. Fold the wraps up gently and serve immediately.

To make the Salad Wrap, arrange the lettuce leaves, alfalfa sprouts, tomato slices, cucumber slices, red onion, and basil or parsley on the wraps. Fold the wraps up gently and serve immediately.

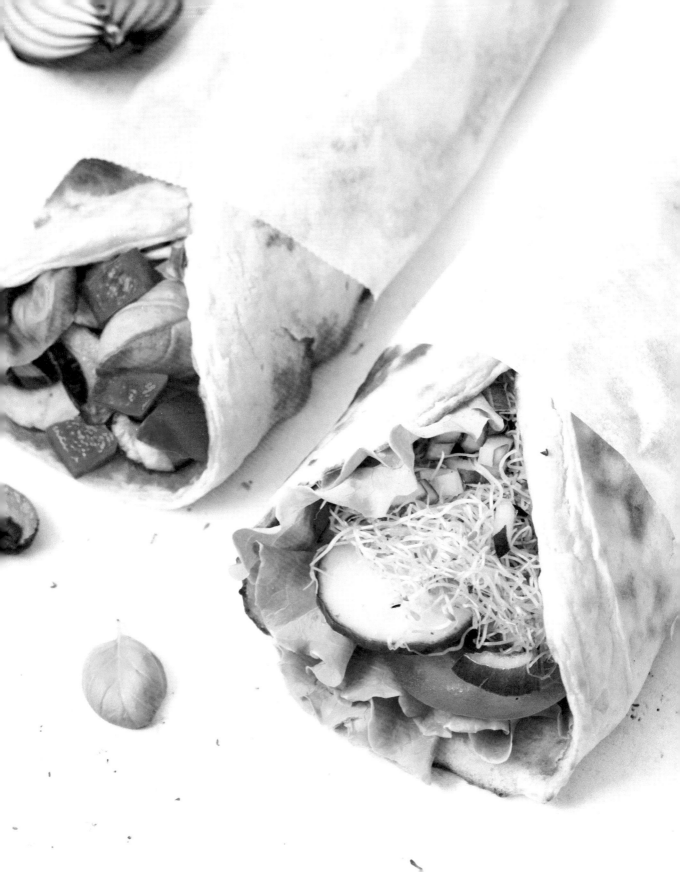

SWEET AND SOUR STIR-FRY

Enjoy the flavor of Sweet and Sour Sauce in this recipe without the processed ingredients that are often used in these sauces. This stir-fry comes together easily and quickly so you can sit down to a beautiful meal in no time!

½ cup chopped green onions

1 cup sliced carrots

2 cups broccoli florets

2 cups chopped asparagus

1 cup thinly sliced bell peppers (red, orange, and/or yellow)

FOR THE SAUCE

1 cup unsweetened or fresh pineapple juice

2 tablespoons lime juice

1 teaspoon grated ginger

1 teaspoon grated garlic

¼ to ½ teaspoon cayenne or red pepper flakes

2 tablespoons pure maple syrup

2 tablespoons tomato paste

1 tablespoon arrowroot powder

In a medium-sized bowl, whisk together the pineapple juice, lime juice, grated ginger and garlic, cayenne or red pepper flakes, maple syrup, tomato paste, and arrowroot powder. Set aside.

Add the green onions and carrots to a large nonstick ceramic pan. Cook for 3 to 5 minutes, adding a bit of water if needed to prevent sticking, until the carrots are almost tender. Add in the broccoli florets, asparagus, and bell peppers and cook for a further 5 minutes. When all the vegetables are tender, pour in the sauce and bring it to a boil, stirring frequently, until thickened. Remove from the heat and serve immediately.

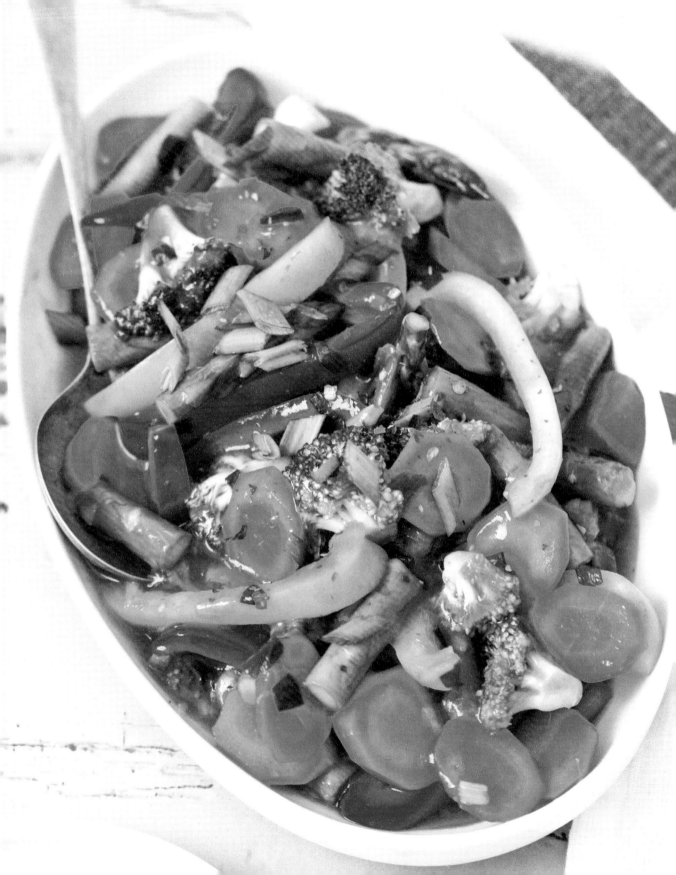

FRIES WITH THREE DIPPING SAUCES

Makes 2 servings

Almost everyone loves a bowl of fries! In this recipe, baked potato fries are the star with your choice of one, two, or three dipping sauces. Pick one or make them all—whatever feels good to you! All the sauces are full of flavor and contain only healing ingredients.

4 to 5 large potatoes, cut into fries

KETCHUP

3 ounces tomato paste

3 tablespoons apple juice

1 tablespoon lemon juice

¼ teaspoon onion powder

¼ teaspoon garlic powder

¼ teaspoon dried oregano

¼ teaspoon cayenne pepper

1 teaspoon raw honey

HONEY MUSTARD

3 tablespoons raw honey

¾ teaspoon mustard powder

2 tablespoons lemon juice

½ clove garlic, finely grated

⅛ teaspoon ground turmeric

PESTO

1½ cups basil leaves, tightly packed

1 cup spinach, tightly packed

1 garlic clove, roughly chopped

4 to 5 cherry tomatoes

1 teaspoon raw honey

1 tablespoon lemon juice

Preheat oven to 430°F/220°C. Line two large baking sheets with parchment paper.

Spread the fries out into a single layer on the baking trays. Bake for 30 to 40 minutes (flipping halfway), or until golden and crispy.

To make the ketchup, combine all the ingredients in a small bowl and whisk until uniform. Set aside.

To make the honey mustard dip, combine all the ingredients in a small bowl and whisk until uniform. Set aside.

To make the pesto, place all the ingredients in a small blender or food processor and process until combined, leaving a little texture. Scrape down the sides as often as needed.

When the fries are ready, remove them from the oven and serve them with the dipping sauce(s) of your choice.

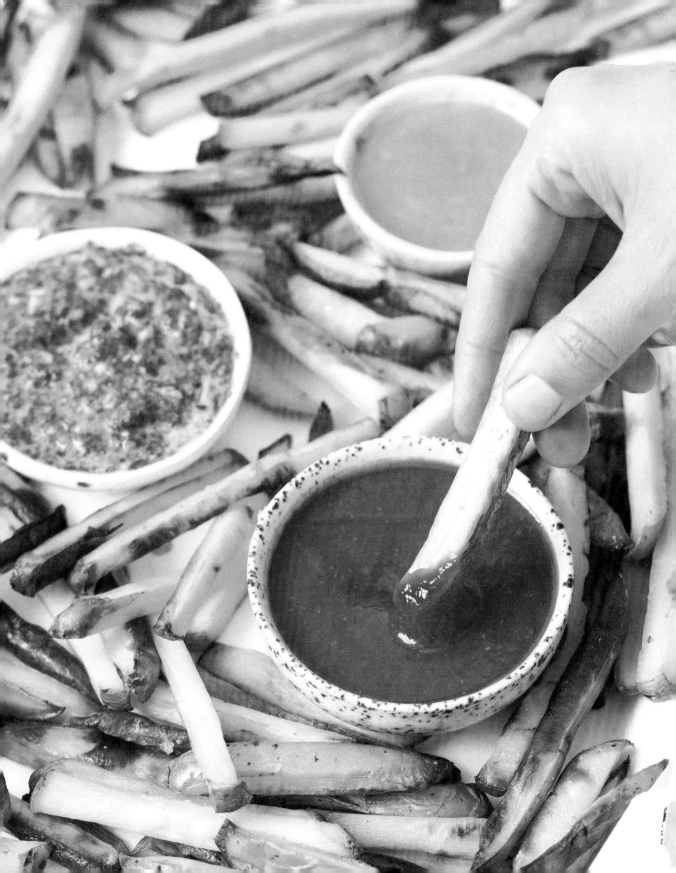

SWEET POTATO TORTILLA SOUP

Makes 2 servings

Full of flavor and with an inviting, rich aroma from the herbs and spices, this delicious twist on traditional Mexican tortilla soup is likely to be a hit. The addition of sweet potato brings extra flavor, satiation, and healing nutrients.

1 cup diced red or yellow onion, extra to serve

4 garlic cloves, minced

2½ cups chopped fresh tomatoes

2 cups Healing Broth (recipe on page 368) or water

2 tablespoons tomato paste

¼ to ½ teaspoon chipotle powder

1 teaspoon ground cumin

1 teaspoon ground coriander

1 teaspoon paprika

1 teaspoon pure maple syrup

1 cup diced sweet potato

1½ tablespoons lime juice

Fresh cilantro, to serve

Place a large ceramic nonstick pot on medium-high heat and add the 1 cup of onion and the garlic. Cook for 3 to 5 minutes, until the onion is translucent, adding a spoonful of water if needed.

Add the chopped tomatoes, Healing Broth or water, tomato paste, chipotle powder, ground cumin, ground coriander, paprika, and maple syrup. Place the lid on and simmer for 20 minutes.

Add in the sweet potato and lime juice and cook for a further 10 to 15 minutes, until the sweet potato is very tender.

Divide between bowls and top with the extra onion and fresh cilantro. Serve immediately.

TIPS

- When you're choosing between water and Healing Broth for the ingredients, keep in mind that the broth will produce a richer flavor. Store-bought vegetable stock isn't called for because it's very difficult to find a variety that's free of oil, salt, natural flavors, and/or other additives. For convenience, make a batch of Healing Broth in advance and freeze it (consider ice cube trays for easy thawing) so you have it on hand for recipes like this.

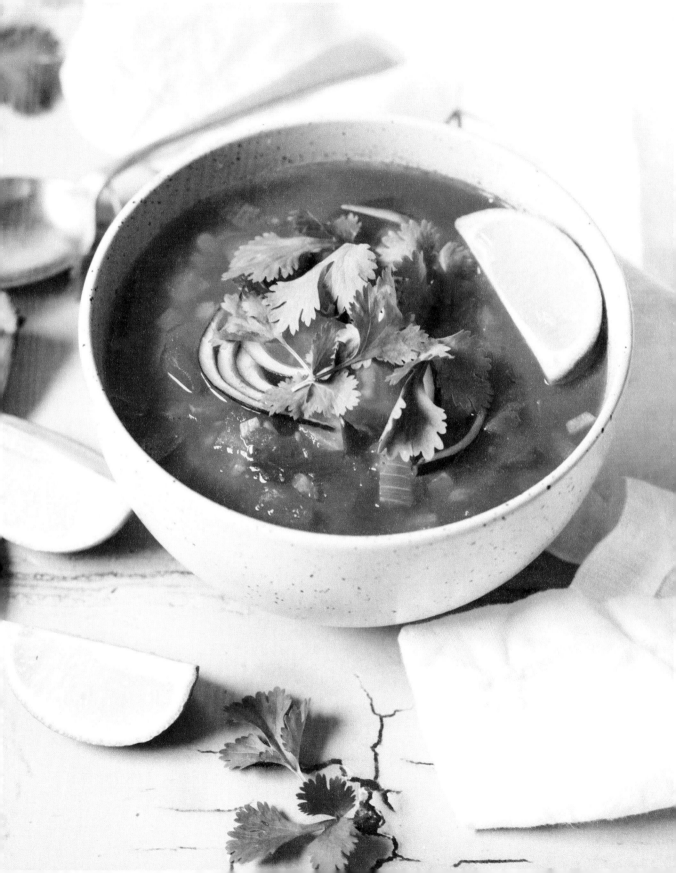

POTATO CAULIFLOWER MASH

Makes 2 to 3 servings

Mashed potatoes are a beloved comfort food for many people. Thankfully, you can enjoy them—without the butter or milk—and still help yourself heal! In this recipe, the potatoes are joined by cauliflower to make a creamy and nutrient-rich mash.

4 to 5 medium-sized potatoes, peeled and roughly chopped

1 small head of cauliflower, cut into large florets

2 teaspoons garlic powder

2 teaspoons onion powder

1 tablespoon chopped chives, parsley, or green onions, to serve

½ teaspoon paprika, to serve

Add 3 inches of water to a medium-sized pot, bring it to a boil, and add a steaming basket. Place the potatoes and cauliflower florets in the basket, cover, and steam for 15 to 20 minutes, until both are very tender.

Remove the potatoes and cauliflower and place them in a large bowl or pot. Add the garlic powder and onion powder. Mash until smooth using an immersion blender or potato masher. Serve topped with chives, parsley, or green onions, and paprika.

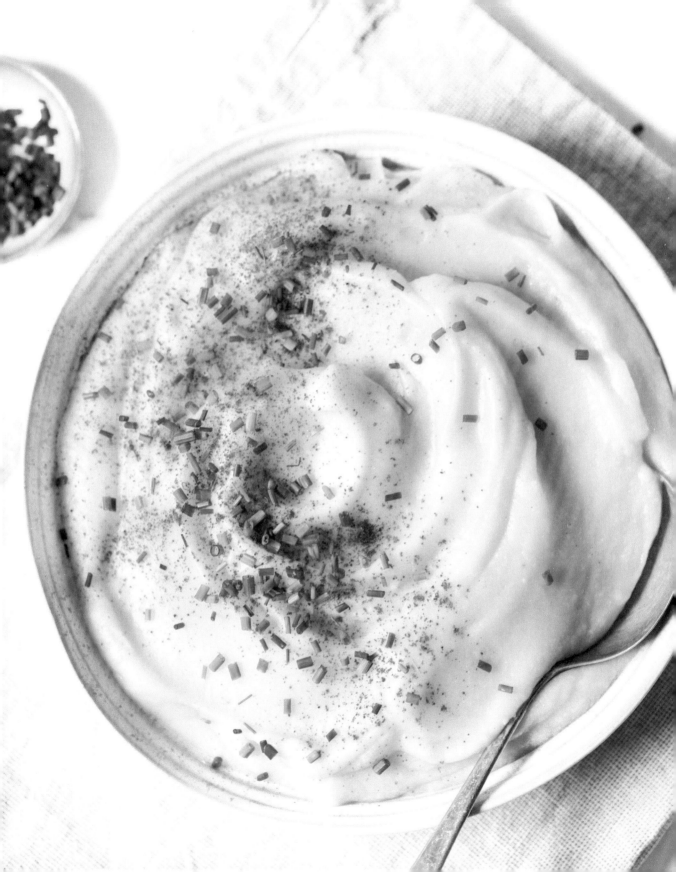

ESTONIAN STEW

This rustic vegetable stew is delicious and warming. It's the perfect nourishment for a cold night or when you want a bowl of simple, home-cooked comfort.

1 cup diced onions

1 cup chopped mushrooms (optional)

1 cup chopped carrots

4½ cups roughly chopped potatoes

2½ cups Healing Broth (recipe on page 368) or water

3 cups roughly chopped cabbage

¼ cup loosely packed fresh dill, roughly chopped

¼ cup loosely packed fresh parsley, roughly chopped

Place a large ceramic nonstick pot on medium-high heat and add the onions, mushrooms (if using), and carrots. Cook for 3 to 5 minutes, until the onions and carrots start to soften, adding a spoonful of water if needed.

Pour in the Healing Broth or water, place the lid on, and bring to a simmer. Cook covered for 10 minutes, until the potatoes and carrots are almost soft, and then remove the lid and cook for a further 5 minutes uncovered.

Add the chopped cabbage and stir until evenly mixed. Cook for 2 to 3 more minutes, until the cabbage is soft. Remove from heat and stir in the dill and parsley. Serve immediately.

TIPS

- When you're choosing between water and Healing Broth for the ingredients, keep in mind that the broth will produce a richer flavor. Store-bought vegetable stock isn't called for because it's very difficult to find a variety that's free of oil, salt, natural flavors, and/or other additives. For convenience, make a batch of Healing Broth in advance and freeze it (consider ice cube trays for easy thawing) so you have it on hand for recipes like this.

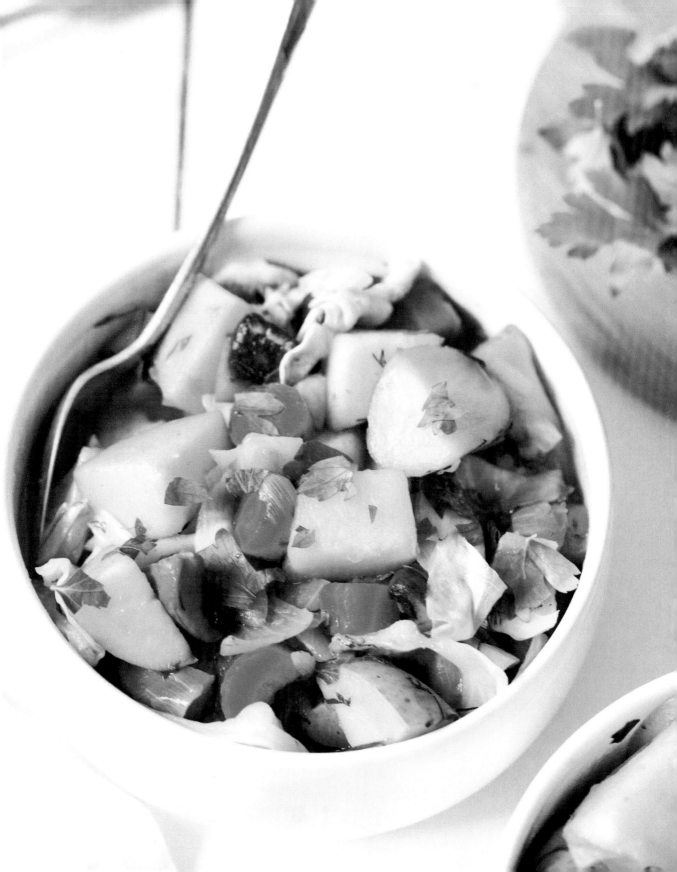

CURRIED CAULIFLOWER SOUP

Makes 1 to 2 servings

There's nothing quite like a creamy soup recipe that you can come back to over and over again. You may just find you turn to this Curried Cauliflower Soup regularly for an easy and tasty dinner. Enjoy it alone or alongside a beautiful, big salad of your choice.

1 cup diced onion

4 garlic cloves, finely minced

1-inch piece of fresh ginger, finely chopped

1 teaspoon ground cumin

1 teaspoon ground coriander

½ to 1 teaspoon red pepper flakes (optional)

½ teaspoon ground turmeric

2 teaspoons curry powder

1 medium-sized cauliflower, cut into florets

3 cups Healing Broth (recipe on page 368) or water

2 teaspoons raw honey or pure maple syrup

2 teaspoons freshly squeezed lemon juice

Fresh cilantro, to serve

Place a large ceramic nonstick pot on medium-high heat and add the onion, garlic, and ginger. Cook for 3 to 5 minutes, until the onion is translucent, adding a spoonful of water if needed to prevent sticking to the pot.

Add the ground cumin, ground coriander, red pepper flakes (if using), turmeric, curry powder, and cauliflower and cook for a further 2 to 3 minutes, until the spices are fragrant.

Add the Healing Broth or water, raw honey or maple syrup, and lemon juice. Place the lid on and simmer for 10 to 15 minutes, or until the cauliflower is very tender.

Ladle the soup into a blender and blend until smooth (you may need to do this in batches). Alternatively, you can use an immersion blender. Pour the soup back into the pot and bring it to a simmer.

Divide between bowls, garnish with fresh cilantro, and serve.

TIPS

- When you're choosing between water and Healing Broth for the ingredients, keep in mind that the broth will produce a richer flavor. Store-bought vegetable stock isn't called for because it's very difficult to find a variety that's free of oil, salt, natural flavors, and/or other additives. For convenience, make a batch of Healing Broth in advance and freeze it (consider ice cube trays for easy thawing) so you have it on hand for recipes like this.

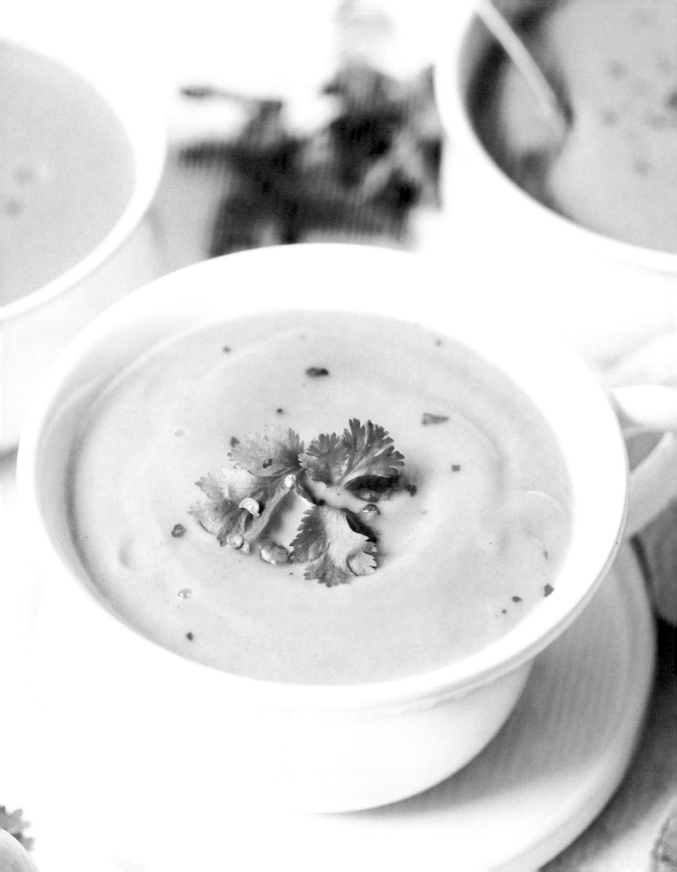

EGGPLANT AND ZUCCHINI PARM

Makes 2 to 3 servings

This fat-free version of Eggplant and Zucchini Parm features delicious Mediterranean flavors without the drawbacks of the traditional ingredients such as cheese and a lot of oil. Enjoy this wonderful meal alongside a salad of your choice, such as the Chopped Salad or Israeli Salad, for a fantastic meal.

1 small eggplant, cut into 1-inch-thick slabs

1 medium-sized zucchini, cut into 1-inch-thick slabs

1 teaspoon dried oregano

1 teaspoon dried thyme

¼ cup fresh basil, to serve

CAULIFLOWER POTATO SAUCE

1½ cups cauliflower florets

1½ cups roughly chopped potatoes

1 teaspoon garlic powder

1 teaspoon onion powder

1 tablespoon water (optional)

MARINARA

⅓ cup finely chopped onions

1 garlic clove, finely chopped

1½ cups roughly chopped cherry or plum tomatoes

¼ cup tomato paste

½ tablespoon raw honey

1 teaspoon dried oregano

Preheat oven to 350°F/180°C. Line a large baking sheet with parchment paper and arrange the eggplant and zucchini slices on top.

Sprinkle them with dried oregano and dried thyme and bake for 15 to 20 minutes, until tender when pierced with a fork. Remove from the oven and set aside.

While the eggplant and zucchini are in the oven, make the cauliflower potato sauce: Add 3 inches of water to a medium-sized pot, bring it to a boil, and add a steaming basket. Place the cauliflower florets and potatoes in the basket, cover, and steam for 15 to 20 minutes, until both are very tender. Remove and place in a blender. Add the garlic powder and onion powder and blend until very smooth, adding a bit of water if needed to blend.

To make the marinara, combine the onions, garlic, tomatoes, tomato paste, raw honey, and dried oregano in a saucepan. Cook for 10 to 15 minutes, stirring frequently, until the tomatoes are soft. Remove and place in a blender. Blend until the sauce is smooth yet still has some texture to it.

Spread 1 to 2 tablespoons of marinara on each eggplant or zucchini slice. Top with the cauliflower potato sauce and place back in the oven for 5 minutes. Remove from the oven and serve immediately with fresh basil leaves.

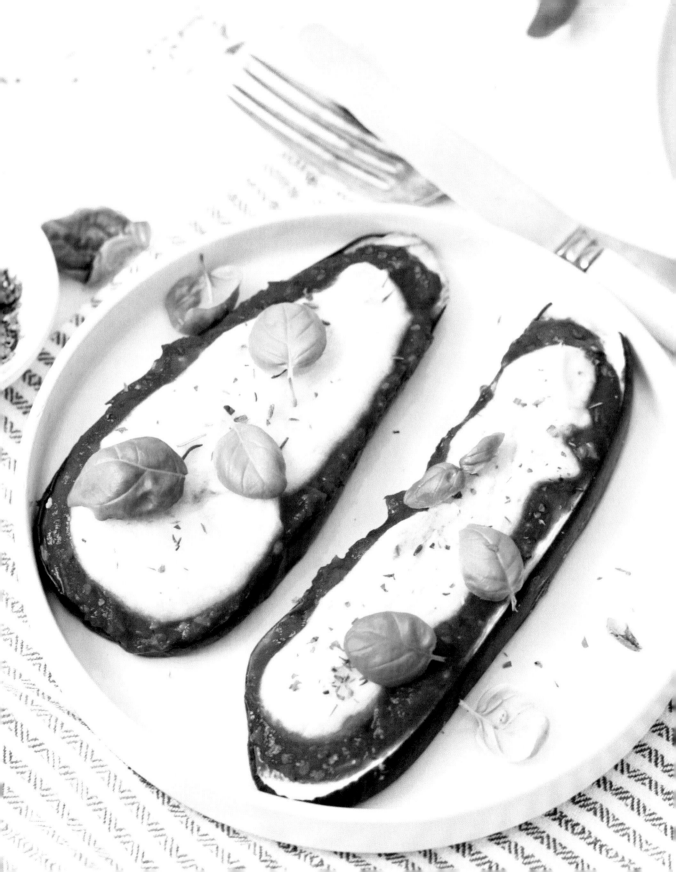

STEAMED ARTICHOKES
WITH TWO DIPPING SAUCES

Artichokes are one of the most healing vegetables on this planet. When steamed, they retain most of their nutrients and make a delicious and healing snack or meal. In this recipe, you'll find two tasty options to enjoy with your artichokes: Mustard Maple Dipping Sauce and Zucchini Herb Dipping Sauce.

4 artichokes

1 lemon, cut in half

MUSTARD MAPLE DIPPING SAUCE

2 tablespoons pure maple syrup

2½ tablespoons lemon juice

1 tablespoon water

½ teaspoon mustard powder

½ teaspoon cayenne

½ teaspoon fresh thyme leaves

1 teaspoon finely chopped parsley

ZUCCHINI HERB DIPPING SAUCE

1½ cups chopped zucchini

1 tablespoon lemon juice

2 teaspoons raw honey

1 teaspoon onion powder

½ garlic clove

3 to 4 tablespoons water

¼ cup loosely packed herbs, such as dill, parsley, thyme, and/or chives

To prepare the artichokes, use a knife to carefully slice off the top quarter of each artichoke as well as the end of each stem. Use scissors to cut off the tips of the artichoke leaves to remove the thorns. Rub the whole artichoke immediately with the cut lemon.

Place a steaming basket in a large pot filled with water until it reaches the basket. Place the prepared artichokes in the basket and cover. Bring to a boil and steam until the artichoke leaves can be removed by gently pulling. This should take about 30 to 40 minutes depending on the size of the artichokes.

To make the Mustard Maple Dipping Sauce, whisk together all the ingredients in a small bowl. Serve immediately.

To make the Zucchini Herb Dipping Sauce, combine all the ingredients in a blender and blend until smooth. Serve immediately.

Once the artichokes have slightly cooled, peel off the leaves, dip them in your dressings, and nibble the "meat" from the base of each leaf. Next, scrape off the choke from each artichoke and enjoy the hearts.

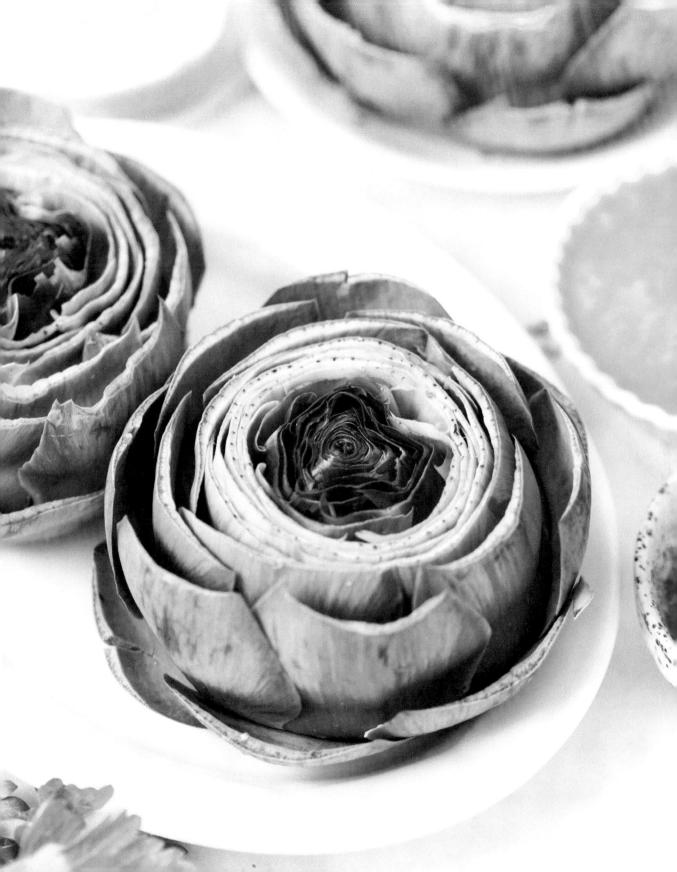

"You may have heard the false theory that illness is just a cry for attention. You may have heard that when bad things happen to us, we caused them by thinking the wrong thoughts, or that something about who we are is wrong.

If you are ill or going through a trial like a loss, you did not manifest it. You did not attract it. It is not punishment or payback. You do not deserve to be sick or unhappy. It is not your fault.

You don't need to travel the world trying to find yourself. Soul healing is about reclaiming who you are. Because who you are already is good enough. Who you are already means more than you know.

You deserve to heal. You deserve to be happy. You deserve to feel whole."

— Anthony William, Medical Medium

CHAPTER 24

Soul-Healing Meditations and Techniques

Everybody is soul-searching. Even if they don't know it, even if they don't call it that, it's what they're doing.

We soul-search because part of us feels lost, or we don't feel whole, or because we feel like we're not living up to our soul's potential. We soul-search because of life's hardships.

Often a negative experience, or a series of them, will prompt a person to feel broken or depleted and want to feel complete again. That's soul-searching. It can take the form of attending retreats, going to hear inspirational speakers, seeking advice from loved ones, enrolling in therapy, or any number of other activities. It's what we do when we're looking to heal and elevate our souls, to strengthen our purpose in life.

Your soul resides in your brain, where your soul stores your *memories* and *experiences*. When you pass from this mortal realm, your soul carries those memories as it moves onward. Even if someone has a brain injury or brain disease that keeps her or him from remembering certain things, the soul will bring all the memories with it when that person passes on.

Your soul also stores your hope, faith, and trust, all of which help keep you on the right path.

Ideally, we would all have fully intact souls. Over the course of life's hardships, though, a soul can become fractured and even lose pieces of itself. This can be caused by traumatic events, such as the death of a loved one, betrayal by a loved one, or betrayal of oneself, as well as ongoing traumas, such as the loss of freedom and trust that comes with experiencing chronic symptoms and illness.

When I scan someone who has been through hardship, fractures in her or his soul resemble cracks in a cathedral window. I can tell where the fractures are, because that's where the light comes streaming through.

As for a soul with missing pieces, it's like a house at night that's meant to have all of its lights on . . . except some of its rooms are stuck in the dark.

When soul injuries are fresh, they can result in the feeling of being lost, or in loss of connection with oneself, loss of desire or inspiration to persevere or thrive, or even loss of life force. That's why it's important to be aware of our soul. Wounds from hardship, betrayal, broken trust, or emotional hurt often exhaust a person's immune system, adrenals, and other body defenses, triggering a physical issue that could be residing deep within our organs and body.

Sometimes a person's soul injury and resulting emotional state isn't a physical problem . . . yet. Symptoms often take time to build quietly in the background, so a soul injury at an earlier time in life could be the trigger for future symptoms or full-blown conditions to come—if you don't have the right knowledge, tools, and resources to care for your soul and physical body.

Let's be clear: emotional wounds and soul wounds are not the *reason* for physical suffering. They are not the cause. Rather, they can act as *triggers* for underlying susceptibilities, which are caused by the pathogens and poisons we're up against in this world. *You* are not weak. You are stronger than you know to have battled this long and gotten yourself this far in life. Now you get to rise above.

A person with soul injury is vulnerable. If you ever hear a friend say, "I'm not ready for another relationship, I'm still hurting from my breakup," she's acknowledging that her soul needs time to heal before she risks putting herself out there again.

Along the same lines, if you ever observe someone who's sick with symptoms or a condition and hasn't been able to find answers, you may see this person hungrily pursuing spiritual learning in any form: religion, spiritual gurus, self-help books, meditation retreats, breath work . . . It's likely because that person's soul

has been injured from all the trust lost along the way, and she or he is instinctively searching for ways to make the soul healthy and complete again. When we fall ill with symptoms that won't go away or that continue to come and go, we lose trust in our body and in others to help us. There are people who have been sick for years who turn to soul-searching when they can't find answers. They find themselves at the best retreats in the world, still in pain or sick.

Sometimes soul-searching will bring people closer to themselves. Many times it will leave them feeling more lost than ever. Under the guise of "help," you may have heard the false theory that illness is just a cry for attention. You may have heard that when bad things happen to us, we caused them by thinking the wrong thoughts, or that something about who we are is wrong.

I've said it before, and I'll say it again: If you are ill or going through a trial like a divorce or a loss, you did not manifest it. You did not attract it. It is not punishment or payback. You do not deserve to be sick or unhappy. It is not your fault.

You don't need to travel the world trying to find yourself. Soul healing is about reclaiming who you are. Because who you are already is good enough. Who you are already means *more than you know.*

You deserve to heal. You deserve to be happy. You deserve to feel whole.

So far in this book, we've focused on the very real, physiological reasons for chronic suffering, as well as the knowledge and tangible tools you need to protect yourself and your loved ones. Those safeguards and the physical healing they bring about create one of the most powerful forms of soul healing, too.

When you use the previous chapters to work on your physical health, you're repairing your adrenals and your nervous system from all they've been through. That, along with all the other physical improvements from getting to the root of your symptom or condition, can mean you start to get your life back. And as your quality of life and the freedom you lost start to return, your soul can gain profound relief, rejuvenation, and liberation.

At the same time, you can bring in the special techniques in this chapter to enhance your healing on every level. Here, you will understand what happens to our souls when we encounter hardship and how to bring healing to your own soul. The exercises I describe are the true answers for soul-searchers.

These techniques are also here to bring healing to your heart and spirit. As I mentioned at the beginning of this book, your soul, heart, and spirit are three separate parts of you. They are still connected. They all still speak to each other.

Your *heart* serves as the compass for your actions, guiding you to do the right thing when your soul becomes lost. Your heart is also a kind of safety net that can compensate for soul injury. This means you can have a tattered soul and a warm, loving heart. When your soul suffers fractures and losses, a strong heart will get you through with *selfless love*, *compassion*, and *joy* until your soul has managed to heal. (Superficial love: that's a matter of the mind. Selfless love: that comes from the heart.)

It also works the other way: having a healthy soul doesn't necessarily make you complete. You can have an uninjured soul, and a broken heart can still hinder you.

Your heart keeps a record of your good intentions. In fact, it's common for someone's heart to grow more loving and accepting as a result of the roller-coaster ride her or his soul has gone through. It's that reaction of "I get it now" after you've experienced a challenge that shows you how hard life can be on this planet. Great losses can lead to deeper understanding of others and what they have gone through, and a deeper understanding of what you yourself have gone through . . . and greater love and compassion.

Then there's your *spirit*—which in this context refers to your *will* and *physical strength.* Your spirit is not your soul. They are two separate parts of you. It's your spirit that enables you to climb, run, and fight.

You can have an injured soul and still have what's left of a strong spirit. Many people, when they experience a breakup, will start exercising or traveling more. That's an example of using your spirit to push through heartache and soul confusion or injury. Even if, at first, that breakup has you lying around in the fetal position, not wanting to eat, work, or do any self-care as you mourn the relationship, oftentimes the power of your free will (which is directly connected to your soul) will kick in, which will propel you to use your spirit to help yourself overcome.

As I said in Chapter 1, "Origins of the Medical Medium," even if your soul has been battered and your heart is faint, your spirit can keep you physically going while you look for opportunities to heal. That's part of why going outside for a walk, watching birds, or looking at a sunset can be so valuable: they help you regain your spirit, and that can be the start to rebuilding your heart and soul.

Every human being is different, with individual experiences, feelings, and soul states. At the same time, the techniques to come are powerful spiritual practices that anybody can do, no matter what their individual experiences, feelings, or soul states. You can turn to these for the rest of your life. They are here to support who you are, not change you because you are somehow not good enough. They're here to help your soul, heart, and spirit heal—which supports your physical healing, too—not rewire you because you are somehow faulty on some fundamental level.

You are not faulty. You are precious.

Be proud of any work you've done on your healing process in any way. Let yourself feel a sense of accomplishment in your soul. Taking control of your own recovery before you leave this planet is worth it. When your time here ends, each and every effort you've put into healing will help your soul on its journey beyond the stars, where God will receive it.

So get ready—you're about to learn the secrets to reviving your soul, heart, and spirit, finding peace, and feeling whole again.

EMOTIONAL DETOX

There's a significant emotional aspect to recovering from any injury or ailment—especially mystery illness. As your body cleanses itself of toxins or a viral load, you may find that emotional detox occurs, too.

For example, if you've suffered with chronic fatigue syndrome since college and have learned through this book that a virus was behind your condition, you might feel initial relief and even elation as you follow the chapters' guidelines and watch your body restore itself.

As your cells release those physical toxins—such as neurotoxins and dermatoxins produced by the very viruses behind your symptoms and conditions—emotions may bubble up. You may find yourself angry with the people who told you your illness was psychosomatic, and you may grieve for the years you lost to being unwell. You may feel intense cravings, as well, for foods that fed pathogens responsible for your inflammation and other symptoms.

This emotional aspect is a perfectly natural part of healing. When you went through past emotional hardships, fight or flight may have taken over. Your heart may have accelerated as adrenaline was being released throughout your body. When the fight-or-flight moment passed, this adrenaline, which contained information about the challenging experience, got stored deep in your cells and organs. Once you start cleansing and this old adrenaline gets released, a feeling of sadness can occur, or other emotional sensations. Emotions you were feeling at the time of hardship may resurface.

Take comfort in the knowledge that this is a temporary phase, and you don't have to engage with everything that comes up. You'll overwhelm yourself and risk dwelling in the past if you try to consciously process every tidbit that comes to the surface. That said, validation is essential to your recovery. Consider this whole book to be validation that your pain is real, that you didn't bring your illness or any emotional struggles or hardships upon yourself, and that you deserve to live a healthy life. You deserve to feel at peace.

During physical detox, one of your goals is to release old adrenaline storage bins and old emotions that are attached to painful memories (on a subconscious level when possible), and to replace them with soothing, positive points of reference—whether in the form of newer experiences or aspirations, or in the form of pleasant moments from the past that you've reclaimed. The more at peace you are, the better an environment you're creating for your nervous system, your immune system, your adrenals and endocrine system, and your digestive system to do their jobs. That peace is what this chapter will help you cultivate.

Using the meditations and techniques that follow, you can let go of the past and claim the life that God—the Higher Source, the Light, the Divine—wants for you.

FORMS OF MEDITATION

Meditation is a state of being that rewires your subconscious to be more at peace, which leads to freeing and healing your soul.

Even if you've never tried it, you're probably familiar with traditional methods of meditation, which involve sitting in a quiet room, choosing a single thing to focus on (e.g., a mantra, a lit candle), and entering into a more peaceful state of consciousness, while at the same time trying not to battle your thoughts or emotions—trying to consciously separate yourself from them so you can be in peace.

It's far from the only way to go. Any activity that you find relaxing, that reaffirms your sense of self and helps you recharge, can have a meditative, rejuvenating quality. These activities include bike rides, swimming (especially in "living" water, such as an ocean or lake), exercising in other fun ways (e.g., dancing, jumping on a trampoline), listening to music, reading, praying, getting extra rest, caring for a pet, learning a new skill with new people, spending time with loved ones, getting a massage, and taking baths with Epsom salts and pure essential oils.

That's just a small selection. You may have a unique pastime—like cleaning the lint filter on the clothes dryer, doing longhand arithmetic, organizing your refrigerator, or clearing out your closet—that calms you because it creates order in your universe. Whatever it is that brings you peace—that makes you feel positive and hopeful about the world—if you bring a meditative awareness to it, you'll promote healing for your body and soul. And when you feel grounded and optimistic, you're likely to encounter other wonderful people who love to be around you.

On top of developing your own special hobbies, you can try the following forms of meditation that Spirit of Compassion has shown me to be extremely powerful. These are exercises that may speak to you—and if you understand their depths, they have the ability to enter into your cells, tissue, and organs, as well as your soul, heart, and spirit, helping to give you a new beginning emotionally and spiritually.

You'll find some of these techniques, such as the Moon Meditation, featured as guided meditations on the *Medical Medium Podcast*. You're welcome to seek out those special episodes for an alternate experience of these soul-healing practices.

Waves on the Beach

It's possible to attain a superior meditative state of healing by watching or envisioning the waves on a beach—if you know how to harness the power within the waves. I have seen countless people rid themselves of PTSD, pain, and suffering with this technique.

If you are living with emotional wounds, or experiencing PTSD, anxiety, depression, depersonalization, bipolar disorder, OCD, or any emotional or physical suffering, this meditation technique can assist and strengthen you. This opportunity to overcome and heal emotional wounds in your soul, spirit, and heart allows your body a greater healing opportunity, too.

Here's how it works:

If you're physically at a beach, go ahead and sit, stand, or walk, looking out at the water. You can choose to watch the waves or close your eyes and listen. We'll focus on the ocean here, although a lake, river, or stream is a source of living water with healing effects, too.

You don't need to be at the water to do this meditation. If you're not near a beach, settle anywhere comfortable and call a peaceful beach to mind. It may help to put on a nature video of the ocean or an audio recording of waves.

To begin, envision the water before you as a powerful living body of life. This powerful living body of life harbors a soul-renewing and cleaning strength. Now think about the sea life within the ocean. The whales, the sea turtles, the sharks, the sea lions, the sea horses, the starfish, the octopus, the crabs, the jellyfish, the schools of fish, the seals, and the dolphins. See them not just as living within the ocean; see them as part of the ocean. See the sea life and the ocean as one.

When you are watching a wave (or envisioning one), imagine it's holding both the power of all the sea life and the power of the living, healing water itself. As the wave rolls in, it starts to enter your soul, attaching itself to any war wounds and emotional injuries you may have sustained in your life. The wave begins to scrub loose any damaging emotional thoughts, encompassing all of these past hurtful experiences. The wave saturates the

thoughts inside and out, swirling around hurtful emotions and swirling around soul wounds.

As the wave recedes, it holds onto these emotions and wounds. These impurities of your soul start to leave your body, exiting with the wave as it travels back down to the beach. These hurtful experiences and emotional hardships get absorbed into the vast ocean and carried away.

A new wave—clean, pure, and fresh—starts to head up the beach. Envision it entering your soul and once again scrubbing loose all of those emotional injuries, struggles, and hardships that remain. The wave swirls and tosses and intertwines itself within your bloodstream and your soul, pulling those emotions and thoughts that are holding you back out of your body. Once again, the wave takes them back out to the ocean.

As each new wave rolls in, let yourself be cleansed of the poisonous memories and injuries from the past. Let the ocean water wash any stains on your soul or within your cells that you want cleaned off, purified, and taken away by the powerful, healing, living salt water. See your memories of toxic thoughts, emotional hardships, and injuries wash out to the sea as you feel yourself purified.

When you're ready, you can begin to let each new wave bring strength and renewal to your spirit and soul. The ocean is one of the most grounding sources of energy. Our thoughts that are toxic in nature are not grounded at all—they are radical bits and pieces of toxic, broken energy that surge through our soul and spirit. The waves' grounding power neutralizes the noise, static, and toxic energy from our war wounds. Envision the waves grounding out those emotional wounds and injuries.

If you love the angels, call upon the Angel of the Ocean. She'll help put you in the best frame of mind for the meditation. (You'll learn more about receiving the support of the angels in the next chapter.)

You can also benefit from wading. Understand that any natural water source—be it a lake, a river, a stream, the ocean—is alive. It has a breath to it, as well as a will and a spirit. When you step into living water, envision the things you want to come true in your life.

Surrounded by Trees

To get the most out of nature, it's not enough just to go for a hike. For the most healing effect, here's what you have to do: when you first enter a wooded area, whether a city park or your own property, take a moment to acknowledge the peaceful environment, especially all the trees that rise up around you. If you love the angels, call upon the Angel of Trees.

Turn your mind to their root systems. Think about the minerals and water they're drawing from deep within the earth, up through their trunks, up through their branches. As you let yourself feel surrounded by this deep earth energy, envision roots growing out of your feet and into the Earthly Mother's soil.

When you intuitively feel it's time to end this glorious grounding experience, imagine that you're leaving roots protected and preserved in the earth as you break free and walk away. These roots remain a part of you. Wherever you are, transcending all time and space, you can draw healing energy from their spot in the ground.

This is the most powerful grounding treatment available. It will fortify every aspect of your being. It will reinforce your will to survive,

invigorate your spirit to receive positivity and ward off negativity, and create a strengthening frequency for body and soul. It will prepare you to free yourself from fear and live life at its best.

To receive the benefits of nature, you don't need to be outside. The following meditation, which expands the technique above, puts you in touch with the outdoors even if you do it inside the home.

You can do this meditation exercise either indoors or outside in nature. You can be sitting or standing. Close your eyes. Envision trees all around you. The environment is peaceful. There are birds on branches chirping and singing. You can hear the wind gently rustle through the trees.

Imagine now that you are following the tree trunks down to the ground. Next, you turn your mind to the root systems. You start thinking about the roots going deeper into the earth. You think about the soil that's surrounding each root. There are minerals that are healing within this soil. These minerals listen below the earth and are healing and nourishing the roots. Think about the minerals we have inside our body that match the minerals we have in the earth nourishing these roots. The minerals are part of what keeps us healthy and grounded.

It starts to rain. Envision raindrops hitting the leaves of the trees. The rain is washing and purifying the dust and dirt that is on the leaves. Imagine the rain hitting the top of your head, your face, and your arms. See the rain rolling down the tree trunks and entering the ground, the earth.

Now think about the water these roots are drawing up from deep within the earth, up through the trunks and up through their branches. Envision roots growing out of your feet into the earth as your legs become a tree trunk. The roots that are attached to your feet and going deep in the earth are surrounded by minerals and soil, and now they are soaking up rainwater.

Start to envision roots growing more quickly out of your feet and into the earth. Envision a root growing off each toe, all of the roots going in different directions into the earth below you. These roots are already strong, and you have the power to make them as strong as you need them to be. Say this: "My roots are strong."

Envision growing as many roots as you feel necessary to fully ground you. Feel the strength of these roots as they grow deep into the earth. Understand that this is the most powerful grounding meditation there is. The earth holds tremendous power, and that power is rising up from the earth through the roots and into your body, giving you strength. The strength enters into your body, surging through your veins, and heading to your heart.

Take a deep breath inward and release the breath outward. Envision your heart sending the power of these roots and the earth throughout every blood vessel and organ in your body. Emotional hardship and struggles from the past and the present start to become grounded, and they begin to become defused. The grounding energy engulfs all that is toxic within you and neutralizes and strengthens your deep inner being.

When you intuitively feel it's time to end this glorious healing, grounding experience, get ready to step forward in your mind, breaking yourself away from these roots. Break away one foot at a time. Imagine that you are leaving these roots that have grown out of your feet and legs behind. You are leaving them protected and preserved in the earth below you as you start to walk away.

Even though you're separate from these roots now, these roots remain a part of you. You can call upon their power at any time, wherever you are. This gives you the ability to transcend all time and space, because you can draw healing energy from where the roots were left in the earth to ground you. If you're someone who feels you need continual grounding because of difficult circumstances, stressful situations, or challenging emotions, feel free to repeat the exercise multiple times a week or month.

Free as a Bird

Bird-watching is a healing activity simply because it connects you with nature. When you truly focus on seeing and hearing the birds, though, you elevate it to one of the most enlightening meditations you can perform.

Birdsong is the most sacred form of music; birds sing the songs of the angels and the heavens. Birdsong mends a fractured soul and can aid in healing symptoms and conditions. This is because the frequency of these melodies resonates deep within our DNA, which allows it to help the body heal on a cell level. If you listen to the birds with respect and appreciation and don't take them for granted, there's no doubt that your life will start to transform.

Observing birds is powerful, too. Here on earth, our souls can become caged up and our spirits suppressed. When we witness birds' freedom in flight, it ignites and unleashes the spirit and breaks the cage of the soul. Further, a bird lands only on an area it deems safe—and has the ability to flutter off if that spot doesn't work out. When we pay attention to the way a bird alights on a branch or the ground, it activates our own healing and promotes a sense of safety within our souls.

If it's healing you're seeking, enlightenment, connection to the Divine, spirituality, wisdom, compassion, knowledge, and understanding of your greater purpose, then seek not the owl. Seek the hummingbird. Admire the owl as a blessed and beautiful creature, yet take your cue from the hummingbird, which flies by day and feeds off the nectar of the earth's flowers, pollinating as it goes. This is the most spiritual form of eating and shows the greatest wisdom.

Hummingbirds are light-workers. Every time you spot one, recognize it as a true and sacred symbol of the Light. Witness it as a fairy spreading the holy light of the angels. Let it purify your thoughts and intentions, then send the hummingbird with a wish or a prayer. It will carry your message to the right recipient.

The exercise to follow is for anyone who has become stifled, unheard, or misunderstood in life. It's also for the many who feel cooped up because of our times, unable to travel or get as much time in nature as you'd like.

As we go through life, we can feel so held back, as if something is holding us down and not letting us move forward. So many of us feel trapped, suffocated, stuck, and stagnant. We can feel as if the stress of life is wrapped around our soul. As we keep busy and try to run from it all, we can lose touch with ourselves and feel unable to climb up above the noise. This meditation is a chance to break free and become emotionally strong.

Our soul can pick up on how we feel because how we feel is directly connected to our soul. When we go through emotional hardships, it can feel as if it leaves a residue on our soul, and that residue can become a cage on the outside of our soul, disconnecting us from ourselves or how we feel about others. We can make misjudgments and choices out of emotion because we've been hurt. We can feel held back by how others have perceived us when we've expressed ourselves. We can become protective, reserved, sanctioned in our thoughts—concerned with how someone will view us, or whether or not they will accept us. This can inhibit us from being who we are. Living in this world today is not easy. Anxiety, nervousness, anxiousness, and depression exist among nearly all.

Even if we don't experience these difficulties, we likely know people who are experiencing them. When we care about others, we open our hearts. We can absorb, sense, or even take on their struggles with feeling trapped, held back, or stifled, or with a loss of confidence. In that case, we can envision them in this exercise, and in that way assist our dear ones.

The Free as a Bird meditation provides an escape from the very difficult emotional challenges we face every day within ourselves and with the world around us. It lifts the residue off our soul so we can gain clarity. If you're sick, not feeling well, and living with symptoms, this is a chance to elevate above it while you're working on our healing.

This exercise can be done indoors or outdoors. Choose a comfortable spot to relax, sitting or lying down. When you're ready, close your eyes.

Now envision yourself in a field of tall grass and wildflowers. The air is clean and fresh. The sky is blue. Envision yourself growing wings like a bird. Choose the bird you wish to be. Do you want the wings of a robin? Cardinal?

Hawk? Crow? Heron? Or even the wings of an eagle? Or do the wings you picture not belong to one particular bird? You decide. See the feathers, soft and strong, growing on your arms and chest.

Now take a deep breath in. Release the breath. You are a bird. You are part of nature. You are nature. Your feathers are strong, and they are able to take on any wind or breeze. Imagine yourself as this bird standing among the wildflowers, butterflies, and dragonflies. You are safely looking out, over the distance to the horizon. The sun is growing lower in the sky. When you look down, you see that bird claws have replaced your feet.

Look back up at the horizon, and start to flap your wings. Propel yourself forward and jump into the air. Keep flapping your wings and start climbing in the sky. Let it feel effortless. As you start to take on height as you rise up in flight, the wildflowers below you get smaller and smaller and blend into a beautiful light blue with spots of pink in between.

As you fly, you are headed for a tree line that you see in the distance. You spot one tall oak tree that you admire. You land on its highest branch and look out over the distance again at the horizon. Can you see mountains, trees, clouds? You are high above the ground. It's getting late in the day. The sun is lower in the sky. Do you see the orange-red streaks over the horizon? Take a deep breath in and release.

Envision that your soul is a ball of light glowing in a cage of barbed wire. The difficulties in your life have become that cage of wire. Anything that may have been holding you back that has been seen or not seen is in that cage of wire. These are things you weren't allowed to say or do throughout life without judgment or misunderstanding. Old wounds and even broken friendships over the years are intertwined in that wire cage around your soul. Now envision that wire cage breaking open. It falls away from your soul, out of your body, down to the ground, by the oak's tree trunk. Take a deep breath in and release.

The air is cool and crisp, and you are warm inside, beneath your soft feathers. From your perch high above the ground, you are getting ready to take flight again. See yourself bending your legs, and envision propelling yourself into the sky.

You're in flight and you're free—free from the worldly powers that try to hinder us. As you fly, see the clouds above you. Feel the wind blowing against your feathers. Your soul is free. The wire cage of hurt is no longer wrapped around your soul. As you fly free, nothing is holding you back. Nothing is holding you down.

When you look to your left, you see another bird flying alongside of you. To your right, you see another bird flying alongside you. They are free and with you on this journey. You see green rolling hills, one after another. Everything below you looks so small. You see dirt roads, cattle grazing, barns, and houses. You are free as a bird. You are floating in air, hovering high in the sky. Your soul is so bright and strong and free now.

It's time to start heading back to the field where you started. As you get closer, the wildflowers begin to define themselves, and their blue color gets stronger and brighter. Get ready to land soon. As you start to descend, the wildflowers get closer and closer. You can even count their petals and see the blades of grass between them. Brace yourself as you float down. When you're ready, touch down and land, with your claws now on the field.

See the feathers disappearing from your arms. Take a deep breath in and release. Take another deep breath in and release. Open your eyes.

You are now in touch with a part yourself that you haven't been connected to in years. As we go through life, we can lose a connection to our soul. We can feel like a great weight is upon us, holding us down from flying free and living the life we strive for. In this moment, the cage that was wrapped around your soul is no longer there. It is open, and you are free. Your soul is free of the residue from earthly woes—hardships, betrayals, broken trust, losses, and struggles from others around us.

You are welcome to repeat this meditation as often as you'd like, whenever you feel the confines of life taking a grip once again, building a new cage around your soul. The more you do this meditation, the less the cage can take hold and the less the residue can hold you back. Make this exercise a regular part of your spiritual growth and healing. When you practice flying free, nothing can hold your soul down or get in your soul's way.

Bee Watching

Bee watching is a secretly miraculous meditation. As bees dance from flower to flower, absorbing the sun and distributing pollen along the way, they emit a healing frequency that can help you heal and restore your physical body, soul, heart, and spirit. This is something we can't fully understand on a rational level, but our cells and our soul understand. When you make yourself aware of the bees and ask your body to tune its channels to their frequency, all of the cells in your body will start to resonate with this healing vibration.

Bees individually do not have a soul. Bees *collectively* have one soul amongst all of them. That soul only exists if there's more than one bee. If there were only one bee left on earth, it would not survive, even given an ideal environment. It would need another bee so that the collective soul of the bees would be sustained, which keeps the bees' frequency alive.

Collecting Stones

When you want to cleanse yourself of challenging emotions, take a walk in nature and keep your eye out for small stones that call to you. Over the course of your stroll, select three that feel good to hold in your hands. Name each stone by the label of whatever you're harboring that you'd like to leave you. For example, you might name the stones Guilt, Fear, and Anger. Or Hate, Shame, and Disappointment. Or Frustration, Sorrow, and Despair.

Carry these stones with you wherever you go. Keep them in your pocket, if you'd like, or even in your hands. Get to know each of your three stones. Look at them when you get an opportunity. Study their surfaces, their terrain. Keep the stones on your bedside table. When you go to sleep, say goodnight to these stones. Upon waking, say good morning to the stones. Bring the stones to the kitchen table when you eat breakfast. Keep the stones on you when you walk. Even take them in the shower with you. (Do not worry if the stones get wet.) Develop a relationship with them; become friends. If you would like to introduce your stones to your other friends and family, feel free. When you hold onto these stones, let the heat from your hands warm them up. When some days are harder, you can lean on your stones. Try to believe that they understand you, and that their job is to absorb the emotions you've named them after out of your soul and body. The healing frequency of the minerals will act as an antidote to whatever ails you, whether emotional, spiritual, or physical.

When the time naturally comes that you feel the stones have done their job and you're ready to let them go, carry them back to nature and release them into a body of water, such as a pond, ocean, lake, river, or stream. The living water will purify them of the venom they've drawn from you, and you'll walk away purified, too.

If you lose a stone or even all three, this was not your fault, nor was it a mistake. This is part of your spiritual experience. This exercise is never under your full control. The stones can make their own choosings. When symbiotically working with your emotions, a stone's disappearance is a sign. It may mean that the stone has absorbed as much as it can for now and needs some time on its own for now, or it may mean that the emotion is already in the process of leaving you, so the stone disappeared for good to help rid that emotion from your soul, spirit, and heart. Whether you lose one, two, or all three stones, you can replace them if you would still like to complete the exercise. If you lose *those* stones, you can replace them again. If you're in a situation where it's difficult to get another stone, then allow for the timing to become right, eventually, for a stone to fall into your hands.

Sunbathing

It will be centuries before science discovers all of the healing benefits the sun provides. Not only is it calming and warming, but the sun's rays contain mystery elements and promote biochemical reactions in our bodies that produce more than just vitamin D.

Just look at the way our pets love to find a warm, sunlit patch of the floor and bask in it. Animals love to sunbathe—they know it's a powerful healing tool.

To benefit from the sun, spend time each day letting your skin absorb it. Try to acclimate yourself to 15 minutes at a time (taking care not to get sunburned). If it's a cold time of year, find a peaceful spot inside where the sun comes through a window. If you love the angels, call upon the Angel of Sun to help the rays enter into your being to soothe your soul and heal your body.

You can also try this sunbathing meditation exercise. If you can be in the sun, find a comfortable spot either indoors or outdoors. You can put on sunglasses if you'd like. Don't look directly at the sun. If you can't be in the sun, you can still do this exercise, imagining the sun's rays on you.

To begin, close your eyes. As the sun is warming you, get comfortable with knowing that the sun is covering your entire body. Get familiar with the sun; get familiar with the *feeling* of it.

Once you've established that connection, take a deep breath in and release. Envision that you're inhaling sunlight—in through your nose, in through your mouth, and into your lungs. In your mind, see the sunlight.

Once that connection is secure, focus on the sun hitting your feet. Connect your mind to your feet. If you can, wiggle your feet around a bit to connect even more. After you've established that connection between the sun and your feet, take a deep breath and then release. Again, envision that you're inhaling sunlight in through your nose, in through your mouth, and into your lungs. See the sunlight in your thoughts, in your mind.

Now focus on the sun warming your knees. Once you've established that connection, take in a deep breath of sunlight to your lungs and release.

Continue this process with your stomach, then your chest, then your arms, and then your head—feeling the warmth of the sun on that area of your body, establishing a connection, breathing in sunlight, and releasing.

We often sunbathe without conscious awareness of how much we can achieve when we use the sun to its full extent. This meditation will align your thoughts with the sun's power. When we are aware of how much the sun affects the cells within our body, it allows us to connect to the sun fully so that our cells can access its healing abilities.

As you are resting in the sun, tell your cells that you know they are being nourished by the sun's rays. You are witnessing this process for your cells—all of the cells in your body are being validated, acknowledged, seen, and understood. Ask your cells to be open, to absorb the vast array of mysterious information and life-giving properties that the sun has to offer. Ask your immune system to be willing to accept the sun as an immune system restoring mechanism. Ask your immune system to be ready to take in the sun's strength, to make the sun's strength your immune system's strength.

Next, envision that you are looking at the sun. (Remember, though, don't open your eyes and look directly at the sun.) Within your consciousness, "see" the sun's fiery blaze. Imagine yourself drifting closer to the sun, and say (either in your mind or out loud), "My immune system, and every cell in my body, is receiving the sun's

rays and the sun's power, and its healing energy is revitalizing and restoring my entire body."

Here's a bonus you can try next: Envision the sun's rays crossing the barrier of your soul and entering into it. The warmth from the sun is now reversing emotional injuries from conflicts and past struggles. You do not have to be aware of what they are. Just let the sunrays lighten the way throughout your soul. Say, "My soul will heal. My soul is strong. My soul is safe. My soul is healed, and my soul will not be harmed." It's an option to call upon the Angel of Sun.

Take a deep breath and release. Now open your eyes.

Picking Fruit

Picking fruit is one of the most powerful meditations in existence. It is a sacred act of respect and gratitude to the Earthly Mother for the miracle of food. Even if you do it only once in your lifetime, it will be an experience you can reignite over and over, just by thought, to activate healing in the soul.

Each piece of fruit still on the tree is living food that's connected, via the plant's roots, to living water from deep within the earth. If you visit a pick-your-own apple orchard, for instance, then when you touch an apple on the tree, your cells will resonate with the apple's grounded nature, and peace will spread throughout your body.

On top of that, you'll naturally assume healing stretches and positions as you reach for apples and bend or crouch to collect them. These natural stretches supersede any human-created exercises. The joy in your heart and soul becomes one with each physical fruit-picking position, making it uniquely healing to you.

Picking berries, or even wildflowers, has the same effect. Since humans have existed on this planet, berry picking has been a celebration of abundance. When we follow in this millennia-old tradition, it ignites that ancient celebration of life within our souls and promotes healing.

As you gather strawberries or blackberries or raspberries or apples or peaches, meditate on all the months of development that led to this moment. First the plant started as a seed or root graft and grew to fruiting size. When it reached maturity, it didn't start bearing fruit every month of the year—rather, it developed with the seasons. Picture the tree or bush or vine in its dormant state, when it must have looked like nothing was happening. Next envision the leaves returning, the buds, the farmers tending to it all, the flowers blooming, and the pollinators paying visits. Our lives go through similar cycles. When we take the time to focus on nature's rhythms, we rewire our neurons, help reverse anxiety and PTSD, and activate trust and faith within our souls that our efforts to live a good life will be fruitful.

The meditation exercise that follows is for anyone who does not have access to picking fruit, whether because of time of year or any other circumstance. If you've picked fruit before, this meditation will let you experience it once again. Even if you've never picked a piece of fruit in your life, this meditation is just as powerful. Picking fruit is a part of our soul, spirit, and heart. Reconnecting with fruit picking is like reconnecting to our very soul's existence.

This meditation is best lying down, although you can do it sitting up if that's more comfortable. You can be inside or outside. When you're ready, close your eyes. Take a deep breath in and release, then repeat. Now envision yourself walking down an old country road. The sky is blue, the sun is shining, and the road is made of dirt and pebbles. When you look into the distance, you see an opening at the end of the road. As you get closer, you notice that it looks like a fruit orchard, although you can't tell what fruit. You reach the orchard and notice shiny red fruits all over the trees. As you walk into the orchard and approach one of the trees, you notice it's filled with cherries.

There is a basket under the tree. You lean over, pick the basket up, and then reach out and gently pluck one of the cherries and place it in the basket. You reach out for another cherry, pluck it, and place it in the basket. You see one more cherry, a large one, that's slightly out of reach, so you stand on your tippy toes, stretch your arms out as far as you can, just barely reaching it. Finally you lock onto the cherry, pluck it, and place it in the basket.

It is warm out. At the same time, there's a comfortable breeze that you feel on your face. You look to the right and see another fruit tree. The fruit on this tree is much larger and also red. You walk over and see that these are apples. They're higher up, so you take a hand, place it on a branch, and gently lift yourself up on your toes. You reach as far as you can and grab an apple. As you lower yourself down, you pull the apple from the tree. This allows two more apples to fall off the tree and land on the ground. You place the apple you've just picked in your basket and bend over to pick up a fallen apple and place it in your basket. You walk over a few steps, bend over, pick up the second fallen apple, and place it in your basket. You notice another apple on the ground that you didn't knock off the tree. You grab it and notice it has a worm. That worm represents PTSD, anxiety, hardship, trust broken, and losses. As you are holding the apple, a bird flies onto your hand

and grabs the worm right out of the apple. It flies off your hand into the sky. Something is freed inside you, and you feel light as air.

The sun is shining, and you feel a gentle breeze on your face. The air is clean and fresh. You feel relieved, so you find yourself a comfortable spot to sit down and rest in the grass. You realize quickly you've sat down in a strawberry patch. With one hand on the ground, you lean over and use your other hand to reach out and pluck a ripe, juicey strawberry off a strawberry plant. You add it to the basket. You see a larger strawberry on the other side of you. You lean over, put your hand down as support, reach out, and pluck that strawberry. You put it in the basket.

You notice the sun is starting to set. You get up and reach your arms out in a gentle stretch, then bend back down, pick up your fruit basket, and head out of the orchard, down the dirt path. You see, along the sides of the road, wild blueberries growing. You step off the road and walk into a blueberry patch. You crouch down in a squatting position and start picking the wild blueberries two or three at a time and placing them in your basket. You reach out again, take two to three more, and you can't help yourself—you put them in your mouth. You pick a handful more and place them in your basket.

You walk out of the blueberry bushes, back onto the dirt road, and head home. As you are walking, you get hungry, so you pick up one of your strawberries from your basket and place it in your mouth. You bite into it, chew, and swallow. You take a few more steps and then grab a cherry and gently bite into it. You feel the pit in the center, and you spit the pit on the ground. The juicy, sweet cherry is unlike any cherry you've ever eaten. Then you grab an apple, a beautiful, red blush apple. You bite into it.

Sweet and juicy, it's the best apple you have ever eaten.

As the sun goes down, you feel nourished. You feel safe. Your soul feels renewed. Your spirit is strong. Your heart is revived.

It's dusk. You get to the end of the dirt road and see an old wooden sign. You read it in the light that is left as the sun sets. It says, "Come back anytime."

Take a deep breath in and release. See cherries, apples, strawberries, and wild blueberries. Take another deep breath and see the sun setting over the road and orchard in the distance. Take one more deep breath in and release. When you're ready, open your eyes.

This experience can begin to help reverse PTSD, anxiety, broken trust, and anything that stands in the way of your becoming a fruitful, empowered, stronger, enlightened being. The wounds we have come to know push us up, just like a fruit tree grows. Over time, all the weather we've been through allows our beauty to show. With this meditation, your soul begins to spark as you bring back the essence of yourself so you can find your way and live free.

Watching Your Garden Grow

Along similar lines, a wonderful form of meditation is tending your own garden. Getting your hands in the dirt for the sake of growing new life grounds your body, strengthens your spirit, and rejuvenates your soul. Further, the soil carries the soul of the Earthly Mother. Getting (literally) in touch with that puts you in sync with divine natural rhythms. If you grow vegetables or fruit, you get the added benefit of eating the toxin-free and super-fresh results of your labors. And if you grow flowers, you get to eventually arrange them in a vase or basket—which is itself a great way to meditate.

As you garden, you'll be absorbing the sounds of nature, which are very healing. Even if you can hear lawn mowers and cars at the same time, the effects of the nature sounds won't be lessened. The chirps of the birds, the buzzing of bees, the wind rustling through the trees—this is a sacred soundtrack that, if you attune your mind to it, will bring peace to your body and soul.

Weeding can have a profound effect on your life, too. If you envision each weed you pull from the soil as an ill thought, difficult emotion, earthly war wound, instance of betrayal, or painful memory that you're simultaneously removing from your soul and mind, you'll make room for abundance in your life. Just as weeds crowd out your special plants—hog the water and nutrients in the soil, and overshadow seedlings below—these "weeds" of the consciousness keep the positives in your life from getting a chance to flourish. This exercise will make room for new opportunities to come into your life, seemingly from out of nowhere.

If you live in an apartment with no plot of land, then grow plants on your windowsill or balcony. Take frequent trips to the park and attune yourself to the cycles, beauty, and abundance of nature. And the city equivalent of pulling weeds is cleaning your apartment. If you turn it into a meditation, then as you straighten up clothing, vacuum up dust, and donate unused items, you'll be clearing detritus from your mind and soul.

Let's be clear, though: your physical world does not have to be in order for you to have a good life, a happy life, or for you to be able to heal, restore, or recover. You may be at your limit, too busy or fatigued or in too much pain

to tend plants or a garden or keep your living space tidy. Making celery juice in the morning and completing a work assignment so you can support your family may be your wins for the day. Getting a healing food in your kids and working on your own healing protocols may be your wins. Let any wins be triumphs. As therapeutic as it can be to bring growth and order to our physical lives, we don't always have that privilege of time, space, resources, or energy. Don't get downhearted if right now, life isn't giving you an opportunity to weed or organize—don't worry that this will block your healing.

With the garden meditation exercise to come, anyone can tap into the healing benefits of tending a piece of land. Whether you don't have access to a garden, can't work on one, or it's the off-season, you can turn to this meditation.

Get yourself settled either sitting or lying down. Close your eyes and envision yourself sitting on a grassy lawn. The sun is shining above. Now envision garden beds with nothing in them surrounding you.

To your left, envision cucumber plants sprouting out of the soil. They are growing quickly into cucumber vines. Yellow buds appear and blossom. A bumblebee flies by, lands on a yellow flower, and starts to pollinate it. A butterfly lands on another flower and begins to pollinate it. A hummingbird flies to another cucumber flower and drinks its nectar, pollinating it at the same time. You see baby cucumbers start to grow where the flowers were as the blooms fade away. The cucumbers are light green and small at first. The green deepens as they grow quickly, within moments, to their full size. With your left hand, you reach over and pick one. These cucumbers are attuned to your body's energy and cells, and they want to nourish you. They understand what your struggles are.

To the right of you, tomato plants start to sprout out of the soil, their vines growing quickly and yellow flowers starting to blossom. Once again, you see a bumblebee land on one of the flowers and pollinate it. You see a butterfly land on another flower and start to pollinate it. You see a hummingbird fly up to a flower and drink its nectar as it pollinates the tomato plant. Small tomatoes start growing. Some ripen to orange; some become red; some become yellow. You reach out with your right hand and touch a ripe tomato. Cells in your body connect to that tomato. The tomato's nutrients and minerals are meant for you. Your cells want to receive them.

Now by your feet in the garden bed, some kale starts to grow. The leaves get larger. The trunks of the kale stems get thicker. Its dark green leaves grow big and beautiful and practically glisten in the sunlight. You lean over and touch one of the kale leaves. You feel its strength and its vulnerability. It speaks to your organs, cells, and soul.

Behind you in the garden are lettuces peeking up from the soil. These lettuces start to grow quickly. They are beautiful and green, crisp and crunchy. You turn around and touch the lettuce leaves. They feel like feathers upon your hand. You can feel their cleansing power, and their minerals and nutrients as they connect to your cells and organs.

In this perfect garden, weeds start to rise up from the soil. You see them sprouting in different places. The first weed is to the left of you, next to your cucumber plant. You reach down, grab onto the weed, and pull it up by its roots. That weed is an old wound within you, one that lies deep within your garden mind.

It's tied to emotions from old relationships, hurt from new relationships. You throw the weed off into the distance, into a compost bin.

On your right, another weed is growing quickly. You grab onto the weed and pull it up by its roots. This weed is about broken friendships, losses, betrayals. You throw that weed off into the distance, into the compost bin.

In front of you, you see another weed popping out. It's a big weed, growing fast. This weed is about broken trust, emotional injuries, soul wounds, and other hardships. You grab onto the weed at the base, pull it out by its roots, and throw that weed off into the distance, into the compost bin.

Behind you is the biggest weed of all, starting to tower above you. That weed has pricklies. It's the weed of fear, insecurities, guilt, loss of self-worth, and judgment. You grab onto that weed with both hands, pull it up with all your might, and throw it in the compost bin.

These are the weeds that are inside your garden mind, inside your garden soul. These are the weeds that sprout up and crowd the garden inside us, that rob and steal our life force.

When you picture the plants throughout this meditation, whatever you envision works fine. Your cucumber, tomato, kale, and lettuce varieties can look however you'd like them to look. However you see them is right. The same goes for these weeds.

Say this: "My garden is now strong and unbreakable. My garden is undamaged, thriving with life, teeming with energy. My garden is surrounded by bumblebees, hummingbirds, butterflies, and dragonflies." This healthy garden is inside your soul, always there. This is a healthy garden you are now strengthening.

Say this: "I will not let weeds take over my garden. Weeds of the past will not stay in this garden." This garden is your sanctuary within your body.

Now open your eyes.

Exercising Creativity

Art can be enormously beneficial for the meditative state, sense of agency, and cathartic effects that it promotes. There's a whole other aspect of creativity that you have to know about for maximum healing benefit: when you create art, you have an audience all around you on an angelic level.

When you paint, angels follow every stroke of the brush. When you write, they read every word. When you sing or play a musical instrument, the angels listen to every note. The angels witness every time you're being creative, in any way. Even if no human sees or hears what you make, your creative acts are never lost to the void. Creativity cannot die. It has a force all its own that lives beyond us and becomes written into the universe. When you become aware that the Angel of Creativity and other heavenly beings are watching you sculpt or dance or sew, it takes on new meaning.

The next time you sit down to make a sketch or even a doodle while taking notes— or the next time you sing a song to yourself, come up with an inventive way of packing your kids' lunches or making their dinners, or think of an idea for starting a new business— imagine the angels cheering you on. Making something beautiful or useful or therapeutic (or all three) is a divine act that becomes imprinted in the heavens.

MOON MEDITATION

Remember, I offer a guided version of this and other meditations from this chapter on the *Medical Medium Podcast*.

For those of us who experience hardships in this world—because Planet Earth is not an easy place to live—we can think of the moon as a sanctuary with no worldly troubles. This Moon Meditation connects us to the moon's powerful ability to heal our soul.

It's not easy for any of us when we get let down by others we trusted, when we have been betrayed, or when we feel hurt by someone, whether on purpose or not. It's not easy when we feel ignored or not heard, insecure, less-than, or when we don't feel whole. It's not easy when we feel we are not understood, when we feel someone has purposely wronged us, when we feel lost and can't see straight because our thoughts are replays of emotional trials, and we start losing touch with who we are as a person deep down inside.

When we feel like anxiety is getting the best of us or depression is ruling our lives— when we feel disconnected from ourselves because we've been so distracted by the hurt we've experienced throughout our lives—we can turn to help from beyond our world. We can use the Moon Meditation to assist in pulling out the venomous poison of hurt and hardship from years past or even the present. This poison hinders us without our even realizing it. During this meditation, you'll use the moon's magnetic power to remove this poison from the center of your soul, which puts you back in touch with your essence. As you mend the soul fractures from hurt, pain, and suffering, your soul strengthens. It gets a new start.

To begin, find a comfortable position—in the presence of the moon, if possible. Here are a few tips for getting settled:

- You can be inside or outside.

- You can be lying down, sitting, or even standing. If you're standing and this meditation becomes too strong, you're welcome to sit or lie down. (Do not perform this meditation, or any other meditation in this chapter, while driving or operating machinery.)

- Try to get at least a glimpse of the moon, even if only for a moment. If you can't see the moon itself because it's behind a cloud, building, or other structure, don't worry. Seeing the light of the moon is powerful enough.

- During this meditation, you do not have to look at the moon. If the moon seems super bright, don't stare at it and hurt your eyes. Do whatever is comfortable. If you do this meditation during an eclipse, do not look at the moon (or sun).

- The moon does not have to be full. It can be a half or partial moon. Keeping track of the moon cycles can be very helpful when the Moon Meditation is a part of your life. Awareness of the lunar phases will connect you more to the moon.

- You can also do this meditation during a sighting of a daytime moon. Many times, you can catch the moon in the late morning and early evening.

- If your eyesight is impaired, that's perfectly fine. As long as you are aware the moon is out.

Once you're ready, look at the moon or its rays, if they're within sight. If you cannot see the moon or moonlight, that is okay. Imagine seeing the moon.

Now close your eyes. Take a deep breath in and release. Do not see the moon as separate from you. See it as part of you. There is already a connection between the moon and your soul. For thousands of years, human beings have lived by the moon cycles. Your soul is aware of this. It's already etched into your being, a part of you.

With your eyes closed, see the moon in your mind. Welcome the moon with open arms. You can even raise your arms as if you are about to hug a friend. You can stretch your arms out, allowing the light rays of the moon to shine upon your whole body, strengthening and reigniting that long-lost connection. Take a deep breath in and release.

The moon has a powerful magnetic pull. This is not to be confused with the moon's gravitational pull. The moon's *magnetic* frequency is what you're accessing in this meditation to draw out darkness and give you a fresh start. The moon's magnetic pull affects our lives in many ways. When we are aware of how to activate its healing power, it will help us heal deep emotional wounds.

As you are staring at the moon in your mind, envision and start to feel the moon's magnetic pull moving through you. This can feel as if your body has become very heavy or even very light. Connect to this feeling. Notice movement inside of you. See colors swirling within you, many colors, and look for the elusive dull yellow hiding in them. This dull yellow is poisonous hurt that hides within the shadows of your soul. Feel the moon's magnetic pull start to take hold. Envision the light rays of the moon going through your body, entering your soul, and attaching to the yellow poison. This poison that emotional wounds leave inside of us can sit in our soul, spirit, and heart for a lifetime if we don't tend to it.

Feel this dull yellow poison start to move around as it's swirling throughout your soul. Feel it entering your organs and blood as it's uprooting. See the yellow poison move through your body. Within this yellow poison, there are hardships, losses, broken relationships, broken friendships, misunderstandings, judgments, injustices, confrontations, sorrow, guilt, shame, insecurities, and sadness—on all levels, mild to extreme. Each person is different in their experiences. You may carry a milder form of betrayal, for example, yet an extreme form of loss. Your set of experiences is unique.

Within this swirling yellow poison, there is freedom to be found because you are letting the moon remove it from your soul. The moon's magnetic power is what identifies that poison and gives it the yellow color. The poison can't hide from the moon's extraction power.

As the poison starts to surface, you will feel it. Perhaps it will give you a cool sensation, some tingles or chills down the spine. Or perhaps it will give you a warm sensation, with your face or stomach heating up. Your hands and feet can feel cold. A form of sadness or loneliness may start to arise, and underneath it all, a feeling of joy trying to peek through. Try to connect to these sensations. Your mind will become grounded, balanced, solid, and strong. That sadness or loneliness will no longer be a part of you as the poisons are leaving your soul and body.

As the poisons are exiting, say, "I am solid and strong. I no longer need to hold onto this poison. No one can harm my soul anymore." Take a deep breath in and release.

The yellow poison and your emotional wounds are leaving your soul and body, the old wounds attached to the dull yellow poison. Those emotional wounds were comfortable living inside of you—even as they were creating discomfort. Now the moon's magnetic pull is extracting this poison from your soul. Your cells and organs are happy this poison is uprooting and leaving. You are taking control of your life. You are not letting these emotional wounds control you or who you are.

See the rays of light shining from the moon as arms extending, reaching into you and scooping the poison out of your soul. When it comes to affecting our soul in this way, the light rays coming from the moon are more powerful than the direct rays of the sun.

Your soul is relieved this yellow poison of hurt has now left. The yellow poison is rising above your body and drifting toward the moon. Take a deep breath in and release.

Now open your eyes. The relationship you now have with the moon is like nothing you've had ever before. You can see that the moon looks different than it did moments ago. And if you can't see the moon, you can feel how different it is. The moon has drawn out years of poison from your soul. It's a brand-new start. You have now removed a portion of the emotional wounds that have been buried deep inside your soul.

Repeating the Moon Meditation regularly will make its benefits and effects on your life more profound. If you can, repeat this exercise every day or every night, especially during the week of a full moon. Each time, you succeed in removing portions of the old hurt. Between meditations, you can come back and read this passage at any time to stay connected to how it works.

The moon is your old friend. When you understand it and know how to lean on it, the moon won't let you down. We don't let anything toxic control us; we take control. With our own free will, we can use this practice to help ourselves rise above the hurt and the pain, the fog and the smoke. When you apply the right tools, freedom is in your hands. You can rise out of the ashes.

RESTORING TRUST WITH SUNSETS

We all go through experiences that limit our ability to trust. Up to a point, that's helpful for survival. An abundance of innocence can lay the foundation for a major betrayal.

And as this book has explained, we can lose faith when we go from doctor to doctor, realizing that medical research and science don't have all the answers to why we are sick.

If you endure a personal struggle or hardship, are let down or even betrayed, it can diminish your ability to trust *anyone*. And perhaps worse, it can endanger your belief in yourself and your judgment.

Along similar lines, if you've been told incorrectly that you're sick because your immune system has gone haywire and is attacking you in an autoimmune response, you may lose the ability to trust even your own body. Further, if you've been given incorrect information because—as is the case in many conditions in this book—the real culprit is a virus or bacteria, you may lose faith in your internal senses, too.

Such emotional blows injure the soul. They also hinder your ability to completely believe that you can overcome illness and recover your health.

A simple yet profoundly effective way to heal such wounds is to become aware of the sunset. Toward the end of the day, take a few minutes to watch the sun go down (while never looking directly at the sun, which is damaging to the eyes). Or if you're in a building that blocks your view of the sky, be mindful of the sun during the time it's setting. If you're usually glued to a device at this time of day, set a reminder to shift your mental focus.

As the sun goes down, you may feel a sense of loss, as if a friend you love has gone away . . . with the promise of returning tomorrow. That's what makes this technique resonate on such a deep level: you face the falling darkness with the absolute, irrefutable knowledge that the light will return. Performing this exercise at least three times a week will change how you experience life—in the best way. If you have a love for the angels, summon the Angel of Trust.

When the sun appears above the horizon the next morning, even if you're asleep when it happens, your body will be attuned to the earth's rhythms. You'll click with the fact that as promised, your friend has returned. The sun has risen every day of your life. It will continue to do so for the rest of your time on earth. Connecting with this truth that the sun will never let you down, the soul will relearn critical trust, which will activate healing energy on the deepest level.

GAZING BEYOND THE STARS

You can experience this exercise as an expanded and guided meditation on the *Medical Medium Podcast*.

It's not uncommon for a person's soul to become injured by adversity or distress, especially when that person has been dealing with mystery illness for years on end. Spirit of Compassion has taught me that this is why

God created a built-in safety mechanism for our souls that I'll share here.

Your soul is here, within you, on earth. Far up in the ether, though, beyond the stars, God has safeguarded the essence of your soul. That's where your soul came from originally. The angels protect it there in the heavens so that no matter what happens down here, your soul will be safe and secure. It's a little like giving a beloved neighbor a second key to your house or apartment so that if your regular key goes missing, you can still get back into your home. In a similar way, God keeps the essences of our souls up beyond the stars in case we lose ourselves.

And there are so many ways for people to lose themselves here on earth. People's souls can fracture as they go through life, or pieces can even go missing. Injuries—whether physical or emotional, from work, childhood, or relationships—send people soul-searching. Addiction, too, comes in every shape and size—and can rob people of their souls. Addictions can be a poison that can take people so far away from themselves that they become almost soulless.

Yet you can never really lose yourself. You always have the ability to reunite with your soul because of God's safekeeping method, which Spirit of Compassion has asked me to reveal here. You don't have to search for that sense of wholeness anymore.

To strengthen or reclaim your soul, spend time each night gazing up at the sky. First get familiar with the stars themselves. Your soul has a direct telepathic connection to them. Let their light and the wonder of their existence resonate for a few moments. You can go outside or do this through a window. Even if you only see a few stars because of cloud coverage or light pollution, or if you can't see any stars at all, still look up and envision stars above you, knowing they're there.

Then shift your focus to the space *beyond* the stars—far beyond the stars. This is where our soul comes from originally. Envision that your true home lies way up there, beyond the stars, in a place free from suffering, judgment, misunderstandings, hatred, and injustice. It's the place some call Heaven, God, the Light, or the Infinite. You may prefer not to name the destination. Either way, remind yourself that part of you resides in this sanctuary, unharmed by the earth's adversities and toxic noise. When we eventually pass from this earth, that's where we'll go. Tell yourself, *This is a home I belong to, and will someday warmly return to.*

Spend as much time on this exercise as you like. The goal is repetition and reinforcement. Whether you stargaze (even if only in your mind's eye) for just three minutes a night or you make it a longer nightly ritual, you'll find that your soul rejuvenates in dazzling ways.

WHO DO YOU WORK FOR?

Whatever kind of work you do—whether you're a nurse, a therapist, a bank teller, a truck driver, an attorney, a teacher, an artist, a volunteer, a stay-at-home parent, an executive, a postal worker, a waitperson, an editor, or a landscape crewmember—there may be certain reasons you do it. You work for a paycheck, benefits, to support your family, to serve your clients, to please your boss. That's the part everyone knows.

If your job feels like a burden, though— if you have a demeaning supervisor or a grueling schedule, if you feel like your work has no meaning or no one appreciates you, if the inspiration or passion for what you do is disappearing and you feel lost—then it's time to shift your mind-set: no matter what you do, no matter where you do it, you work for God. Repeat this aloud—using whatever term feels most comfortable for you—each day, connect to it, and *everything* will change.

When you wake up in the morning and open your eyes or sit up in bed, open the door to the day, and say it: "I work for God." (Or, "I work for the Higher Source," "I work for the Light," or "I work for the Divine.") If you don't remember to say it when you first wake, it's fine to say it later in the day.

Maybe you're a cashier at a grocery store. You usually arrive for your shift to a harried manager and harried shoppers, and it's all you can do to get through until your break without crying because this isn't what you pictured for your life. You'd planned to change the world.

If you start the day by affirming that you work for God, you'll have a different perspective when you get to the store. Maybe your manager is still harried, yet it's not such a big deal—you know he's not your *real* boss. Then as the customers start to put their groceries on the conveyor belt, as you process food stamps and credit cards, you understand that you're making it possible for people to nourish themselves and their families, even if they don't show their appreciation. You're a hero on the frontlines. You *are* changing the world. Maybe someone in the checkout line will notice your glow and ask for advice—you could change a life, or many lives, without realizing it. Before long, your manager may see you in a whole new way and ask you to join the store's community outreach team or help strategize about stocking the store with the best healing foods.

Even if you have a very different job with very different responsibilities, you may be able to see yourself in this story. Maybe you're facing the challenge of working from home while caring for family, constantly navigating the boundary between the two, constantly pulled in both directions. Maybe your work is gig to gig, and that ongoing hustle and uncertainty has you exhausted. Maybe you're in a position that didn't turn out to be what you'd hoped. Maybe you feel disillusioned with your work or disconnected from how it affects others. Maybe you're having trouble finding or keeping a job, and you feel directionless or worried. Maybe you're taking time away from work or school to focus on healing or raising a family, and you feel anxious about the future.

Whatever you're facing, you're not alone in it—and it's not meaningless. You work for God. Always remember: you have a life ahead of you, years to come. Everything can change in the days ahead.

When you understand that you have a divine role in the world, you'll shine with the light of purpose. More opportunities that require your unique strengths will start to come your way. And if you feel overloaded with helping the world, then affirming that you work for God each day will help you find new ways of approaching the work, or connect you with others to help share the load. No matter what your challenge, if you remind yourself whose work you really do, your life will change in untold ways.

CHAPTER 25

Essential Angels

You were born with the God-given right to reach out to angels whenever you need them. If you've struggled with your physical or emotional health, they've been your witness. Angels want to help ease our minds, rebuild our spirits and souls, and heal our bodies.

They want to guide us in our most purposeful direction. Since humankind began, angels have existed to help us adapt and survive here on earth.

When you're searching for a partner, can't find work, or feel like new opportunities aren't coming your way, that's a *drought*. Angels are there to help us adapt to the circumstances and survive until they can bring the cool rains of the right partner, financial support, or exciting change.

When your cup is overflowing, and you have too much work, too many opportunities, or a relationship so abundant you can't keep up with it, you're in a *flood*. The angels are there to buoy you, to help you stay afloat and nurture your relationships as you balance out your commitments and turn down the spigot on projects.

A *heat wave* is when you have too much stress and too many demands upon your time,

confrontations, responsibilities, or issues with loved ones. In this case, the angels are available to intervene in confrontations, help alleviate stress, lower demands, and strengthen you for any remaining responsibilities.

Finally, an *earthquake* is the name for when unexpected problems and disruptions arise—accidents, illness, getting laid off, losing loved ones. There are angels you can call upon to help loved ones pass on to the right place, to resolve loss, to recover from accidents (emotionally or physically), sustain a job, or heal from sickness.

Just like a weather map can display totally different conditions in different parts of the country or world, you can experience any combination of the categories above. You can even experience all four at once. For example, you could have a drought of support, a flood of work, a heat wave of responsibility, and then suffer an earthquake of loss.

You're not alone, though.

And your life and path are not set in stone. You can use your free will to choose a new direction.

To say it another way: when our souls arrive here on earth, we can decide to play a certain role and not stray from that . . . or we can use our free will to write our own part. Everything is not already written. Everything hasn't all happened already.

We all have the option to break out of the mold. We have a say in our destiny.

The angels are here to help guide us in our decision-making, to make the most of our free will. They're here to intercept trouble and present opportunity. They're here to help us grow, change, and handle what life brings our way. They're here to help us see the light, guide us, and pull us out of darkness. However you need to envision or interpret the angels, whether as light beings or animals or another type of creature unique to your inner vision, they will take that form to help you. Angels don't exist to fulfill our every wish and desire. They're here to help us do God's work, whether that's healing ourselves from illness, reclaiming our souls, or helping others in need.

They've been doing it for millennia.

The angels want to help you. It's important to know the right angels to ask and *the right way to ask*. Having faith, being open, and wanting to work with them is key, too. That's what I'll cover in this chapter.

THE TRUTH ABOUT ANGELS

Angels are sometimes best known by their individual names. Everybody loves Archangel Michael, for example, and Archangel Gabriel. They're powerful angels who have fought darkness for God for millennia.

Here's what you have to understand about these guys: they're so popular, they are cherry-picking their jobs at this point. Because they're so busy and revered, they like to choose gigs that really speak to them.

The three basic facts of angels are that they work for God, their powers are vast but finite, and they have free will.

Because of that last fact, they're susceptible to ego. (Any being with free will, whether human or angelic, is vulnerable to it. If you've ever heard of fallen angels, those are the ones whose egos got so big, they felt they were mightier than God and tried to overthrow Him—which caused a fall from grace.)

So since everyone knows about Archangels Michael and Gabriel, and they're flooded with requests for help from all over the globe, they may not be able to meet everyone's demands. I'm not trying to deter you from calling upon them. They are named and loved by God and hold extreme power. It's just that the need for God's angels is great right now—greater than ever before. Archangels Michael's and Gabriel's phones are ringing off the hook.

There are other, more powerful angels we can call upon, ones who can be more useful in our lives and who will hear our prayers. These angels are female and rarely called upon. Each is best known by a word of power that represents her essence.

THE 27 ESSENTIAL ANGELS

This book was first published with a list of the 21 essential angels who are critical for your times of need. Though there are many other known angels, these were the ones most powerful and beneficial in that moment's trying times. Because of the changing times and the threat of plagues and environmental distrust,

Spirit of Compassion told me this was the moment to bring in more angels.

The number 21 stands for rebirth, new beginnings, reclamation, rising out of the ashes, and fresh starts. That still holds true. The first 21 angels in this list continue to represent all of this, and they are still needed today. This time around, you'll find more information on how each of them can help you and your loved ones.

You'll also find that the list keeps going. Altogether, you'll now find 27 essential angels. You can call upon any of these angels alone, or you can call on two or more as a team.

(For a list of even more angels, turn to the second book of the Medical Medium series, *Life-Changing Foods*. Those life-changing angels offer us critical support around food and our food supply, on both an individual and global level.)

Now for the 27 essential angels. The number 27 stands for a strong foundation. It means home, finding home, settling down. It means seeing things how they truly are. It's about finalizing, especially as it relates to personal commitments. The number 27 is about sustaining long-term peace after hardship, conflicts, and spiritual wars. It's about staking a claim in your life. It's about the light—a rising of the light, a brightening of the light. It's about fulfilling prophecy for the light to destroy darkness.

- **Angel of Mercy:** by far the most powerful angel to call upon in your darkest hour—more powerful even than the archangels. She is one of the strongest angels in God's Angelic Realm. God has summoned her many times to battle darkness. Darkness holds no mercy for humankind. The Angel of Mercy will not relinquish her holy powers to evil and its darkness in any way. Her powers are only for human and animal suffering, however that suffering has transpired. Oftentimes we come across conflicts where we wish the other party would be more open and understanding—would have more mercy in their actions. When you encounter this, you can call upon the Angel of Mercy to be sent to someone who isn't accessing compassion enough to have mercy.

- **Angel of Faith:** call upon her with whatever words suit you. If you make this a daily practice, the rhythm will help you transition the habit into full-blown conviction. Tell the Angel of Faith you are finally ready. We all have a spark of faith deep within us. You can ask the Angel of Faith to grow that spark, allowing you to feel the healing liberation faith has to offer.

- **Angel of Trust:** for help when you're struggling to recover from a betrayal, loss, letdown, disappointment, or thinking you can't do anything right. Call upon the Angel of Trust when you feel so untrusting of anything that it starts to dominate your life, to the point where you can't even trust your own decisions. It's very healthy not to trust everyone and everything in order to protect yourself. The Angel of Trust will help you discern what could be a safer avenue when venturing outside your own world of safety. She is also one of the angels you can call upon when you're meeting new people or starting a new job.

- **Angel of Healing:** to provide temporary relief and/or to heal a loved one. (For long-term healing, you must call on other angels to help build you up to a point where you can heal yourself.) The Angel of Healing is versatile. You can also call upon her as the Angel of Soul Healing if needed. For many people who have been wounded emotionally, healing of the soul is an important facet. This angel can help strengthen your soul, allowing you to feel less blocked and scattered, while also helping to ground your soul, organize your thoughts, and calm down any anxiousness and fear.

- **Angel of Restitution:** she understands how the spirit and soul can be beaten down, and she can help you recover from emotional trauma. This angel will help you to resolve deep-seated issues. She will also help you resolve how you feel about what has happened to you. Often we get confused when we go through emotional abuse, trauma, or any kind of hardship. We don't understand why or how it happened. This can lead us to feel unrested. The Angel of Restitution can help us understand why something could have happened, in the hopes that we can gain some peace. She is also good for situations where, whether or not you are confused, you are craving the sense that something has been returned to you. When others have done us wrong or harmed us through painful words or actions, we may feel we're drained by it and losing energy. The Angel of Restitution can help restore what has been drained out of us or taken from us.

- **Angel of Deliverance:** this angel provides relief to someone who's going through an earthly judgment— for example, one's spouse filing for divorce, or a school board unjustly firing a teacher. She can also help free your soul from the imprisonment of fear and anger, and from the injury of deception. If either side of a misunderstanding or argument will not give in, you can ask the Angel of Deliverance to help those involved come to terms and mend the relationship. When a couple is fighting, for example, it can feel very hurtful and saturating. Call upon the Angel of Deliverance to help an understanding occur, to get a fresh start with someone you care about or love. Also call upon the Angel of Deliverance if you feel you need assistance in getting your message out to the other angels through your thoughts because of an obstacle with speech.

- **Angel of Sun:** call for her while you're in the sun to open up your body's cells so they fully take in the healing power of the rays, and so that those rays deliver so many of the mysterious benefits the sun has to offer. Many people take the sun for granted and don't oven know what it's doing for them. The Angel of Sun is there to connect your consciousness to the sun hitting your body. The sun has immune system building properties. If you ask for the Angel of Sun, she will assist in making those properties stronger; as the sun rays are warming your body, focus on her helping to strengthen your immune system. The sun also stimulates a very mild and gentle detox of poisons and toxins from organs throughout your body. As you're warming in the sun, ask the Angel of Sun to enter deep into your organs and assist in uprooting those poisons and toxins. When the sun isn't out, you can ask the Angel of Sun to help you remember the joy of a sunny day and connect to what it offered you. This is especially helpful if you're doing the sunbathing meditation from the previous chapter on a cloudy day.

- **Angel of Light:** name her in order to be bathed in restorative angelic light given to her by God. The Angel of Light is more powerful than any light on earth, and more powerful even than the light of the sun. Use the Angel of Light if you fear you're in danger, or if you fear someone may be trying to deceive you. The Angel of Light is to shine upon and expose what is not in your favor. If you wake from a bad dream, you can call upon the Angel of Light. If you're swimming in unproductive or troublesome thoughts, call upon the Angel of Light

and envision her light within your mind, within your soul, saturating your thoughts. (It can help to close your eyes when you do this.) You can also call upon the Angel of Light and imagine her bringing light into the air you breathe into your lungs.

- **Angel of Water:** you can ask her to change the frequency of the water you bathe in to make it more cleansing, nourishing, and grounding. If you're soaking a wound, you can call upon her to quicken its healing. Also call upon the Angel of Water to assist with the water you consume: before you drink water, you can ask her to assist in your cells' absorption of that water—of its minerals and trace minerals—and to assist you with flushing toxins out of your body. When you're driving in a rainstorm, call upon the Angel of Water to help minimize downpours and puddling on the road in hopes of making you safer.

- **Angel of Air:** right after a frustrating encounter such as an argument, ask for the Angel of Air to cleanse the negative vibration that person passed on to you. Her special, purifying energy will change the frequency of the air around you to promote harmony. This is a powerful technique to change your frame of mind. You can also use the Angel of Air if you're stuck breathing in what feels, smells, or seems to be toxic air. If you're concerned about your air having contagions in it, call upon the Angel of Air to hopefully shift the air enough that you can stay out of harm's way. If you're doing any type of breath work, call upon the Angel of Air as air is entering into your lungs to help you get the most oxygen and detoxification from it.

- **Angel of Purity:** when you want to rid yourself of an addiction, this angel can help you break free from the poisonous chains of habit. She can also help you break addictive thoughts. Use the Angel of Purity to help navigate or disarm temptations in any realm of your life. Perhaps that's the temptation to stay up past your bedtime, the temptation to prove to someone how right you are, the temptation to continue with an argument that could have subsided otherwise, or the temptation to overthrow your body's natural abilities by pushing it too hard with your desires to accomplish physical goals.

- **Angel of Fertility:** for aid in conception and carrying a baby to term. You can ask her to help stimulate and waken the reproductive system, to get it to optimal capacity for conception. You can ask her to disarm and remove toxins away from critical reproductive organs so they don't interfere with fertility. Call upon the Angel of Fertility to help protect you and your baby, as well: You can ask her to help with anything you may be doing that could affect the baby, such as eating certain foods. You

can ask her to make an environment even safer for the baby. You can ask her to help minimize exposure. You can also ask the Angel of Fertility to help another person who's having fertility issues—you could pray to her every night to help with the fertility of a friend or loved one. The Angel of Fertility can assist after birth as well, aiding in a quicker recovery. Keep in mind: Fertility doesn't always have to be within the womb. It can be related to caring for a project or other venture, or it can signify rebirth, even within the soul. Turn to the Angel of Fertility for anything in your life that you want to be fertile.

- **Angel of Birth:** for health of mother and child during delivery. This applies to any living creature. You can call upon the Angel of Birth when an animal is delivering a litter, for example, or when baby birds are hatching. The Angel of Birth can also help when you've finished a project and you're handing it in or sharing it with others. Call upon the Angel of Birth if you're trying to unlock the experience of your own birth, to bring you back to that moment of time when you were born, to help you remember the first time you opened your eyes as a baby, or to get in touch with the journey of your soul from above down to earth.

- **Angel of Peace:** to help heal your mental distress and bring new seeds of hope and positivity. You can also use the Angel of Peace for the outer aspects of life—call upon her for causes that mean a great deal to who you are and your soul's belief. Or when you are trying to quiet your mind before you fall asleep, when you are still thinking about the events of the previous day or those of the day to come, you can call upon the Angel of Peace to come sit by your bedside. Ask her to place her hand on your body, wherever is comfortable for you, and envision her doing so.

- **Angel of Beauty:** if you feel closed off to the beauty of nature that surrounds you—the sun, the trees, the hills or rivers—summon the Angel of Beauty. She'll open you up to appreciate and absorb your surroundings in powerful ways you didn't think possible. This angel is also your ally when a romantic partner is obsessed with talking about people's physical appearance, when a coworker's good looks have turned him vain, or when a sibling's physical beauty earns her all the attention and adoration. Ask the Angel of Beauty to shift people's mind-sets to recognize true beauty: the beauty of a shining soul. Further, you can ask the Angel of Beauty to help you see what others see in something. Say a companion tells you, "Look how beautiful that horizon is." The Angel of Beauty can open your eyes and connect you to what that person is experiencing.

- **Angel of Purpose:** call upon her if you're struggling with your purpose here on earth—if you're numb or

confused or worried you're not useful to others or even yourself. If you've lost confidence in something or everything, the Angel of Purpose will be by your side. You can also turn to her if an overabundance of stress is inhibiting you from working with your purpose in any given moment. Some people lose sight of their purpose midway through pursuing it. The Angel of Purpose reignites the value of whatever your purpose is.

- **Angel of Knowledge:** when a loved one needs advice and you're at a loss, or you want to give more than just a pat on the back, you'd be surprised at the healing, soothing words that come out of your mouth when you call upon this angel. You can also ask her for help when you need information or advice for yourself and don't know where or how to find it. Call upon the Angel of Knowledge if you're having difficulty understanding what a friend, loved one, or other source has to offer with their advice— if you know the knowledge at hand could be valuable or fruitful, yet you're not ready to hear or receive it. When you have up that wall of righteousness or doubt because someone's knowledge doesn't seem appetizing or applicable to the moment, you can ask the Angel of Knowledge to give you insight so you don't stay closed off and miss a critical piece of information. She will help you become more open to the teachings that you receive or read, to discern if they could be helpful.

- **Angel of Wisdom:** for guidance when you're about to make an important decision. The Angel of Wisdom helps bring the bigger picture into your decision-making process. In every decision, there are other decisions to be made. That's true even when it doesn't seem so, or when those other decisions come much later. Making one sound decision doesn't guarantee that we'll make a good or healthy decision the next time. To avoid difficulty with future decisions, keep the Angel of Wisdom close to your heart. The Angel of Wisdom can be very helpful when the decisions you are making involve another person's life, not just your own. She can help you see what kind of effect a decision could have on the ones who care about you.

- **Angel of Awareness:** people are always trying to be more present and mindful. It's critical to summon the Angel of Awareness to make this intention complete—only then will you be fully in the moment. Also, if you want the people around you to be less judgmental and better communicators, you can call upon this angel to help open their minds. You can use the Angel of Awareness to become more aware of who you are, too. What often gets in the way of awareness is how we think about ourselves. We tend to judge ourselves, not value our intentions or accomplishments. We are often not compassionate toward ourselves, do not see our own value or believe we

hold worth. The Angel of Awareness helps us see truly who we are. This world is a hard world. Many of us are continually trying to please others and get lost in it. We tend to see others as living their truth and yet feel as if we are not. We lose track, lose awareness, of who we are. We become unaware of the goodness within us. Call upon the Angel of Awareness to show you your inner value. She is also a great one to call upon in order to see what someone else has gone through in life. Without true awareness, we tend to become self-absorbed. The Angel of Awareness allows us to get a sense of what someone has sacrificed and given up, how they have suffered or struggled in life.

- **Angel of Relationships:** if you're having a problem with your spouse or someone you're dating, or if you're single and looking for a good match. Call upon the Angel of Relationships for help with partnerships of any other kind, too, whether work-related or friendship. If you're feeling at a loss, like you're not being heard within that partnership, or encountering another difficulty, you can ask for this angel's help. You can also turn to her if you're not listening to the other person in a relationship, if you need a more level playing field in hopes that communication can strengthen.

- **Angel of Dreams:** you can pray to her to enter your dreams and help you sort out and resolve emotional turmoil. So many have experienced the Angel of Dreams when they were younger—she was the one who could make them fly when they were asleep. Even if your waking life is troubled, you can call upon her to help you re-experience that soul freedom in your dreams. Oftentimes, there is a meaningful message in our dreams that we forget by morning. Call upon the Angel of Dreams if you want to remember your dreams. Also call upon the Angel of Dreams if you are someone who doesn't dream and you want to experience dreams, learn, and grow from them. If you're struggling with harsh dreams because of difficult life experiences, ask the Angel of Dreams to make the dreams more peaceful while still allowing you to process and heal through those dreams. The Angel of Dreams goes beyond our sleeping state. We can also try to use the Angel of Dreams for our dreams and aspirations in our waking lives.

- **Angel of Time:** for help remembering events in your life. You can use the Angel of Time to go back to a moment so you can remember or pick up on parts of it you'd forgotten or critical aspects of what was happening that you weren't aware of in the moment. These may be happier events that you'd like to revisit, learn, and grow from or unresolved situations. Use this angel to help free you of any guilt from a sad time—to see elements in play that really weren't your fault or discover that a situation wasn't what it seemed. The Angel of Time can help take you back there so you can realize, "Hey, wait a minute," and find resolve. Keep in mind, this isn't about retraumatizing yourself. Not every difficult time in life needs to be remembered. For help moving on without revisiting a painful moment, call upon the Angel of Restitution.

- **Angel of Free Will:** many feel they are trapped in some type of conformity, not able to choose their own path or make their own decisions. The Angel of Free Will helps you make decisions that are governed by you rather than anyone who is governing over you. She helps free you up from anyone who has control over you—even if that's underlying, subconscious, or subliminal control—and helps guide you to your own path. She assists you with using your free will to define and project your own future without getting persuaded otherwise. For help using your free will for the greatest outcome, ask for the Angel of Wisdom at the same time as the Angel of Free Will.

- **Angel of Promise:** call upon this angel in hopes that promises are kept, or to address the fallout of broken promises. When promises are broken, prayer to the Angel of Promise will help break your fall; she'll aid you in the heartache and letdown. If you have a promise breaker in the family, you can tell that person, "I'm calling upon the Angel of Promise in hopes you don't break that promise. I ask *you* to tell the Angel of Promise you're not going to break it." That will help weed out if someone was actually planning to break the promise, and it will hold them responsible and encourage them to come through for you. For example, when somebody with a history of being late says, "I'll be there at two o'clock," you can tell them, "Look, I'm asking the Angel of Promise to make that happen. Can *you* ask the Angel of Promise?" The Angel of Promise can also help if you're the one who wants help keeping a promise or when you've broken a promise. Many people don't purposely break promises. Certain situations, often outside your control, cause it to happen—a train that never leaves the station, a traffic jam, any number of other obstacles large and small—and you can end up just as heartbroken that you don't come through on your promise. Ask the Angel of Promise to help you figure out a way to make amends and move forward. The Angel of Promise is also for those situations where you see promise in a person or possibility, or when you need help feeling like the future and life itself hold promise.

- **Angel of Inner Vision:** for people to look into and understand themselves. When you're dealing with emotional struggles, sadness, or anxiousness, or when you're feeling lost, like you're not in the right place at the right time, or like you're missing out on something, the Angel of Inner Vision will help you look inside. When you're able to self-analyze, it's priceless. The Angel of Inner Vision is about opening a dialogue with oneself. You're not judging yourself; you're analyzing so you can have that understanding of yourself and your actions. And that true understanding is important—it's actually an antidote to self-obsession. You can ask the Angel of Inner Vision to help you see and understand your behaviors, what drives them, and what effect they have on others around you.

- **Angel of Strength:** call upon this angel when you're looking for the strength to bear what comes your way, or when you need to be strong for others. Whether something happens in someone else's life that affects you, or something happens in your life that affects someone else, call upon the Angel of Strength for both sides of it, both people. The Angel of Strength can be really helpful when a person needs to hold up and be that rock for someone else.

- **Angel of Dimension:** pray to this angel for the awareness that there's more here around us than we can see. The Angel of Dimension brings us outer vision. We tend to become closed off or lost in the bubble we live in, when in truth, there's a lot happening around us that we play a part in without realizing. When something unexpected happens in our lives, or when we witness the unexpected, we can experience shock. It can feel like we can't wrap our head around why it happened. The Angel of Dimension helps you come to a peaceful place about it, understanding there's more happening around and above us that's not in our control. She helps you come to terms—to realize, *There's more at work*, and that the picture is much greater than what it seems in this moment. When the unexplainable happens, when you can't make sense of it, the Angel of Dimension helps light the way.

UNKNOWN ANGELS

There is another category of angels to reach out to in this time of need called the Quickening—an army of angels. These *don't* have names; they're referred to as the *Unknown Angels*. They are here for you when you feel embattled in any form of spiritual war, either within yourself or with outside forces. The Unknown Angels want you to ask for their help.

There are exactly 144,000 of these Unknown Angels in existence. This is a holy number that God reveres.

Because they are unnamed, they have no notoriety or acclaim, and therefore very little temptation to develop an ego, plus their angelic powers are all equal. The Unknown Angels are some of the most powerful of all. If you have faith in them, they can perform

miracles. They do their work on you while you're asleep, restoring both your body and soul.

This group of angels can be so powerful because life instills a fear of the unknown in us. On earth, nearly everyone and everything is named. It takes some rewiring for us to see the value of anything not known, and to tap into the deep reserves of faith required to believe in these angels. When we do get in touch with that utmost form of trust, it can have a radical effect on our lives.

While you might call upon, say, the Angel of Light, Angel of Restitution, or Angel of Soul Healing to restore your soul while you're awake, when you go to bed, you can call upon the Unknown Angels to aid in your healing and rejuvenation as you slumber. And calling upon Unknown Angels while dealing with chronic illness can be life-changing. You can even ask them to sit by your bedside, to help you heal and keep you safe while you sleep. You can ask for just one Unknown Angel, or you can ask for a group of them—say, three or four—together.

The Unknown Angels are eager for the chance to work on us. If you summon the Unknown Angels, you'll find yourself tapping into a resource of profound power for healing your body, mind, heart, spirit, and soul.

HOW TO ACCESS ANGELIC AID

Here's the most important thing I'll say about angels in this chapter: *You have to ask for their help aloud*. You can't just think it. (Unless you are deaf or unable to speak—in which case, the angels are attuned to that. See more below.)

This is huge. Angels are dealing with so much darkness on the planet—violence, epidemics, pandemics, corruption—that we need to be active (and proactive, whenever possible) in calling their attention. Our minds are spiderwebs of thought and emotion: obsessions, fear, anger, insecurities, guilt, worry, pain, music, imaginary conversations with people we're mad at, and even happy thoughts . . . angels don't want to get stuck in all of that; it's too difficult to disentangle the genuine requests for help. On top of which, humans believe their thoughts are a sanctuary, where they have the freedom to think what and how they want. They put up boundaries and barriers. Angels respect this. It's part of why they want to hear you ask for help.

Remember that angels have free will. It takes a little work on our end to show that we are sincere, honest, and committed. Angels don't like to be toyed with or tested; they want us to take them seriously.

In order to get a response from an angel, you must fully set your mind to her and say her name out loud. You don't have to scream or shout—even a whisper works. As long as it comes out of your mouth, that will separate it from everything else in your consciousness and signal it as a clean message, not one clinging to anything else.

And if you are deaf, have a speech impairment, or are too weak to speak, again, the angels are attuned to that. You can use sign language or your thoughts to ask for the Angel of Deliverance. She will express your soul's wishes to the other angels. The angels will take it upon themselves to read your thoughts in order to help.

This is the secret truth that will change your relationship with angels. People who have lost faith in angels, who haven't seen results from their prayers, who think the concept of angels is hogwash—this is what they have yet to learn.

The truth of how to contact the angels is similar to how you make a phone call. You don't just look at the phone and silently will it to call a dear friend in times of need. You pick up the phone—or you use voice activation to dial her, or an interpreter relay service. However you do it, you make the effort to make that call. Then you wait until she can answer. When you reach her and express yourself about your situation, she listens with compassion. That may be all you needed. Or maybe you called your friend asking for a specific favor, and she has a better idea of how to help. Maybe you were hoping she'd come right over, and instead, you're going to have to be patient because it's going to take some time for her to put her plan in motion. Even if all you called for was a comforting conversation, you have to remain open. From her outside perspective, she may see more possibility for you than you see for yourself, and that may require you to put in work or expand your thinking. The process takes will and intention. That's okay. The compassion your friend gave you and the sense of being aligned with someone dear will be enough to get you through until you start to see change in your life.

If you wanted to contact the Angel of Healing, you'd turn your attention to her and then humbly say, "Please, Angel of Healing, I need your help." If you do this with focused intention and you're willing to receive her, that will be enough. If she's not too busy helping others—an angel's powers are impressive, but finite—the Angel of Healing will arrive within anywhere from a few seconds to a few minutes to aid and comfort you. A miracle may not happen overnight. If you keep calling for her, though, she will sustain you until you get where you need to be.

You can access the Angelic Realm in this way anywhere, and at any time, as long as you're sufficiently focused on what you're calling for and truly open to receiving help and have faith that it will work. (And if you're short on faith, you may want to make the Angel of Faith your first call, or try the faith meditation in the final chapter of this book.)

You can talk to the angels about specific outcomes you think would be most helpful in your life, but be open. It's important to note that an angel's response may not be what you expect. If you're praying to the Angel of Relationships to give you space from your spouse, the angel might surprise you instead by changing your spouse's vibration and prompting her or him to apologize for the wrongdoing that made you want distance.

Another scenario is if you pray to the Angel of Fertility to give your daughter a little sibling—and yet you don't get pregnant. This doesn't mean the angel didn't hear your call. It just means that you may not have been destined for this exact outcome. Perhaps the angel knows that it isn't the right time for you or the baby, or she knows of an underlying health issue. Perhaps your sister or a friend will give birth to a child who ends up being just like a sibling to your daughter.

Don't be afraid to ask the angelic forces for help with your problems. Needing help doesn't mean you're weak. You don't have to frame your requests in only positive terms, or only use affirmations. You're not perpetuating the negative in your life by saying, "My body is weak. I can't even get out of bed to open the curtains and see the day. Please, Angel of Light, I'm desperate for help and hope." You're just stating the facts. And you're showing great strength and honesty by accepting the truth in your life and wanting to move forward.

You *get* to move forward with your life. You get to heal and have good things happen to you. If you start tapping into the angels' power in the ways I've outlined above, your life will change.

CASE HISTORY:
A Miracle from the Angel of Mercy

One evening when her husband was out of town, Edith was looking after their sick four-year-old daughter, Emma, when Emma's fever spiked to 105 degrees. Edith rushed to the emergency room, but before any doctors were available, Emma lost consciousness. The hospital admitted Edith's daughter into the intensive care unit, where she lay in a coma.

Doctors told Edith that a blood test had determined Emma had a vicious and rare form of meningitis. It was the worst case they'd seen in a long time. An MRI showed that brain damage had occurred, and the doctors said it would probably mean at least paralysis, if not death. They warned Edith that even if Emma came out of the coma and survived, she would need permanent care.

Edith dialed her sister, Valerie, who was my client. Valerie begged her to call me. My assistant reached me on my emergency line, and I got on the phone with Edith. Spirit told me this was a case for the Angel of Mercy, so I told Edith what she needed to do.

For the next hour, Edith sat by Emma's side in her hospital room, pleading aloud for the Angel of Mercy to come and save her daughter's life. Nurses tried to quiet her, but Edith just kept chanting: "Angel of Mercy, Angel of Mercy, please help, please help." Edith's husband arrived sometime in the middle of it all, but she didn't stop.

At one in the morning, Edith was slumped over her daughter's hospital bed, still calling to the angel. Out of nowhere, a light flashed. Even though Edith's hands were covering her eyes and her face was buried in Emma's blankets, it blinded her for a moment—that's the kind of light we're talking about here. Edith rushed to the window to see where the light had come from, yet saw nothing unusual in the dim parking lot. Reflected in the window, though, she also saw a figure standing over Emma's bed. Edith turned quickly—and instead of finding a nurse in the room, as she'd expected, saw another, smaller flash of light. The figure had vanished. Just then, Emma coughed. Edith shouted for a nurse and sent her husband racing down the hallway to bring someone back. When a nurse returned with him, they were both stunned to see Emma blinking back at them. She was out of the coma.

Two days later, Emma was released from the hospital. She made a full recovery—and the doctors still can't explain it.

That's the power of the Angel of Mercy.

CASE HISTORY:
A New Frame of Mind from the Angel of Faith

Jill was a single mom who'd long ago lost her faith in God. She'd believed as a child, but a college boyfriend had argued that faith in God was as naïve as believing in Santa Claus. What gave her the right to believe in a benevolent, almighty force when so much suffering existed in the world? Didn't she watch the news?

Jill sat in her dorm room one day and tore up the book of prayers her Uncle Al had given her when she turned twelve.

When Jill came to me years later, her faith was at an all-time low. She'd been laid off from her job at a nonprofit, and after months of searching was now up for a position as the marketing director at a food bank—but she was one of 100 applicants. Her unemployment was about to run out. If she didn't get the job, she'd have to break the lease on her apartment, uproot her children from their school, and move in with her uncle, who was already supporting his grown son.

I brought up the need to believe that things could turn around, and Jill objected. That sounded too much like the type of thought process her ex-boyfriend had told her was narrow-minded, she said. If things could go so terribly in the world, what made her so special? As much as she wanted and needed the job, she didn't feel she deserved it. Maybe she should set her sights lower.

Spirit told me, first of all, that Jill was the best candidate for the position, and second of all, that the Angel of Faith was the only one who could help her see that. I coached Jill on speaking aloud to the angel. She was to ask the Angel of Faith to help her see that she works for God, that God does exist, that when we close ourselves off to Him, it's like drawing a shade against the sun. It doesn't mean the sun doesn't exist—it just means that we don't benefit from its light.

Later, Jill told me that after we got off the phone that day, she was ready to write off the whole conversation. But then she got to thinking about the good she could do for the food bank. She had a top degree in marketing and connections all over the city. She was probably better qualified than any of the other applicants to shape the charity's message and spread it far and wide, which would ultimately mean more hungry people fed. On top of that, Jill would be providing for her son and daughter and sparing Uncle Al the burden of looking after them.

That night she knelt by her bed like she had when she was a girl and asked, "Angel of Faith? If I get this job, I'll make the best of it. I will do God's work. Please help me believe that I can do this—that I deserve to do this."

Jill got called back for a second interview the next day. She whisper-prayed to the Angel of Faith just before she went into the meeting room—and proceeded to blow everyone away with her vision and conviction. Before she left, they told her she had the job.

When I talked to Jill that afternoon, she was elated—but feeling a little shaky, like she'd somehow asked for her needs to be put above others' and "messed with the order of the universe." I assured her this wasn't the case. If she hadn't been the best candidate, her prayers wouldn't have catapulted her above someone else. The Angel of Faith knew Jill would mastermind the rebranding that the food bank desperately needed to bring in the right donors. If this hadn't been the job for her, her prayers would have helped her keep the faith that some other plan would work out.

Jill absorbed this for a minute. "I guess it's time I pray to the Angel of Quit-Your-Whining-and-Say-Thank-You."

I assured her that no one, least of all the angels, thought she was a whiner. Faith is complex, and God loves it when we engage with these questions. I did tell Jill I was positive the Angel of Gratitude would love to hear from her.

CASE HISTORY:
A Renewed Connection from the Angel of Relationships

Ever since Nicole's parents divorced when she was in second grade, she'd had a difficult time keeping friends. Each time she made a new bond with someone, she was afraid she'd lose the person—just like she lost her dad to his new wife in another state. So rather than risk the pain of Jordan or Maya or Caroline blowing her off, Nicole would play it cool. If anyone asked her to hang out after school, Nicole would give a "maybe" and only show up half the time. The invitations trickled off before too long.

As Nicole got older and started dating, she noticed the same pattern with men. Even if she really liked a guy, she'd tell him his haircut was dorky or "forget" to call him when she got off work.

By the time she was 30, she'd been through a series of flings, each lasting only a few dates—if that. She was tired of holding potential relationships at bay with her noncommittal act.

When she met Ethan through a dating app, she decided she wanted this to be a real relationship—her first. It was time she tried to trust someone, she told herself. And for two years, things worked out. Then they didn't. Over brunch one Sunday, Ethan told Nicole that he felt she'd become codependent, and he wasn't the type to be tied down. "I think it's time for you to get your own life," he said.

Now Nicole was convinced she'd never feel safe in a relationship again—if she could even attract someone. She felt broken and unlovable. Over time, she did start to go out again here and there, but she couldn't find anyone who made her feel comfortable in her own skin. Whenever a guy asked her out a second time, even if she liked him, she declined. She was too afraid to get attached and end up with another broken heart.

At this point, Nicole came to me for help with her chronic stress stomachaches, which had started when her parents divorced and had gotten worse in the last year. The topic of relationships inevitably came up in our conversation. Nicole told me that commitment gave her the heebie-jeebies, and she didn't know how to feel safe taking that step with a new man.

Spirit said it was time for Nicole to learn about the Angel of Relationships. I coached her on how to ask aloud for assistance, and for the next few months off and on, Nicole practiced talking to the angel in the car. While running errands and during her commute, Nicole would speak to the Angel of Relationships about her fears and insecurities, as though the angel were a pal sitting in the passenger seat. "How am I ever going to find someone who gets me?" she'd always ask.

One day, Nicole stopped at the natural foods store to replenish her supply of aloe leaf and papaya, which Spirit had recommended for her stomachaches. As she parked the car, she changed her tune: "Angel of Relationships, what if there really is a guy out there for me? Please, please help me find him."

In the store, Nicole picked up her groceries and stood in line to pay. A magazine headline about couples who had met at yoga retreats grabbed her eye. Maybe, she thought, this was the Angel of Relationships trying to communicate with her. She flipped to the article and started to read. After a minute, though, someone tapped her on the shoulder. She turned to see a man she didn't know.

"Nicole!" he said.

The man introduced himself as Tyler, a former high school classmate, and asked if she'd like to meet for coffee sometime to catch up. Nicole hesitated. He didn't look familiar, and she wasn't sure if this was a scam. Then again, he looked genuinely happy to see her. She agreed to meet somewhere very public with a lot of exits—and somewhere with good herbal tea, since coffee made her stomach hurt.

At home, Nicole pulled out one of her yearbooks and found Tyler in a photo of the bird-watching club. She *did* remember him—as a scrawny boy the year below her who had always carried binoculars and barely hit puberty before she graduated. The Tyler she met at the store had really grown into himself, she realized. She texted him back to say so.

Two days later, as Nicole walked into the café they'd picked, she called to the Angel of Relationships under her breath. Maybe this could actually go well.

Before they'd even gotten to the counter to order tea, Tyler confessed he'd had a crush on Nicole back in high school. This gave her just the confidence boost she needed to be herself. Tyler shared about the fiancée who broke up with him a week before they were supposed to get married, and Nicole talked about her own relationship trials. She felt free as she spoke, not distracted like she usually was by insecurities. By the time they said goodbye that day, they had their next three dates planned.

The night before Tyler and Nicole got married, Nicole prayed aloud to the Angel of Relationships from the hotel room where she was spending her last single night. Nicole had checked in with the angel here and there over the last few years with Tyler, to ask for help with their occasional misunderstandings. This time, Nicole wanted to say thanks: "I just wanted you to know I don't feel spooked about this commitment. You changed everything for me."

CHAPTER 26

Keep the Faith

Faith is tremendously lacking here on earth. Even if people believe in God, in a higher source, so many lose faith that they can heal from illness and other afflictions and go on to succeed in life.

It's understandable. Bad things happen in the world, from personal betrayals, to disease, to war. It's not easy to reconcile. Almost three and a half billion people on the planet don't have faith.

Yet part of the reason things go wrong is *because* of this lack of faith. When a person doesn't believe in the good of the world, it can cause her or him to behave recklessly—which can have extremely negative consequences for everybody else. One such action can cause countless people to question the good in humanity, to doubt their faith.

Sometimes this recklessness happens in the form of violence. Other times it's hidden—like the industries at the turn of the 19th century that started releasing toxic chemicals and heavy metals into our environment, causing people to get sick left and right with conditions such as goiters and cancers and mental illness. It didn't happen because the world is an inherently bad place. It happened because

people in positions of power lost their faith and higher purpose somewhere along the way, and so they took a gamble and exposed factory workers and townspeople to untested chemical brews in the interest of profit.

So many people today struggle with their health. When you are ill, or your loved ones are, and you keep hearing more disheartening stories of people coming up against health issues, it's easy to get mad at life. It's easy to feel unsafe, unprotected, trapped in a world of disappointment and fear.

Always come back to this truth, though: You are allowed to live a good life. You *deserve* to live a good life. *A good life exists for you.* And the foundation of a good life is good health. You deserve to heal, to tap into your body's restorative mechanisms. You deserve to be happy and well.

It is not life itself fouling things up; it's people who lose touch with their essence and conviction, then make heedless choices as a result.

The most powerful thing you can do in the face of this is to have faith.

People without faith walk around with their eyes technically open, yet remain blind to the helping hands of God and the universe trying to reach out to them. They may make a compelling argument for the reasons they don't believe and convince others of the bleakness of the world—in which case, it's the blind leading the blind.

As we, too, walk through life and experience difficulties, adversities, hardships, judgments, injustices, losses, emotional injuries, emotional abuse, and struggles, so many of us look for answers above. We question our faith. We question who we are. We question if our soul has a connection to the heavens. We question if we are connected to the universe. We question if anybody hears us or knows our pain—if anybody has witnessed what we are experiencing. When times are difficult, we question our existence. We lose faith, if we even had any to start with.

We can't let the news headlines or our physical trials make us stop believing. And we have to nurture our belief so that it becomes a part of our soul, building up to become faith that saturates our very being. It takes practice. It takes patience. It may take some help from the Angel of Faith.

Faith is a light that leads the way. Faith is a burning torch that allows us to see far ahead of what we are feeling or living with in this moment. If we let it, faith can lead the way to the hope of positive outcomes. It can lead us to fruitful experiences, fruitful relationships, and new friendships. If we hold onto faith—access it, carry its torch—we can use it to find new health, gain new inspirations, and see and envision new dreams.

Still, so many of us lose faith, get lost, and don't know where to turn. If faith feels impossible to access, this powerful practice will give you strength and allow faith to re-saturate your soul:

Try lying down on your bed, on a couch, or on the floor, in a comfortable position. Close your eyes. If you are indoors, imagine that you are looking up through the ceiling, through the roof, straight up to the sky. If you're lying outside, still keep your eyes closed and envision that sky above you.

See yourself traveling upward. Rise up above the buildings around you toward the clouds, and as you rise, take a moment to look down and notice how high you are. (If you're afraid of heights, remind yourself that you're safely lying down.) You reach the cloud line, and there, starting to peek out from the bottom of the clouds, you see a golden rope. You reach for it and grab onto the golden rope with your hand. If you choose, you can even lift your arm from your position lying down, as if you really are reaching for that rope. Keep hold of the rope, with both hands if you'd like. Hold onto it as you let the rope start to lower you down, and know that this glistening, glittering rope is the golden rope of faith.

Now come back to earth, still holding the rope. Pull on that rope, and as you do, feel the weight of a bell on the other end, a bell that starts to ring in the heavens above. As the bell begins to swing, gently ease off the rope. Then pull it again. Each time you ring that bell, its sound will vibrate throughout your soul and body, purifying fear, chaos, guilt, sadness, and shame—and vibrating those emotions and feelings *out* of your soul and body.

The sound of the bell is heavenly. It harbors peace, power, and sanctuary. It clears the slate of how others have shamed or judged you. It clears the slate of what others have thought of you. The sound of the bell brings out the true being of your soul. The sound of the bell brings back faith that starts to restore your soul, your heart, and your spirit.

Ring this bell for as long as you feel you need during this meditation. You do not have to keep your arm up—only if you'd like to. Once you are finished ringing the bell, envision the rope heading off above you, up to the sky. When the rope is out of sight, take a deep breath inward and release. Repeat this breath two more times. Then open your eyes and slowly sit up.

You are now in the process of rebuilding your faith. Over time, come back to this exercise periodically to strengthen faith as needed.

Sometimes in the moments we need faith most, we don't have time to stop what we're doing and lie down to meditate. Between faith meditations, you can also try this simple visualization: Imagine faith as that golden rope—a lifeline—trailing down from the sky. Picture yourself grasping it, then pulling on it as though you were ringing a bell in the heavens above. Let the golden rope come to your mind's eye whenever you need it, and let that bell's ring bring you strength. Over time, if you have faith that faith will come to you, it will enter your heart, soul, spirit, and body. When you finally experience an ignition of faith, and start to live in its glory and virtue, so much more becomes visible. Your conviction lights the way, and you can finally see how to leave the path of despair. You can restore yourself to health.

If you take the lessons in this book to heart, you will watch your life transform and understand that God, Spirit, and the Angelic Realm really want us to thrive. Then, just as one candle can pass its flame to thousands more, you'll be a light in the world that can ignite the faith of countless others.

Many blessings on your journey.

"Always come back to this truth: You are allowed to live a good life. You *deserve* to live a good life. *A good life exists for you.* And the foundation of a good life is good health. You deserve to heal, to tap into your body's restorative mechanisms. You deserve to be happy and well."

— Anthony William, Medical Medium

CONVERSION CHARTS

The recipes in this book use the standard United States method for measuring liquid and dry or solid ingredients (teaspoons, tablespoons, and cups). The following charts are provided to help cooks outside the U.S. successfully use these recipes. All equivalents are approximate.

Standard Cup	Fine Powder (e.g., flour)	Grain (e.g., rice)	Granular (e.g., sugar)	Liquid Solids (e.g., butter)	Liquid (e.g., milk)
1	140 g	150 g	190 g	200 g	240 ml
¾	105 g	113 g	143 g	150 g	180 ml
⅔	93 g	100 g	125 g	133 g	160 ml
½	70 g	75 g	95 g	100 g	120 ml
⅓	47 g	50 g	63 g	67 g	80 ml
¼	35 g	38 g	48 g	50 g	60 ml
⅛	18 g	19 g	24 g	25 g	30 ml

Useful Equivalents for Liquid Ingredients by Volume					
¼ tsp				1 ml	
½ tsp				2 ml	
1 tsp				5 ml	
3 tsp	1 tbsp		½ fl oz	15 ml	
	2 tbsp	⅛ cup	1 fl oz	30 ml	
	4 tbsp	¼ cup	2 fl oz	60 ml	
	5⅓ tbsp	⅓ cup	3 fl oz	80 ml	
	8 tbsp	½ cup	4 fl oz	120 ml	
	10⅔ tbsp	⅔ cup	5 fl oz	160 ml	
	12 tbsp	¾ cup	6 fl oz	180 ml	
	16 tbsp	1 cup	8 fl oz	240 ml	
	1 pt	2 cups	16 fl oz	480 ml	
	1 qt	4 cups	32 fl oz	960 ml	
			33 fl oz	1000 ml	1 L

Useful Equivalents for Dry Ingredients by Weight		
(TO CONVERT OUNCES TO GRAMS, MULTIPLY THE NUMBER OF OUNCES BY 30.)		
1 oz	1/16 lb	30 g
4 oz	1/4 lb	120 g
8 oz	1/2 lb	240 g
12 oz	3/4 lb	360 g
16 oz	1 lb	480 g

Useful Equivalents for Cooking/Oven Temperatures			
PROCESS	FAHRENHEIT	CELSIUS	GAS MARK
Freeze Water	32° F	0° C	
Room Temperature	68° F	20° C	
Boil Water	212° F	100° C	
Bake	325° F	160° C	3
	350° F	180° C	4
	375° F	190° C	5
	400° F	200° C	6
	425° F	220° C	7
	450° F	230° C	8
Broil			Grill

Useful Equivalents for Length				
(TO CONVERT INCHES TO CENTIMETERS, MULTIPLY THE NUMBER OF INCHES BY 2.5.)				
1 in			2.5 cm	
6 in	1/2 ft		15 cm	
12 in	1 ft		30 cm	
36 in	3 ft	1 yd	90 cm	
40 in			100 cm	1 m

INDEX

X

Y

Z

ACKNOWLEDGMENTS

Thank you to Patty Gift, Anne Barthel, Reid Tracy, Margarete Nielsen, Diane Hill, everyone at Hay House Radio, and the rest of the Hay House team for your faith and commitment to getting Spirit of Compassion's wisdom out into the world so it can continue to change lives.

Hilary Swank and Philip Schneider, your dedication to the healing truth and wisdom is remarkable, and I am deeply honored. Your support is immensely powerful.

Helen Lasichanh and Pharrell Williams, you are extraordinarily kindhearted seers.

Sylvester Stallone, Jennifer Flavin Stallone, and family, your support has been legendarily game-changing.

Kate Hudson, Danny Fujikawa, Erinn and Oliver Hudson, and Elisabeth Stassen, having you guys on my side with your love and support is a blessing.

Miranda Kerr and Evan Spiegel, it's so amazing to have your hands of light and compassion behind the healing movement.

Laura Dern, thank you for spreading your light and changing the world for the better.

Novak and Jelena Djokovic, you are pioneers in advancing health and teaching the world how to thrive.

Gwyneth Paltrow, Elise Loehnen, and your devoted GOOP crew, your caring and generosity are a profound inspiration.

Uma Thurman, I deeply value and treasure our friendship.

Robert Downey, Jr., you're truly all heart and soul.

Sage and Tony Robbins, it's an honor to be part of your world that's helping so many.

Martin, Jean, Elizabeth, and Jacqueline Shafiroff, thank you for always being there, believing in me, and helping to spread the message so that others can heal.

Dr. Alejandro Junger, life would not be the same without you, brother.

Dr. Ilana Zablozki-Amir, your willingness to support the Medical Medium cause is epic.

Dr. Christiane Northrup, your inexhaustible devotion to the health of womankind has become its own star in the universe.

Dr. Prudence Hall, your selfless work to enlighten patients who need answers renews the true, heroic meaning of the word doctor.

Craig Kallman, thank you for your support, advocacy, and friendship on this journey.

Caroline Fleming, you're truly a blessing because you have the gift to always care about everyone around you as you share your light.

Chelsea Field and Scott, Wil, and Owen Bakula, how did I get so blessed to have you in my life? You are true crusaders for the Medical Medium cause.

Kimberly and James Van Der Beek, there's a special place in my heart for you and your family. I'm truly thankful to have crossed paths with you in this lifetime.

Kerri Walsh Jennings, you truly amaze me with your hopeful nature and endless positive energy.

John Donovan, it's an honor to be on the planet with such a peace-seeking soul.

Nanci Chambers and David James, Stephanie, and Wyatt Elliott, I can't thank you enough for your dear friendship and everlasting encouragement.

Suze Orman and KT, your determination and commitment are exceptional.

Lisa Gregorisch-Dempsey, your acts of kindness have been deeply meaningful.

Grace Hightower De Niro, Robert De Niro, and family, you are precious, gracious beings.

Liv Tyler, it's such a great honor to be a part of your world.

Jenna Dewan, your fighting spirit is an inspiration to behold.

Debra Messing, you are bettering people's lives with your vision for a healthy planet.

Alexis Bledel, your strength in this world is extraordinarily heartening.

Lisa Rinna, thank you for tirelessly using your influence to spread the message.

Jennifer Aniston, your kindness, caring, and support are on another level.

Taylor Schilling, what a joy to know you and have your support.

Marcela Valladolid, knowing you is a gift in my life.

Kelly Noonan and Alec Gores, thank you for always looking out for me. It means so much.

Jennifer Meyer, I'm beyond grateful for your friendship and how you're always spreading the word.

Calvin Harris, you've changed the world with a powerful rhythm.

Courteney Cox, thank you for having such a pure, loving heart.

Hunter Mahan and Kandi Harris, I'm proud of you for always being game to take on a challenge.

Kidada Jones and Rashida Jones, the deep care and compassion you bring to life mean more than you know. Your mother was a treasure who lives on in you.

Andrew Kusatsu: love you, brother, for persevering past the pain and fighting for health freedom.

To the following special souls whose loyalty I treasure, my thanks go out: Naomi Campbell; Eva Longoria; Lewis Howes; Carla Gugino; Mario Lopez; Renee Bargh; Tanika Ray; Maria Menounos; Michael Bernard Beckwith; Jay Shetty; Alex Kushneir; LeAnn Rimes Cibrian; Hana Hollinger; Sharon Levin; Nena, Robert, and Uma Thurman; Jenny Mollen; Jessica Seinfeld; Kelly Osbourne; Demi Moore; Kyle Richards; India.Arie; Kristen Bower; Rozonda Thomas; Peggy Rometo; Debbie Gibson; Carol, Scott, and Christiana Ritchie; Jamie-Lynn Sigler; Amanda de Cadenet; Marianne Williamson; Erin Johnson; Gabrielle Bernstein; Sophia Bush; Maha Dakhil; Bhavani Lev and Bharat Mitra; Woody Fraser, Milena Monrroy, Midge Hussey, and everyone at Hallmark's Home & Family; Morgan Fairchild; Patti Stanger; Catherine, Sophia, and Laura Bach;

Annabeth Gish; Robert Wisdom; Danielle LaPorte; Nick and Brenna Ortner; Jessica Ortner; Mike Dooley; Kris Carr; Kate Northrup; Ann Louise Gittleman; Jan and Panache Desai; Ami Beach and Mark Shadle; Brian Wilson; John Holland; Jill Black Zalben; Alexandra Cohen; Christine Hill; Carol Donahue; Caroline Leavitt; Michael Sandler and Jessica Lee; Koya Webb; Jenny Hutt; Adam Cushman; Sonia Choquette; Colette Baron-Reid; Denise Linn; and Carmel Joy Baird. I deeply value you all.

To the compassionate doctors and other healers of the world who have changed the lives of so many: I have tremendous respect for you. Dr. Masha Kogan, Dr. Virginia Romano, Dr. Habib Sadeghi, Dr. Carol Lee, Dr. Richard Sollazzo, Dr. Jeff Feinman, Dr. Deanna Minich, Dr. Ron Steriti, Dr. Nicole Galante, Dr. Diana Lopusny, Dr. Dick and Noel Shepard, Dr. Aleksandra Phillips, Dr. Chris Maloney, Drs. Tosca and Gregory Haag, Dr. Dave Klein, Dr. Deborah Kern, Dr. Darren and Suzanne Boles, and Dr. Robin Karlin—it's an honor to call you friends. Thank you for your endless dedication to the field of healing.

Thanks to David Schmerler, Kimberly S. Grimsley, and Susan G. Etheridge for being there for me.

A very warm, heartfelt thanks to Muneeza Ahmed; Kimberly Spair; Amber Stone; Lauren Henry; Kayla Botelho; Tara Tom; Bella; Victoria and Michael Arnstein; Nina Leatherer; Michelle Sutton; Haily Cataldo; Kerry; Amy Bacheller; Michael McMenamin; Alexandra Laws; Ester Horn; Linda and Robert Coykendall; Setareh Khatibi; Heather Coleman; Glenn Klausner; Michael Monteleone; Bobbi and Leslie Hall; Katherine Belzowski; Matt and Vanessa Houston; David, Holly, and Ginnie Whitney; Melody Lee Pence; Terra Appelman; Eileen Crispell; Kristin Cassidy; Calvin Stebbins; Catherine Lawton; Alana DiNardo; Min Lee; and Eden Epstein Hill.

Thank you to the countless people, including those in the Medical Medium communities, whom I've had the privilege and honor of seeing blossom, heal, and transform.

Sally Arnold, thank you for shining your light so brightly and lending your voice to the movement.

Ruby Scattergood, your masterful patience and countless hours of dedication have heroically formed the true spine of this book. The Medical Medium series would not be possible without your writing and editing. Thank you for your literary counsel.

Vibodha and Tila Clark, your creative genius has been astoundingly instrumental to the cause of helping others. Thank you for standing with us throughout the years.

Friar and Clare: *Behold, he cometh with clouds; and every eye shall see him, and they also which pierced him: and all kindreds of the earth shall wail because of him. Even so, Amen (Rev. 1:7).*

Quincy: Thank you for your invaluable support and hard work.

Sepideh Kashanian and Ben, thank you for your warm, loving care.

Oliver Niño and Mandy Morris, so proud of you for all you do for so many.

Jeff Skeirik, thank you for the best pictures, man.

Alyssa Degati, you are changing lives with your voice.

Jon Morelli and Noah, you two are all heart.

Robby Barbaro, your unwavering positivity lifts up everyone around you.

For your love and support, as always, I thank my family: my luminous wife; Dad and

Mom; my brothers, nieces, nephews, aunts, and uncles; my champions Indigo, Ruby, and Great Blue; Hope; Marjorie and Robert; Laura; Rhia and Byron; Alayne Serle and Scott, Perri, Lissy, and Ari Cohn; David Somoroff; Joel, Liz, Kody, Jesse, Lauren, Joseph, and Thomas; Brian, Joyce, and Josh; Jarod; Brent; Kelly and Evy; Danielle, Johnny, and Declan; and all my loved ones who are on the other side.

Finally, thank you, Spirit of the Most High (aka Spirit of Compassion), for providing all of us with compassionate wisdom from the heavens that inspires us to keep our heads up and carry the sacred gifts you've been so kind to give us. Thank you for putting up with me over the years and reminding me to keep a light heart with your never-ending patience and willingness to answer my questions in search of the truth.

ABOUT THE AUTHOR

Anthony William is the originator of the global celery juice movement, host of the *Medical Medium Podcast*, and #1 *New York Times* best-selling author of the Medical Medium book series:

- *Medical Medium Cleanse to Heal: Healing Plans for Sufferers of Anxiety, Depression, Acne, Eczema, Lyme, Gut Problems, Brain Fog, Weight Issues, Migraines, Bloating, Vertigo, Psoriasis, Cysts, Fatigue, PCOS, Fibroids, UTI, Endometriosis & Autoimmune*

- *Medical Medium Celery Juice: The Most Powerful Medicine of Our Time Healing Millions Worldwide*

- *Medical Medium Liver Rescue: Answers to Eczema, Psoriasis, Diabetes, Strep, Acne, Gout, Bloating, Gallstones, Adrenal Stress, Fatigue, Fatty Liver, Weight Issues, SIBO & Autoimmune Disease*

- *Medical Medium Thyroid Healing: The Truth behind Hashimoto's, Graves', Insomnia, Hypothyroidism, Thyroid Nodules & Epstein-Barr*

- *Medical Medium Life-Changing Foods: Save Yourself and the Ones You Love with the Hidden Healing Powers of Fruits & Vegetables*

- *Medical Medium: Secrets Behind Chronic and Mystery Illness and How to Finally Heal*

Anthony was born with the unique ability to converse with the Spirit of Compassion, who provides him with extraordinarily advanced healing medical information that's far ahead of its time. Since age four, Anthony has been using his gift to see into people's conditions and tell them and their doctors how to recover their health. His unprecedented accuracy and success rate as the Medical Medium have earned him the trust and love of millions worldwide, among them movie stars, rock stars, billionaires, professional athletes, and countless other people from all walks of life who couldn't find a way to heal until he provided them with insights from above. Over the decades, Anthony has also been an invaluable resource to doctors who need help solving their most difficult cases.

Learn more at www.medicalmedium.com

Hay House Titles of Related Interest

YOU CAN HEAL YOUR LIFE, the movie, starring Louise Hay & Friends
(available as a 1-DVD program, an expanded 2-DVD set, and an online streaming video)
Learn more at www.hayhouse.com/louise-movie

THE SHIFT, the movie,
starring Dr. Wayne W. Dyer
(available as a 1-DVD program, an expanded 2-DVD set, and an online streaming video)
Learn more at www.hayhouse.com/the-shift-movie

***

MEDICAL MEDIUM LIFE-CHANGING FOODS: Save Yourself and the Ones You Love with the Hidden Healing Powers of Fruits & Vegetables, by Anthony William

MEDICAL MEDIUM THYROID HEALING: The Truth behind Hashimoto's, Graves', Insomnia, Hypothyroidism, Thyroid Nodules & Epstein-Barr, by Anthony William

MEDICAL MEDIUM LIVER RESCUE: Answers to Eczema, Psoriasis, Diabetes, Strep, Acne, Gout, Bloating, Gallstones, Adrenal Stress, Fatigue, Fatty Liver, Weight Issues, SIBO & Autoimmune Disease, by Anthony William

MEDICAL MEDIUM CELERY JUICE: The Most Powerful Medicine of Our Time Healing Millions Worldwide, by Anthony William

MEDICAL MEDIUM CLEANSE TO HEAL: Healing Plans for Sufferers of Anxiety, Depression, Acne, Eczema, Lyme, Gut Problems, Brain Fog, Weight Issues, Migraines, Bloating, Vertigo, Psoriasis, Cysts, Fatigue, PCOS, Fibroids, UTI, Endometriosis & Autoimmune, by Anthony William

All of the above are available at your local bookstore,
or may be ordered by contacting Hay House (see next page).

***

We hope you enjoyed this Hay House book. If you'd like to receive our online catalog featuring additional information on Hay House books and products, or if you'd like to find out more about the Hay Foundation, please contact:

Hay House, Inc., P.O. Box 5100, Carlsbad, CA 92018-5100
(760) 431-7695 or (800) 654-5126
(760) 431-6948 (fax) or (800) 650-5115 (fax)
www.hayhouse.com® • www.hayfoundation.org

———

Published in Australia by: Hay House Australia Pty. Ltd.,
18/36 Ralph St., Alexandria NSW 2015
Phone: 612-9669-4299 • *Fax:* 612-9669-4144
www.hayhouse.com.au

Published in the United Kingdom by: Hay House UK, Ltd.,
The Sixth Floor, Watson House, 54 Baker Street, London W1U 7BU
Phone: +44 (0)20 3927 7290 • *Fax:* +44 (0)20 3927 7291
www.hayhouse.co.uk

Published in India by: Hay House Publishers India,
Muskaan Complex, Plot No. 3, B-2, Vasant Kunj, New Delhi 110 070
Phone: 91-11-4176-1620 • *Fax:* 91-11-4176-1630
www.hayhouse.co.in

———

Access New Knowledge.
Anytime. Anywhere.

Learn and evolve at your own pace
with the world's leading experts.

www.hayhouseU.com

Listen. Learn. Transform.

Listen to the audio version
of this book for FREE!

Unlock endless wisdom, fresh perspectives, and life-changing tools from world-renowned authors and teachers—helping you embrace vibrant health in your body, mind, and spirit. With the *Hay House Unlimited* Audio app, you can learn and grow in a way that fits your lifestyle . . . and your daily schedule.

With your membership, you can:

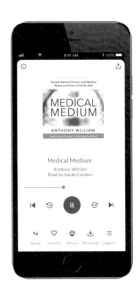

- Develop a healthier mind, body, and spirit through natural remedies, healthy foods, and powerful healing practices.

- Explore thousands of audiobooks, meditations, immersive learning programs, podcasts, and more.

- Access exclusive audios you won't find anywhere else.

- Experience completely unlimited listening. No credits. No limits. No kidding.

Try for FREE!

Free e-newsletters
from Hay House, the Ultimate
Resource for Inspiration

Be the first to know about Hay House's free downloads, special offers, giveaways, contests, and more!

Get exclusive excerpts from our latest releases and videos from *Hay House Present Moments*.

Our *Digital Products Newsletter* is the perfect way to stay up-to-date on our latest discounted eBooks, featured mobile apps, and Live Online and On Demand events.

Learn with real benefits! *HayHouseU.com* is your source for the most innovative online courses from the world's leading personal growth experts. Be the first to know about new online courses and to receive exclusive discounts.

Enjoy uplifting personal stories, how-to articles, and healing advice, along with videos and empowering quotes, within *Heal Your Life*.

Get inspired, educate yourself, get a complimentary gift, and share the wisdom!

Visit www.hayhouse.com/newsletters to sign up today!

HAY HOUSE

HAY HOUSE
online learning

"Our bodies love us unconditionally. They do not judge or blame or hold on to resentment. Day in and day out, all of our body systems are working for us without complaint.

The immune system is constantly ready for battle, patrolling every part of the body looking for invaders.

Let's make it crystal clear: Nobody wants to be sick or compromised. Nobody has a fear of healing. I believe in you. With the knowledge and power, I know you can heal."

— Anthony William, Medical Medium